Opioid Dependence

Heath B. McAnally

Opioid Dependence

A Clinical and Epidemiologic Approach

Springer

Heath B. McAnally, MD, MSPH
Medical Director
Northern Anesthesia & Pain Medicine, LLC
Eagle River, AK, USA

Clinical Instructor
University of Washington School of Medicine
WWAMI Program
Anchorage, AK, USA

ISBN 978-3-319-47496-0 ISBN 978-3-319-47497-7 (eBook)
DOI 10.1007/978-3-319-47497-7

Library of Congress Control Number: 2017948662

Printed on acid-free paper

This Springer imprint is published by Springer Nature
The registered company is Springer International Publishing AG
The registered company address is: Gewerbestrasse 11, 6330 Cham, Switzerland

Preface

The physician's oath begins with a commitment to risk reduction—*primum non nocere*. The physician's responsibility also includes the fundamental duty to relieve suffering whenever possible. Opioids are a powerful and dangerous tool in the therapeutic armamentarium. Much like the homesteader's chainsaw or the miner's dynamite in the Last Frontier where I reside, opioids can accomplish much in the short term, although untrained and indiscriminate use invites disaster. As with most decisions in medicine, opioid therapy involves ongoing risk-benefit ratio analysis. At the beginning of the twenty-first century, we are in a position to better evaluate previously underappreciated risks and potentially overstated benefits (of chronic opioid therapy).

At an individual level, we are seeing prevalent recalcitrant (and likely increased) chronic pain and depression and dysfunction associated with chronic opioid use. We are becoming aware of immunosuppressive and endocrinopathic effects of this drug class that have not yet made it into standard pharmacology textbooks. We are being told that more people die today in America from opioid overdose than from automobile accidents. And unlike many other intervention decisions the physician must make, there are societal "ripple effects" of chronic opioid therapy. Opioids prescribed by even the best-informed and best-intentioned clinicians are diverted into the wrong hands. No other therapeutic intervention (besides benzodiazepines) even comes close to sharing the public health liability of opioids.

This book is intended to "bring the practitioner up to speed" on:

- Opioid basic science
- Current areas of drug improvement research and development
- Alternatives to opioid therapy
- Evidence-based indications for opioid therapy
- Evidence-based indications against opioid therapy
- Clinical strategies for preventing and overcoming opioid dependence

Part I of the book provides an overview comparing (and contrasting) classic infectious disease epidemiology concepts with what has been labeled the opioid epidemic in America. A paradigm categorizing our current understanding of basic science and best clinical practices in terms of agent (opioid), vector (prescriber), and host (patient) factors is offered. The remainder of the book is organized according to these three arenas.

Part II of the book is devoted to understanding the agent and potential means of attenuating its "virulence." Chapter 2 surveys the current state of our basic science knowledge concerning opioids. While attempting to be as comprehensive as possible in scope (under the constraints of maintaining clinical relevance), no single work can survey the vast research into opioids that has amassed over the past half century. Every decade brings more answers into mechanisms of action that beget more questions. The complexity of opioid receptor activity on an enormous array of biochemical processes is only beginning to be unraveled. Heteromerization of receptors with alterations in function and effect and regulatory interactions between these receptors and other systems are apparently protean. Traditional concepts of pharmacokinetics and pharmacodynamics are constantly being revised by new understanding of these interdigitating systems and also by pharmacogenetics which confer another level of clinical variance altogether.

Chapter 3 examines the adverse effects (or "harms" as they are increasingly described as in the literature) of various opioids, organized by physiologic systems. A literature review of opioid adverse effects follows, based upon recent systematic reviews.

Chapter 4 presents agent-specific pharmacology for the commonly prescribed opioids in America (arranged in alphabetical order). While the generalist certainly does not need to be an expert in all of the agents available, the growing scope of the problem of opioid abuse in this country necessitates some familiarity with all of the commonly used agents, regardless of specialty. The old injunction to "know a few agents really well" is certainly reasonable; however, staying abreast of the current knowledge base is essential when prescribing potentially lethal agents and those that can otherwise ruin a life.

Chapter 5 looks at historic, current, and potential future means of altering currently available drugs and adjunctive therapies—attenuating agent virulence—to reduce the risks of adverse effects, especially as they pertain to psychological and physical dependence and addiction.

Part III of the book examines the vector, and while the entire book is obviously intended to educate prescribers about best clinical practices, this section focuses on presenting guidance to providers for reducing their contribution to the epidemic or attenuating vector transmission.

Chapter 6 introduces the section with a primer on acute and chronic pain assessment and treatment. It is not intended to serve as a textbook on pain; vast works (e.g., Bonica's, Waldman's, Deer's) provide excellent resources for pain management and other specialists and generalists. This chapter is intended to provide a scaffold for thinking about pain which (despite aggressive campaigning to label as a disease in its own right) remains a symptom, and a cardinal one at that, for many underlying pathologic states—including emotional and cognitive disturbance. It also offers a brief survey of multimodal approaches to explore with patients or consult with colleagues in other specialties.

Chapter 7 discusses *why* (or *why not*) and *when* (or *when not*) to prescribe opioids. An initial discussion of acute pain, and the special situation of postoperative pain (which increasingly represents "acute-on-chronic" pain), is followed by an evaluation of the evidence for or against opioid therapy for chronic pain. Currently available systematic reviews examining the efficacy of chronic opioid therapy are organized by categories of both "nociceptive" pain and neuropathic pain. Finally, a survey of both national and international clinical practice guidelines on opioid therapy for cancer pain is presented.

Chapter 8 presents *how* to prescribe opioids, arranged by regulatory and advisory oversight. Federal and state laws are discussed, followed by a synthesis of recommendations from the major current national clinical practice guidelines on opioid therapy, arranged loosely to follow the well-established Federation of State Medical Boards' Model Policy.

The book's final section is centered on an attempt to better understand and prevent opioid misuse and dependence in the host population—our patients and their families and associates.

Chapter 9 begins with a review of addiction theories. Choice and compulsion models are compared and contrasted in an effort to illuminate these complex self-destructive human behaviors that science will likely never fully explain nor address. An introduction to social models of addiction follows. The chapter closes with a brief acknowledgment that the understanding of motivation lies at the heart of comprehending addiction.

Chapter 10 examines specific risk factors for opioid use disorder/addiction based upon current research and also presents guidance on risk assessment when considering opioid therapy. The more commonly used standardized clinical instruments are discussed along with a literature review of their validation. This is followed by a brief overview of compliance/aberrancy monitoring using standardized and validated questionnaires and urine drug testing.

Chapter 11 concludes this section on addressing host factors—likely the most important and difficult to effectively intervene upon in this epidemic—arranged by the common public health schema of primary, secondary, and tertiary prevention. Primary prevention will most effectively occur if we are able to confer "behavioral immunity," i.e., reducing or eliminating the desire to seek and use the drug. Negative motivation includes education as to the risks and diminishing benefits of opioid use. Enlightening patients that pain is not in fact their worst enemy, but biologically and teleologically perhaps the most important protective sense we possess, is vital to overcoming disproportionate focus on and dread of pain, with potentially escalating sensitization and/or hyperalgesia (which is often accelerated by opioid use). Positive motivation includes promotion of healthy lifestyle choices, non-opioid pain management options, and above all self-efficacy. The environment comprises a crucial and to this point unaddressed component of the standard "epidemiologic triangle" and is introduced in this section.

Secondary prevention assumes that the process can be reversed. Education is not confined to primary prevention. It has been said that there are two things that will reliably bring people into the physician's office—bleeding and pain. If we can convince the patient that chronic opioid use in most situations is worsening their pain (via opioid-induced hyperalgesia, depression, and overall health reduction), we may achieve more risk reduction than attempting to convince them about morbidity and mortality. As a sidenote, while I still preach cardiovascular, pulmonary, and oncologic risk reduction as more than adequate reasons for smoking cessation, increasingly, I appeal to data showing that cigarettes increase pain; patients seem to care more about that issue oftentimes. Opioid weaning and a brief introduction to Rollnick and Miller's motivational interviewing techniques are introduced.

Tertiary prevention is traditionally equated with damage control, but I do not hold the completely pessimistic viewpoint that "once an addict, always an addict." Despite the discouraging statistics on relapse, there are too many success stories from people who have decided that there is something they want more than voluntary slavery to a substance—be that alcohol or oxycodone—and have sought and found the help they need in achieving recovery and abstinence. An overview of clinical practice guidelines from the American Society of Addiction Medicine, with its biopsychosocial-spiritual "multidimensional assessment" focus, is given, along with a discussion of medication-assisted treatment, organized by the three currently FDA-approved pharmacotherapeutics (methadone, buprenorphine, and naltrexone). The chapter concludes with an examination of evidence and recommendations for overdose education and naloxone distribution.

Each of the chapters in Parts II through IV begins with a case study, some of which are drawn from the author's practice and some from the literature or popular news. Josef Stalin reportedly once said that the death of one man is a tragedy, while the death of millions is a statistic. While espousing none of his political viewpoints, this quote serves to remind us that the epidemic we face and the strategies and policies we implement affect individual human beings as well as our nation.

Eagle River, AK, USA Heath B. McAnally, MD, MSPH

Acknowledgments

Thank you, Wendy Shaw, for your help in editing. I'm sorry your anti-bombast campaign met with such limited success.

Thank you, Drs. Andrea Trescot and Paula Colescott, for your mentoring and encouragement along the way.

Thank you, Philip Licht, for your friendship, partnership, and vision.

Thank you, Pastor Todd Michero, for your friendship, prayer, counsel, and heart for the hurting and the addicted.

Thank you to my patients, who have entrusted their best interests to my fallible mind and hands.

Thank you to my friends, the staff and "Special Ops Care Team" of NAPM, and Set Free Alaska for their camaraderie and prayers.

Thank you, Jules, my wife, for putting up with the many months of my preoccupation and emotional absence during the tedious evening and weekend hours and for always believing in me. Thank you for always having my back and always looking ahead.

Above all, I thank You, Jesus Christ, whom I rely on for my life in this world and the next.

Contents

Part I
Overview of the Epidemic

"...when in all these thousands of years has there been a time when man has acted only from his own interest? What is to be done with the millions of facts that bear witness that men, consciously, that is fully understanding their real interests, have left them in the background and have rushed headlong on another path, to meet peril and danger, compelled to this course by nobody and by nothing, but, as it were, simply disliking the beaten track, and have obstinately, willfully, struck out another difficult, absurd way, seeking it almost in the darkness....

"You see, gentlemen, reason is an excellent thing, there's no disputing that, but reason is nothing but reason and satisfies only the rational side of man's nature, while will is a manifestation of the whole life, that is, of the whole human life including reason and all the impulses...."

--Fyodor Dostoevsky, *Notes from the Underground*

Chapter 1
An Epidemiologic Perspective

Twenty years is a very long time in epidemiologic terms. It's generally impossible to pinpoint an exact time and place of origin for most epidemics; sometime between 1996 and1999 is the commonly accepted inception of what the Centers for Disease Control (CDC) has labeled the opioid epidemic in America [1]. That puts us at nearly 20 years at the time of this writing.

Most epidemics run their course or are controlled within a handful of years. The influenza pandemic of the early twentieth century, often described as "the greatest medical holocaust in history," lasted less than 2 years. Known at the time as the "Spanish flu," this worldwide disaster infected an estimated 500 million people and killed as much as 5% of the world's population. Yet it began and ended within a relatively short time period, within the closing years of the First World War (Fig. 1.1).

Cholera ravaged the world for the greater part of the nineteenth and twentieth centuries, but the majority of the component epidemics lasted 10 years or less (Fig. 1.2).

An epidemic is classically thought of as a widespread communicable disease affecting a significant percentage of a population; however in recent years noncommunicable diseases have been granted epidemic status, such as cardiovascular disease, chronic pulmonary disease, obesity, and the like.

The United States at the beginning of the twenty-first century is squarely in the middle of an epidemic of prescription opioid drug abuse. Hardly a community in America is untouched by this crisis. Very few people in our country do not have family or friends or close associates who have not fallen prey to the scourge of opioid dependence. The tragedy of an individual life lost or ruined, along with the devastating ripple effects on loved ones, is certainly the most heartbreaking consequence of opioid abuse. But the magnitude of this problem is perhaps better appreciated by stepping back and taking a "bird's-eye view" of the issue. The CDC reports that drug overdose deaths, the vast majority of which involve prescription opioids, are now the leading cause of injury death in the United States—surpassing motor vehicle crashes (Fig. 1.3) [2].

H.B. McAnally, *Opioid Dependence*, DOI 10.1007/978-3-319-47497-7_1

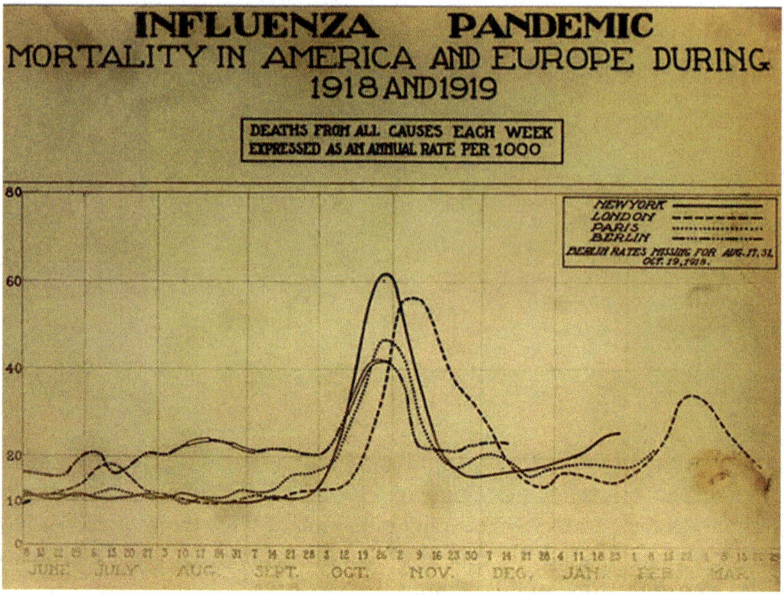

Fig. 1.1 The death count from the 1918/1919 influenza pandemic is not known, but estimates range from 40 to 100 million people worldwide, with as many as 25 million in the first 6 months killed from the disease. It remains the most staggering microbial victory over mankind to date

Opioid dependence and abuse are not limited to any one geographic region; they are truly a nationwide issue, and recent trends indicate that the fastest spread of this problem is in rural states without a significant history of illicit drug problems [3]. Nor is opioid dependence a problem impacting a limited demographic—every race and socioeconomic classification is touched (although certain groups are less affected).

Nearly 2.6 million people in the United States are reported [4] to be dependent on either prescription opioids or heroin. Over 1000 emergency room visits every day occur due to complications of opioid use and abuse [5]. More than 165,000 people in this country died between 1999 and 2014 due to prescription opioid overdose (not including heroin deaths)—with the rate quadrupling over that 15-year period (Fig. 1.4) [6].

How Did We Get Here?

The scope of epidemiology encompasses far more than simply generating descriptive statistics. The analysis of associations between various factors and the disease comprises the main role of the discipline, with the ultimate goal being the understanding of causal factors that can be intervened upon.

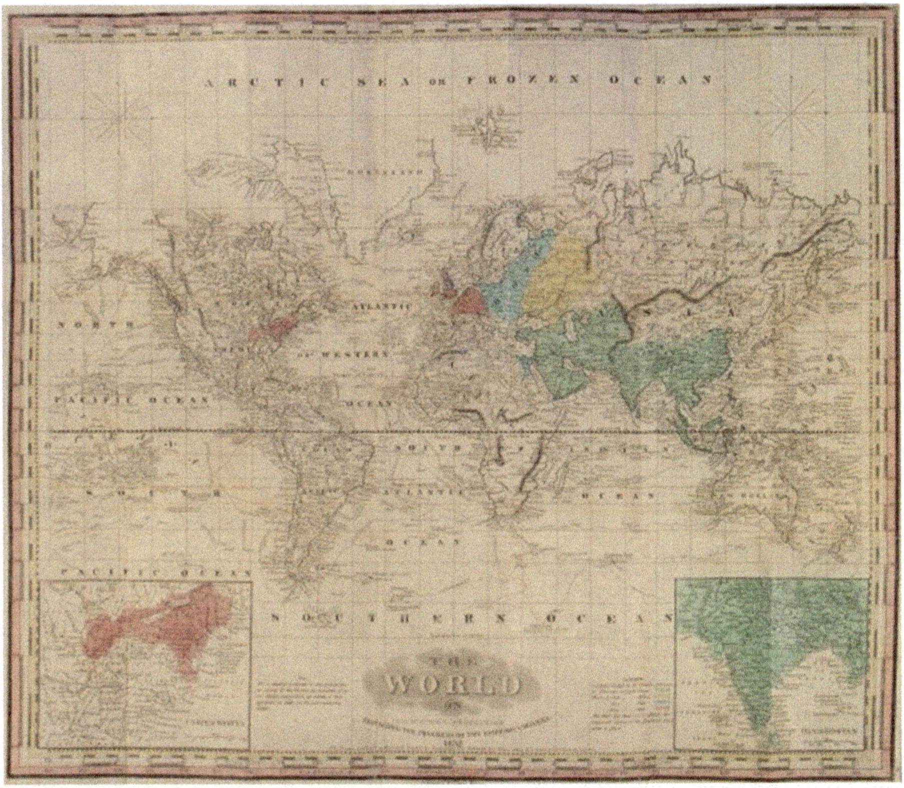

Fig. 1.2 Henry S. Tanner's world map depicts the spread of cholera prior to 1830 (*green*), in 1830 (*yellow*), in 1831 (*blue*), and in 1832 (*red*). Courtesy of the New York Academy of Medicine

In terms of a simple "point-source" outbreak, where a single agent-vector combination is responsible for causing an epidemic (e.g., hantavirus and deer mice in the famous 1993 *Sin Nombre* outbreak in the Four Corners area or *Legionella pneumophila* and air conditioners in the even more famous 1976 Philadelphia Legionnaire's convention outbreak), elucidating the causal factors is a relatively straightforward task.

In the analysis of multifactorial chronic disease states, with numerous contributors, determining true "risk factors" (let alone causation) while weeding out "confounders" becomes a much more involved process. (These terms are defined in the next section.)

The opioid epidemic represents a spectrum of behavioral disease that by its very nature is multifaceted. Beyond easily measured contributors such as pharmaceutical sales, prescribing trends, geographic analysis, and the like, there are elusive factors involving motivation, reward, and the complex neuropsychobiology of addiction.

Numerous analyses over the past two decades have identified characteristics including genetic and psychiatric/psychological (including both Axis I and Axis II

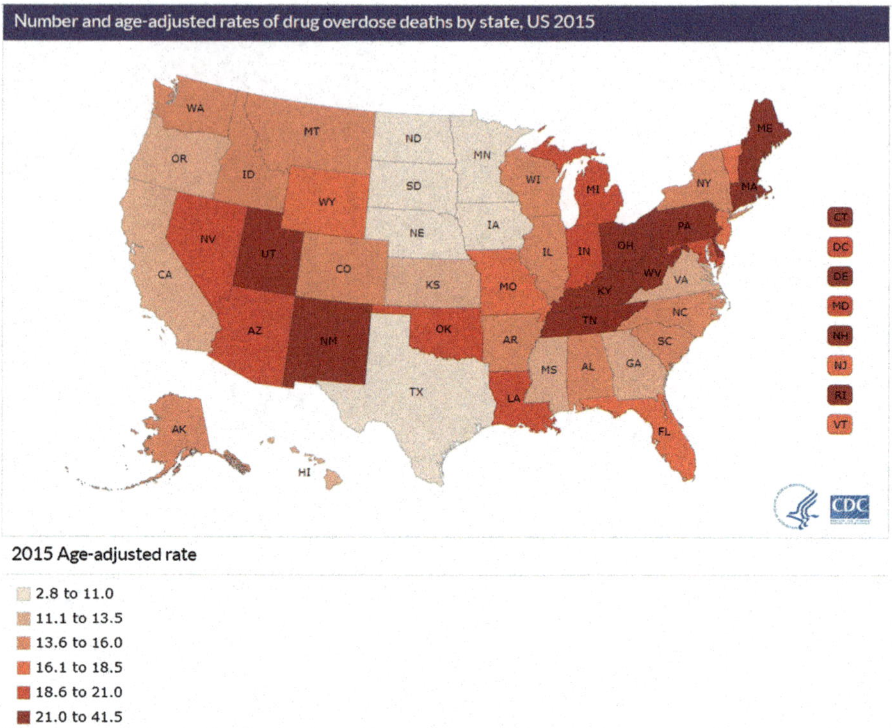

Fig. 1.3 State-by-state mortality figures for opioid overdose deaths, 2015. Source: CDC/NCHS, National Vital Statistics System, Mortality

conditions from pre-DSM-5 schema) that render individuals more susceptible to seeking, using, and developing dependence upon opioids. Chapter 10 presents some of these data in more detail.

The complex interplay between psychological/emotional distress and physical pain adds to the confusion of defining variables.

Societal "norms" in terms of pain perception, tolerance, and coping influence behavior. This is certainly not readily quantifiable, but those who have been practicing medicine long enough can attest to the fact that what is considered intolerable today (or at least, deserving of opioid therapy) was not 15 or 20 years ago. Part of this "pendulum swing" phenomenon discussed frequently in the literature over the past few years was undoubtedly due to aggressive marketing by pharmaceutical companies and also by well-meaning parascientific organizations such as the American Pain Society and their famous "5th Vital Sign" campaign in the 1990s.

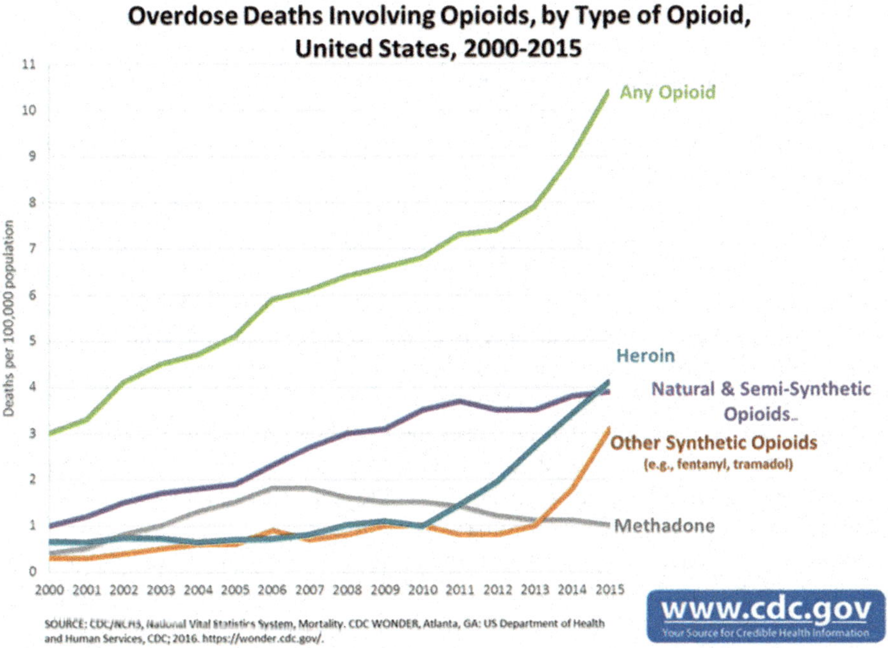

Fig. 1.4 Opioid overdose death rates, 2000–2015. Source: Centers for Disease Control and Prevention. https://www.cdc.gov/drugoverdose/images/data/opioid_deaths_multicolor.gif

Some Basic Definitions

Understanding terms is important to any scientific endeavor or clinical application, and this applies to epidemiology as well as any branch of science.

Epidemiology, the study of epidemics, has been defined as "the study of the occurrence and distribution of diseases and other health-related conditions in populations" [7]. An *epidemic* is defined as "an increase in the number of cases over past experience for a given population, time and place." Classically, as mentioned previously, epidemics have been thought of primarily in terms of spread of an infectious/communicable agent.

The *agent* is the entity that interacts with the host population to cause the disease. While not epidemiologic terms, we should also describe *opioids* and *opiates* here, as they are the agent of interest. An opioid is a chemical compound that acts upon opioid receptors (defined later) to cause various effects, the most well-known of which are relief of pain and also sedation. An opiate is a naturally occurring (or modification of a naturally occurring) compound derived from the opium poppy (*Papaver somniferum*). Chapters 2 and 4 are devoted to describing opioids in much more detail.

A *vector* is a carrier for the agent, such as mosquitoes that carry malaria, or fleas in the case of the plague. The vector in this crisis has been for the most part of the medical profession. "Trickle-down" vectors exist of course; entrepreneurial (and criminal) "diverters" of pills who provide an illegal source of opioids to the population may be patients themselves, family or associates of the patients, or, increasingly these days, thieves.

The *host* is the entity infected or affected by the agent. The *population* of course is the grouping of hosts.

A few other basic epidemiologic terms such as incidence, prevalence, mortality, and case-fatality rates should probably also be discussed here. *Incidence* refers to the number of new cases over a defined time period, while *prevalence* refers to the total number of cases at any given time period. *Mortality* in epidemiologic terms describes the frequency of occurrence of death in the population, while the *case-fatality rate* is a more specific term that describes the proportion of hosts with the condition that die specifically from the condition.

Risk factors are anything that increases the likelihood of the disease state. They are generally variables associated with either the host or the environment that render the host more susceptible, for example, non-sickle cell trait and malaria in Africa or cigarette smoking in the case of coronary artery disease.

Confounders appear to be risk factors but are not. They are factors associated with both the host and the agent that lead to spurious conclusions. A classic example is the apparent risk of developing scurvy from sea travel. Thanks to the work of Dr. James Lind in the 1700s (and subsequent investigation into the twentieth century), we now know that vitamin C deficiency is the cause of scurvy; however, prior to his demonstration of effective prevention by consumption of citrus fruits in British seamen, the real cause lays shrouded beneath an erroneous assumption. Another classic example of epidemiologic confounding is the apparent risk of birth order with Down's syndrome. Until the twentieth century, it was thought that being born later "in the pecking order" was a risk factor for Down's. We now understand that increased chromosomal fragility occurs with advancing maternal age (the true independent variable or risk factor) and a higher birth order is associated with both older mothers and trisomy 21. Common confounders in many epidemiologic studies include age, gender, ethnicity, socioeconomic status, and the like.

Ingredients for a (Successful) Epidemic

Essentially, epidemics require only two ingredients:

1. A virulent/transmissible agent
2. A vulnerable population

Virulence in epidemiologic terms basically means how successful an agent is in attacking and spreading. *Transmissibility* is a slightly different term that measures how communicable the agent is—how readily it is spread from host to host. *Vulnerability* of the population is fairly self-explanatory and has to do with how susceptible people are to the agent. It can be thought of as loosely synonymous with lack of immunity.

Perhaps the most famous of all epidemics was the Great Plague that ravaged Europe in the fourteenth century. Commonly referred to as "the Black Death," it claimed the lives of an estimated 60% of Europe during its course. The agent, *Yersinia pestis*, is a highly virulent and transmissible bacterium that infects a number of rodents; in the case of the Great Plague, rats are thought to have been the primary host population, and fleas the vectors transmitting the bacteria to susceptible humans. (*Y. pestis* can also be transmitted via respiratory droplet from one human being to another.)

The second requirement of a vulnerable population was met in the fact that most of Europe lived in a state of overcrowded squalor with poor hygiene. Fleas didn't have to exert much effort to find a nearby human, and person-to-person spread by droplet was also much more likely in close quarters.

Another well-known epidemic is frequently credited with turning the course of history in the New World. The Spanish invasion of what is now Central and South America in the sixteenth and seventeenth centuries is thought to have been enabled by smallpox. While a significant scourge to the Old World, the devastation wreaked by this virus upon the Aztec and Inca Empires was unparalleled in Europe due to the complete immunonaivete of these peoples to European diseases. This is perhaps the most striking demonstration of a highly virulent organism encountering an utterly vulnerable populace.

In the late twentieth and early twenty-first centuries America, we have apparently arrived at the right set of societal conditions to create the "perfect storm" of a highly virulent agent (opioids) with a substantial population at risk, as the grim statistics bear out.

Striking the Right Balance

In order to be "successful," the responsible agent has to strike the right balance of virulence and imminent lethality.

Too "timid" (i.e., low virulence) and the host population avoids infection (generally by developing immunity or otherwise containing the agent as we have managed to accomplish with antimicrobial agents and vaccines in the twentieth and twenty-first centuries).

Too aggressive (killing off the victims too quickly—e.g., Ebola) and the agent defeats its purpose by eradicating its population—much like a horde of locusts devouring everything in its path and leaving no substrate for its own perpetuation.

Most epidemics don't even come close to a 20-year run due to an inability of the agent to achieve and maintain the optimal intersection (from the standpoint of the agent) of these two extremes:

1. Immunity (natural or artificial—i.e., vaccination) develops.
2. The vulnerable population dies off (the epidemic "burns out") (Fig. 1.5).

The rate (and duration) of spread of the opioid epidemic is evidence that the agent is apparently maintaining highly effective transmission while avoiding excessive

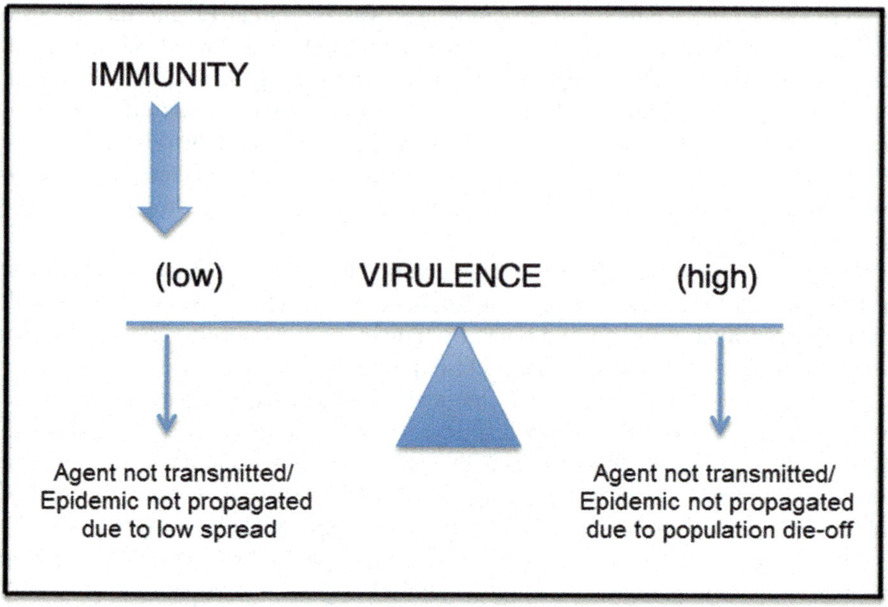

Fig. 1.5 Conceptualization of the balance between suboptimal and overly aggressive virulence

destruction of the host population. Dependence and addiction to opioids (the subject of later chapters) render the development of immunity within vulnerable population extraordinarily difficult. No statistics describing the rate of recovery from opioid dependence and addiction exist at any population level. The estimated rate of relapse to drug abuse in general is between 40 and 60% according to an often quoted study [8]; however, when separating opioids out from drugs in general, the rate climbs to nearly 90%.

While certainly lethal, the fact is that most people who abuse prescription opioids don't die from it—or if they do, it is generally years into their own "infection," and there is ample time for the host to interact with other vulnerable hosts. According to the CDC [9], overdoses involving opioids killed more than 28,000 people in 2014, which is a staggering figure. However, set against a denominator of 2.1 million people estimated that same year to be dependent upon prescription opioids (with almost 500,000 more addicted to heroin) [4], this yields an approximate case fatality rate of almost 11%, which is substantially lower than rates cited for smallpox and plague (30–50%).

Moths to a Flame

There is a third limiting factor, however, that isn't generally considered in most epidemiology courses, perhaps because it is too obvious to us as rational creatures: **the desire of the vulnerable population to avoid the agent**.

Inherent in living creatures is the desire to avoid our own destruction, and as the highest form of biologic life on the planet, we have always been motivated as a species to protect ourselves from our enemies. In the case of addiction, however (which has historically been defined by psychiatrists as persistent/compulsive behavior despite adverse consequences), it is clear that rational self-preservation instincts are surrendered or are conquered by the overwhelming compulsion to seek the substance regardless of the results.

In all fairness, at an individual level, there are both positive and negative reinforcements in this epidemic. Opioids persist in the therapeutic armamentarium for treating pain for a simple reason: they are effective. (Or at least, they are effective initially—prior to the onset of tolerance and hyperalgesia, which is covered in detail in Chap. 3.) And as is the case with most addictive substances, once a person has become dependent—physically and/or psychologically—absence of the drug poses a (perceived) threat to the well-being of the host.

At a population/societal level, the issues influencing our deadly affair with opioids are complex and protean, but one of the factors that has been shown repeatedly in epidemiologic investigations of substance abuse is lack of perceived danger. The opioid epidemic has finally captivated the attention of our nation at a media and governmental level, but until recently awareness of the problem has been limited. Twenty years spans the formative period of a generation, and it remains to be seen whether the next one looks upon our current predicament as normative or aberrant.

Strategies in the War Against Opioid Abuse

The analogy of infectious disease breaks down, of course, at some point when analyzing the opioid epidemic and constructing a strategy for victory for our species. Opioids are not truly "virulent," as inanimate, non-replicating substances.

However, there is a substantial population at risk, and the framework remains useful as a starting point for both individual and collective thought regarding how to address this issue at a population level.

Addressing the Agent

Even in the case of infectious epidemics, eradicating the agent itself is generally impossible due to the ubiquitous nature of microbes. In the case of opioids, eradication is similarly impossible and, furthermore, would be irrational (and some say immoral) as we lack suitable alternatives at present to treat severe pain from cancer or acute trauma, etc.

Similarly, attenuating (decreasing) the virulence of infectious agents is not generally feasible outside laboratory conditions; however, in the case of noncommunicable diseases, this approach has been attempted to some degree in the case of the obesity epidemic, with public campaigns to reduce the appeal of foods with poor nutritional to caloric ratio.

Extended release/long-acting (ER/LA) opioids were developed and are often prescribed not only to provide greater stability of opioid blood levels ("round-the-clock") and analgesia or pain relief but also out of the concept that less variability in those blood levels (with less rapid swings) confers less dramatic surges in striatal dopamine—the issue currently thought to be at the biologic core of addiction. Decades of evidence support the evidence that the more rapidly a drug exerts its effect, the more addictive it is. Many prescribing guidelines over the past two decades advocated the use of ER/LA opioids in chronic pain conditions under the paradigm that "chronic pain deserves round-the-clock coverage." Ironically, however, OxyContin, which is an extended-release opioid, is credited in large part with the rapid spread of prescription opioid dependence and addiction in the late 1990s at the outset of this epidemic. This was likely due in part to the exceedingly addictive nature of the compound itself and also due to the fact that the large amounts of oxycodone contained within higher-dose OxyContin pills could be rapidly accessed by various means of defeating the extended-release mechanism (e.g., crushing and snorting or injecting it).

In response to this, over the past few years, the FDA has issued a directive to pharmaceutical manufacturers requiring abuse-deterrent ("tamper-proof") formulations of new opioid products, which should reduce activities such as crushing and snorting or dissolving and injecting pill contents. This is discussed in much greater detail in Chap. 5.

While efforts to reduce virulence are laudable, to date—as evidenced by the statistics—they have not been shown to be effective. Nonetheless, the second section of this book is devoted to understanding the agent in hopes that as we better "know [our] enemy" both vectors and hosts will be better equipped to make rational decisions about exposure to and control of the agent. Knowledge, after all, is power.

Addressing the Vector

Attenuating transmission has been a disease control measure almost since recorded history began. Long before the understanding of microbes and the "germ theory," lepers and other people infected with various infectious diseases were exiled from society or quarantined in later centuries within their homes or certain quarters of the city. Public campaigns to reduce droplet and other means of transmission by improving personal hygiene and the wearing of masks began in large scale in the early twentieth century during the influenza pandemic.

Until recently, addressing the "vector" has been the sole focus of controlling opioid misuse by governmental oversight (ranging from the federal government all the way down to state medical boards). Efforts to reduce the "transmission" of opioids began to some extent long before this epidemic. Local and state laws controlling the distribution and use of opiates have been extant in this country since the

1800s. Federal laws exerting societal control over the prescription and dispensing of opioids began in earnest in 1914 with the Harrison Narcotic Act, and multiple subsequent legislative efforts (including the sweeping Controlled Substances Act of 1970) have followed since. Among other things, the Controlled Substances Act (CSA) established the current system of "scheduling" controlled substances based on potential for abuse and currently accepted medical use. The drug's schedule determines how tightly it is regulated in terms of allowable means and duration of prescription, refills, and the like.

Establishing rational prescribing guidelines and educating clinicians about responsible opioid prescribing are essential to turning the tide of this epidemic. Many such resources exist (and are proliferating) and are covered in more detail in the third section of this book. The recent CDC guidelines [10] are perhaps the most well publicized of these as of late and echo sound practice advice from prior documents such as the Federation of State Medical Boards' model policy [11] and the American Society of Interventional Pain Physicians' guidelines [12].

More aggressive oversight has been instituted in various forms around the nation. Over the past few years, many states now require physicians to complete annual or biannual continuing education courses on opioid prescribing. Several states have recently enacted legislation limiting either quantities, doses, or duration of prescribed opioids, and some require consultation from pain management specialists depending on dose thresholds, etc. Most states now require that prescribes register with and utilize their State Prescription Drug Monitoring Program (PDMP) prior to writing controlled substance prescriptions.

PDMPs have proven to be one of the most recent and useful tools at a prescriber level in the "war against opioids" so far. These federally and state-funded databases exist in 49 states at the time of this writing and provide relatively current information to prescribers regarding controlled prescriptions filled by patients within that state. The primary purpose of the PDMP is to reduce the incidence of successful "doctor shopping"—a drug-seeking strategy whereby individuals travel in quick succession from prescriber to prescriber obtaining multiple controlled substance prescriptions by placing information into the hands of the healthcare provider.

Prescribers are of course not the only source of prescription opioids; patients, family members, and thieves/illicit dealers can all divert the drugs. Federal agencies such as the Office of National Drug Control Policy (with a mission "to lead the Nation's counternarcotics efforts by developing policies and coordinating, promoting, and implementing initiatives to successfully reduce the supply, the use, and the social acceptance of Drugs in the United States") and law enforcement agencies such as the Drug Enforcement Agency and the Federal Bureau of Investigation work tirelessly to attempt to curb the appeal and availability of illicit opioids regardless of the source.

Ultimately, from a pragmatic standpoint, economics continues to be the driver of much of how healthcare is delivered. Unfortunately, those who pay medical bills (from government to commercial insurance plans) generally do not cover (labor-intensive) comprehensive interventions for chronic pain and instead reward brief office visits and hastily written prescriptions. The US Department of Health and

Table 1.1 Approaches to containing/reducing the opioid epidemic

Addressing the agent	Addressing the vector	Addressing the host
• (Elimination not feasible, as prescription opioids often currently practically and morally necessary to treat severe pain) • ER/LA opioids • Tamper-proof opioids	• Prescriber education regarding dangers of/ alternatives to opioids • Prescriber education on best prescribing practices • Tighter regulation of prescription by state medical boards or government • PDMPs • Reimbursement-driven changes in treatment models	• Prevention of painful conditions • Patient/population education regarding dangers of/ alternatives to opioids • Education on safe storage • Community naloxone • Effective substance dependence/abuse rehabilitation

Human Services' recently released National Pain Strategy [13] highlights the practical difficulties our healthcare system currently faces in implementing satisfactory solutions to addressing an issue as complicated as chronic pain under current reimbursement schema. It also advocates for a fundamental shift in how chronic pain is treated, beginning with provider education regarding current pain, basic science, and therapeutic options and also a focus upon patient self-efficacy, i.e., equipping them with knowledge and confidence to manage their symptoms and underlying pathology on their own (Table 1.1).

Addressing the Host: Creating Immunity

Addressing the vulnerability of the host comprises the last section of this book. As pointed out earlier, there are significant parallels between opioids and successful epidemic-generating infectious agents including transmissibility, virulence, and chronicity/delayed mortality. As was also proposed previously, a significant departure from historic epidemics, which must inform both clinical and epidemiologic strategy, is the irrational conscious pursuit of the agent by vulnerable hosts. Propensity to misuse and abuse a substance requires some positive motivation, and besides their analgesic qualities (at least in the short term), opioids also confer substantial euphoria and hedonic reward—again at least in the short term. Dependence and addiction do not affect every individual exposed to opioids (or other addictive substances) however, and numerous theories involving varying degrees of chemical compulsion and conscious or subconscious choice have been championed over the decades without rendering a clear answer to many of the basic questions surrounding addiction, such as who becomes addicted. Nonetheless, an understanding of risk factors for misuse, dependence, and addiction is essential for both clinician and epidemiologist, and careful risk assessment by the clinician is one of the most important tactics in the "war on opioids." Risk factor reduction is an invaluable strategy in reducing opioid dependence and aligns significantly with the nebulous concept of instilling host "immunity."

Primary prevention, efforts taken to prevent the problem before it happens, begins with education. Lack of perceived risk (or the risk-benefit ratio) has been shown to play an integral role in persistent use of substances. Lack of understanding alternatives to opioids may be another significant component of host vulnerability. Adequate education regarding "risks/benefits/alternatives" of any therapy is a time-honored component of the informed consent to treatment process that has arguably been lacking in the prescription of opioids over the past two decades.

Education, however, is not enough. Any rational effort at reducing patient proclivity to seeking and using opioids must also include a focus on prevention of the underlying condition that initially drives most hosts to the agent—in this case pain. Such an endeavor requires individual responsibility for health maintenance. Prevention by definition encompasses active steps taken to minimize the risk of an undesirable event, and the prevention of chronic pain must include what are often difficult lifestyle modifications such as smoking cessation, dietary changes, and exercise.

Perhaps the most difficult issue affecting this dynamic is that the motivator is often not merely physical pain; emotional pain is a significant (and sometimes exclusive) contributor to opioid seeking and use. Pain by its very nature is a complex experience involving far more than physical sensation; cognitive and emotional factors are thought to comprise as much as 70% of overall "pain burden" in the majority of people who suffer with chronic pain, and the treatment (let alone prevention) of these problems is no small undertaking.

Such improvement of overall health—mental, emotional, physical, and spiritual—is not confined to the arena of primary prevention. This attenuation of underlying vulnerability/risk factor modification comprises essential efforts during secondary and tertiary prevention phases of intervention as well. Secondary prevention comprises attempts to detect and retard or even reverse nascent pathology and is the battleground where most practitioners work on a daily basis. Vigilance on the part of the practitioner is essential at this stage to identify and confront budding opioid dependence. Effective secondary prevention (like primary prevention) must include palatable alternatives for the patient that address their underlying reasons for seeking opioids in the first place.

Tertiary prevention basically comprises damage control. The ultimate harm that opioids, whether prescription analgesics or illicit agents (e.g., heroin) exert, of course, is respiratory arrest, and the advancing tide of grim statistics shows no sign yet of abatement. As such, a recent population-level strategy to reduce the incidence of fatal opioid overdose has gathered increasing momentum in this country –community/bystander naloxone ("Narcan") distribution. Naloxone is a short-acting antagonist compound that rapidly reverses the effects of opioids by occupying and "blocking" the cellular receptor (mu-opioid receptor) where the drug exerts its effects. It is used worldwide by emergency medical services and emergency departments (and other areas of healthcare) to resuscitate overdose victims. Beginning sometime around 2010, several local and some state governments began efforts to make naloxone widely available to the public, and the FDA approved an "auto-injector" device in 2014, followed quickly by a nasal spray version in 2015. This approach may have merit in that it has the potential to reduce opioid overdose fatality; however, opponents argue that an increased sense of security among opioid misusers will be fostered, thus potentially even increasing virulence, so to speak. Nonetheless data support the efficacy of overdose education and naloxone distribution (OEND) in reducing opioid-related mortality, and the approach is rapidly becoming "standard of care" with recent inclusion in the CDC (and other) guidelines [10, 14, 15].

OEND however does not address the full spectrum of tertiary prevention, however, nor is established disease irreversible. Effective rehabilitation/recovery is possible albeit labor-intensive on all parties and not without significant attrition. "Necessary but not sufficient" skillful multidisciplinary clinical efforts saturated with patience are required, but the crux of the matter is the fostering and facilitating of the patient's desire and commitment to persist in the struggle to refuse what has become an all-consuming pursuit. Once opioid dependence is solidified, cessation of use becomes extremely difficult not so much due to reward as to the motivation to avoid withdrawal symptoms. Complex and overwhelmingly powerful neurochemical alterations take place in the brain, and even more complex and abstruse mechanisms of habit solidify within the shrouds of the mind. The hallmark of addiction is continued compulsive use despite awareness of danger and negative consequences, and simple education is not enough to reduce the vulnerability of much of the population at risk. More than warnings are required for the host to be augmented with effective resources to defend itself.

Medication-assisted treatment (MAT), comprising either agonist (substitution) therapy with methadone and buprenorphine or antagonist treatment with naltrexone, is a valuable and validated ally in the fight against opioid dependence-related morbidity and mortality. Statistically significant reduction of illicit use and comorbidities including HIV transmission and overdose deaths has been documented for decades with substitution therapy, with most of these data coming from methadone which has been in use to treat opioid dependence for half a century at this point. Methadone carries disproportionately high risks owing to unique pharmacologic properties however as discussed in Chap. 3, and more recently buprenorphine has demonstrated comparable efficacy with advantages of incomparably greater safety, as well as much greater accessibility as it can be prescribed outside the confines of federally approved opioid treatment facilities ("methadone clinics"). An even more appealing option by many metrics is extended-release naltrexone, available in this country now as a monthly intramuscular depot injection which improves treatment adherence and retention significantly over oral antagonist therapy.

It must be remembered that these medications comprise the "assistance" component of MAT, and effective behavioral treatment with a broad psychosocial-spiritual focus is required if true recovery/host immunity is to be achieved. While the vulnerability of the population may be the most logical arena to try to intervene upon (akin to vaccination), it remains the most difficult as at every stage the agent provides significant perceived benefit, whether positive (pain and distress reduction) or negative (withdrawal distress reduction). The individual struggling against opioid dependence experiences conflicting desires and motivations, and a cornerstone of behavioral treatment is to assist identification of the underlying factors reinforcing motivations for abstinence vs. use and strengthening the former while eroding the latter. Successful treatment approaches, whether cognitive-behavioral, "third-wave" (acceptance and commitment, mindfulness) therapies, or motivational enhancement, as well as mutual support groups, must effect recalibration of the user's desire for the substance. The experience of countless individuals who have overcome opioid (and other substance dependence) bears witness to the primacy and efficacy of substitution and cultivation of a greater desire, subjugating the appeal and even compulsion to seek and "use." While not appealing nor effective for all individuals, it is well documented in the medical literature, including the National Institute of Drug Abuse (NIDA)—funded "Monitoring the Future" study [16] that religious and spiritual practices are inversely related to alcohol and drug use. Rehabilitation-focused studies have shown that among people involved in attempts to overcome substance dependence (whether volitional or court-ordered), those with a greater spiritual and religious affectation have statistically significantly higher abstinence rates [17, 18].

Regardless of the route(s) chosen and the changes made, effecting recovery from opioid dependence is not a "quick fix," but like all complex chronic conditions affecting mind and body, one that requires ongoing intensive effort on the part of the individual as well as their care team. Addicts who successfully remained in recovery at the 5-year follow-up mark in the Drug Abuse Treatment Outcome Studies (DATOS) sample [17] demonstrated statistically significantly greater perception of self-motivation toward that end; this was in fact the most important discriminating factor in the analysis. Those individuals who maintained sobriety/recovery were almost four times more likely than those who relapsed to perceive improved overall personal growth including:

- Ability to handle responsibility
- Ability to recognize and express feelings
- Improved relational and social skills
- Improved self-efficacy perception in health maintenance
- Ability to lead a constructive and contributing life

It is unlikely that physical and psychological stimuli encouraging/tempting chemical coping via opioids will fully abate, but vulnerability to such maladaptive behavior can be overcome. In essence this is the ultimate effect of vaccination—not elimination of the agent or prevention of contact—but rather the equipping of the host's immune defenses (antibodies, lymphocytes, and natural killer cells) to resist and render impotent the would-be invaders. Thus only will propagation of the opioid epidemic cease.

Summary

The physician's oath begins with a commitment to risk reduction—*primum non nocere*. The physician's responsibility also includes the fundamental duty to relieve suffering whenever possible. Opioids are a powerful and dangerous tool in the therapeutic armamentarium, and like any power tool, untrained and indiscriminate use invites disaster. America's 20-year experiment of sowing liberal opioid prescriptions for chronic non-cancer pain is reaping us the whirlwind of the opioid epidemic, with over 198,000 people dying from prescription opioids between 1999 and 2015. A complex constellation of factors, including increased emphasis on pharmacotherapeutic intervention for chronic pain as well as psychopathology, in concert with a significant national decrease in self-efficacy and health mindset (with concordant increases in fear-avoidance behaviors, disability mindset, etc.), underlies this flawed management paradigm. In order to successfully contain and reverse this epidemic, a radical overhaul of how chronic pain is treated must occur at a national level.

Toward that end, the classic epidemiologic model involving agent, environment/vector, and host has been applied to the opioid epidemic in this book, with the drugs conceptualized as agent, prescribers as vector, and the population as host.

As in most epidemics, attenuating the virulence of the agent (in this case opioids) is of limited utility and efficacy. Nonetheless, understanding pathogenic mechanisms is essential in any public health endeavor, and understanding the complexity of opioids in their native/endogenous role (as well as their demonstrated extreme abuse liability when prescribed indiscriminately) is fundamental to enlightening us as to means of intervening upon the deadly interaction between host and agent, facilitated by vectors and other environmental factors. The second section of the book is devoted toward that end.

Attenuating the vector—addressing the transmission of the agent by prescriber education—comprises the third section of the book. This material however is not without relevance to non-prescribers, as vector and host in this epidemic must work collaboratively. The material presented in this section is in fact essential to equipping patients/hosts with risk factor modification or behavioral defenses against seeking out the agent (which in this epidemic does not exert the survival goals of an infectious agent—i.e., it does not seek out the host for its own subsistence and replication purposes).

The final section of the book focuses on modification of host risk factors and the cultivation of "behavioral immunity" which we contend is essential to the success of containment and reversal of the grim and rising toll of opioid morbidity and mortality.

Alteration of vulnerability and exposure behaviors is a difficult and effort-laden process but remains achievable and the only viable solution.

References

1. CDC Grand Rounds. Prescription drug overdoses — a U.S. epidemic. MMWR. 2012;61:10–3.
2. Center for Disease Control and Prevention. Increases in drug and opioid-involved overdose deaths—United States, 2010–2015. MMWR Morb Mortal Wkly Rep. 2016;65(5051):1445–52
3. Okie S. A flood of opioids, a rising tide of deaths. NEJM. 2010;363:1981–5.

4. Substance Abuse and Mental Health Services Administration. Results from the 2012 national survey on drug use and health: summary of national findings, NSDUH series H-46, HHS publication no. (SMA) 13–4795. Substance Abuse and Mental Health Services Administration: Rockville, MD; 2013.
5. Substance Abuse and Mental Health Services Administration. Highlights of the 2011 drug abuse warning network (DAWN) findings on drug-related emergency department visits. The DAWN report. Rockville, MD: US Department of Health and Human Services, Substance Abuse and Mental Health Services Administration; 2013. Available from: http://www.samhsa.gov/data/2k13/DAWN127/sr127-DAWN-highlights.htm
6. CDC. Wide-ranging online data for epidemiologic research (WONDER). Atlanta, GA: CDC, National Center for Health Statistics; 2016. Available from: http://wonder.cdc.gov
7. Kelsey JL, editor. Methods in observational epidemiology. 2nd ed. New York: Oxford University Press; 1996.
8. McLellan AT, Lewis DC, O'Brien CP, Kleber HD. Drug dependence, a chronic medical illness. Implications for treatment, insurance, and outcomes evaluation. JAMA. 2000;284(13):1689–95.
9. Centers for Disease Control and Prevention. Increases in drug and opioid overdose deaths — United States, 2000–2014. MMWR. 2015;64:1–5.
10. Dowell D, Haegerich TM, Chou R. CDC guideline for prescribing opioids for chronic pain – United States, 2016. MMWR. 2016;65:1–49.
11. Federation of State Medical Boards of the United States, Inc. Model policy on the use of opioid analgesics in the treatment of chronic pain. Available from: http://www.fsmb.org/Media/Default/PDF/FSMB/Advocacy/pain_policy_july2013.pdf. Accessed 20 Nov 2016.
12. Manchikanti L, Kaye AM, Knezevic NN, McAnally H, Slavin K, Trescot AM, et al. Responsible, safe, and effective prescription of opioids for chronic non-cancer pain: American society of interventional pain physicians (ASIPP) guidelines. Pain Phys. 2017,20(2S):S3–S92.
13. The Office of the Assistant Secretary for Health at the U.S. Department of Health and Human Services, National Pain Strategy–A comprehensive population health-level strategy for pain. 2016. http://iprcc.nih.gov/docs/HHSNational_Pain_Strategy.pdf.
14. Center for Substance Abuse Treatment. Clinical guidelines for the use of buprenorphine in the treatment of opioid addiction. Treatment improvement protocol (TIP) series 40. DHHS publication no. (SMA) 04–3939. Rockville, MD: Substance Abuse and Mental Health Services Administration; 2004.
15. The American Society of Addiction Medicine. The national practice guideline for the use of medications in the treatment of addiction involving opioid use. American Society of Addiction Medicine, Chevy Chase, MD; 2015.
16. Miech RA, Johnston LD, O'Malley PM, Bachman JG, Schulenberg JE, Patrick ME. Monitoring the future national survey results on drug use, 1975–2016: volume I, secondary school students. Ann Arbor: Institute for Social Research, The University of Michigan; 2017. Available at http://monitoringthefuture.org/pubs.html#monographs.
17. Flynn PM, Joe GW, Broome KM, Simpson DD, Brown BS. Recovery from opioid addiction in DATOS. J Subst Abus Treat. 2003;25:177–86.
18. Schoenthaler SJ, Blum K, Braverman ER, Giordano J, Thompson B, Oscar-Berman M, et al. NIDA-drug addiction treatment outcome study (DATOS) relapse as a function of spirituality/religiosity. J Reward Defic Syndr. 2015;1(1):36–45.

Part II
Focusing on the Agent

"知彼知己 百戰不殆 不知彼 不知己 每戰必殆"

(If you know the enemy and know yourself, you need not fear the result of a hundred battles… If you know neither the enemy nor yourself, you will succumb in every battle.)

– Sun Tzu, *The Art of War*

Chapter 2
Understanding the Agent, Part I: Opioid Biology and Basic Pharmacology

A Canadian mother was prescribed codeine for post-episiotomy pain in April 2005; the pregnancy and delivery were otherwise uncomplicated, and the infant was born at 90th percentile for weight. One week later, he developed lethargy and difficulty breastfeeding, and on day of life 11, he was brought to a pediatrician for evaluation; he was found to have regained his birthweight and sent home. On day 13, the infant was found cyanotic, apneic, and pulseless, and both field and emergency department resuscitations were unsuccessful. Postmortem analysis included extensive evaluation for inborn errors of metabolism, none of which were found. Toxicologic analysis revealed morphine plasma levels of 70 ng/mL. The mother had been taking acetaminophen 500 mg/codeine 30 mg twice daily, titrating down from the prescribed dose, due to her own sedation and constipation [1].

Opioids, which have enjoyed centuries of therapeutic use and for the most part an unchallenged reign in treating severe pain, are conceptualized in this book as the etiologic *agent* in what has come to be known as the opioid epidemic in America.

Understanding all that we can about any agent in an epidemic is essential to ending its upper hand in the conflict, and this section of the book seeks to invest the practitioner with the essentials of the agent.

In order to understand opioids, however, a solid understanding of the host system that exogenous opioids mimic and affect is fundamental. Knowledge of a bacterium or virus' anatomy and physiology is not enough; understanding its biologic/chemical substrates and tissue "preferences," virulence mechanisms, and transmission is critical to designing strategies for host protection. We also live in the era of elucidating host (and agent) genetic factors that affect pathogenicity, and this may ultimately inform and direct the most rational and effective treatments—and prophylaxis. While much of these concepts are explored in more detail in subsequent sections focusing on vector and host, it is essential to first explore the native

H.B. McAnally, *Opioid Dependence*, DOI 10.1007/978-3-319-47497-7_2

systems which opioids are designed to both mimic and affect in order to understand how they exert their influence both therapeutically and pathologically. As such, we begin our examination of the agent with an examination of ourselves.

Opioid Biology

The opioid system exists throughout the animal kingdom, even within invertebrates [2]. This complex system is apparently designed not only to provide relief of pain but is intimately involved with numerous physiologic functions including neuroimmunoendocrine homeostasis, and in higher organisms both cognitive and emotional processes.

Endogenous Opioids: The Body's Natural Analgesics

Opioids by definition are chemical agents that exert their effects via interaction with opioid receptors located primarily within the central nervous system but to some extent within the periphery as well. Three opioid receptor classes are currently described: the *mu-opioid receptor (MOR)*, *delta-opioid receptor (DOR)*, and *kappa-opioid receptor (KOR)*. The biochemistry and activities of these receptors will be described in more detail in a subsequent section. Endogenous opioids are polypeptides currently classified within four major families: the *endorphins*, *endomorphins*, *enkephalins*, and *dynorphins*. These peptides are cleaved from precursor peptides: pro-opiomelanocortin (POMC), proenkephalin, and prodynorphin, respectively. (Each of these precursors is in turn derived from a longer sequence indicated by the prefix "pre-," e.g., pre-pro-opioimelanocortin [pre-POMC] rendered during the post-ribosomal translation process).

β-Endorphin is the most well studied of the endogenous opioids. POMC (the precursor to β-endorphin) is known to be produced primarily within the pituitary, hypothalamus (arcuate nucleus), and medulla (nucleus tractus solitarius) as well as extraneural sites such as the pancreas, and melanocytes. This widespread distribution mirrors the diverse activity of POMC derivatives, with complex roles in energy homeostasis, stress response, immune function, and also melanocyte stimulation. As POMC travels through the cell's endomembrane system, it is cleaved (primarily within the trans-Golgi network) to various active molecules including β-endorphin, adrenocorticotropic hormone (ACTH), lipotropins, and melanotropins. Discussion of these latter hormones is outside the scope of this work, but is referenced here briefly to bring attention to the fact that the body's natural pain—modulating system—is intricately connected with the neuroimmunoendocrine system as a whole. As a point of interest, the well-known anecdotal observation that redheaded individuals apparently have decreased responsiveness to exogenous opioids and sedatives and/or decreased tolerance to pain may have some biologic possibility in the fact that mutations within the POMC production process are associated with the redhead phenotype [3]. However, the few studies done in this area are contradictory, with some studies showing increased and others showing decreased tolerance to both pain and analgesics/anesthetics [4–6].

β-Endorphins act within both central and peripheral nervous systems to produce analgesia via multiple modes of action, primarily by interaction with the mu-opioid receptor (MOR), In the 1970s and 1980s, most research on endorphin and MOR ligand activity within the brain focused on the *periaqueductal gray (PAG)* region of the tegmentum of the midbrain. It was shown that endorphins/MOR ligands block the release of gamma-aminobutyric acid (GABA) within the PAG which normally acts tonically via projection fibers to inhibit serotonergic activity in the nucleus raphe magnus and other areas of the *rostroventral medulla (RVM)*. These medullary areas provide powerful analgesic activity via "descending modulation" effects upon the dorsal horn of the spinal cord and also within the trigeminal nucleus caudalis and are tonically inhibited by PAG GABA activity (Fig. 2.1).

More recent research, beginning with the work of Fields [7, 8] has focused on direct activity of MOR ligands upon cell populations within the RVM itself, labeled "ON" and "OFF" cells. "OFF" cells are antinociceptive neurons within the RVM that are tonically inhibited by GABA, but upon activation by endorphin (or exogenous MOR ligand) activity work at the level of the dorsal horn of the spinal cord via serotonin to downmodulate ascending pain signals. MOR ligands conversely demonstrate a direct inhibitory effect upon RVM "ON" cells, which tonically act to facilitate ascending pain signals within the spinothalamic and pathway [9].

Inhibition of substance P activity within the RVM may be another mechanism of endorphin/MOR ligand-facilitated analgesia.

Of significant historic and clinical interest is the phenomenon of the placebo effect. First demonstrated (and propounded as an essential control mechanism in prospective trials) by Dr. H. K. Beecher at the Massachusetts General Hospital, the placebo effect has subsequently been shown to be a manifestation of endorphin activity within the PAG (Fig. 2.2) [10–12].

At the level of the spinal cord, endorphins/MOR ligands act in several ways to attenuate pain transmission. First, within the dorsal horn (and more specifically Rexed laminae I, II, and V), endorphins/MOR ligands act directly presynaptically (on the first-order pain afferent traveling from the periphery) to reduce substance P and other tachykinin release, which serve as the primary pain neurotransmitter at this level. This inhibition is thought to occur via suppression of N-type voltage-gated calcium channel activity necessary for the release of substance P [13, 14]. Secondly, endorphins/MOR ligands inhibit the presynaptic release of glutamate, reducing excitatory neurotransmission [15]. Thirdly, endorphins/MOR ligands may act to reduce calcitonin gene-related peptide (CGRP) release from primary afferents. Until recently, this activity had been demonstrated in vitro but in vivo studies consistently refuted the effect [16]; however, newer assaying techniques have shown that CGRP inhibition does occur in a mouse model [17]. Fourthly, MOR ligands at supraphysiologic (and supratherapeutic for most agents) have been shown to directly inhibit voltage-gated sodium channel action potential propagation in a

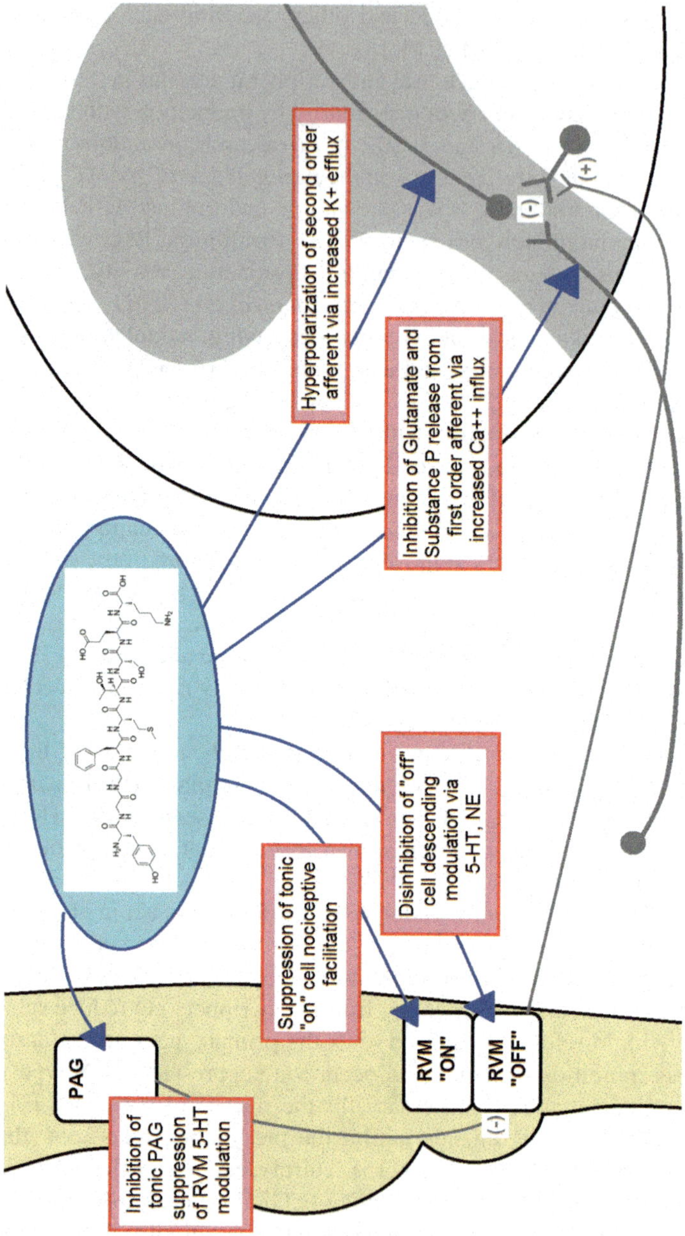

Fig. 2.1 Supraspinal and spinal mechanisms of actions of opioids

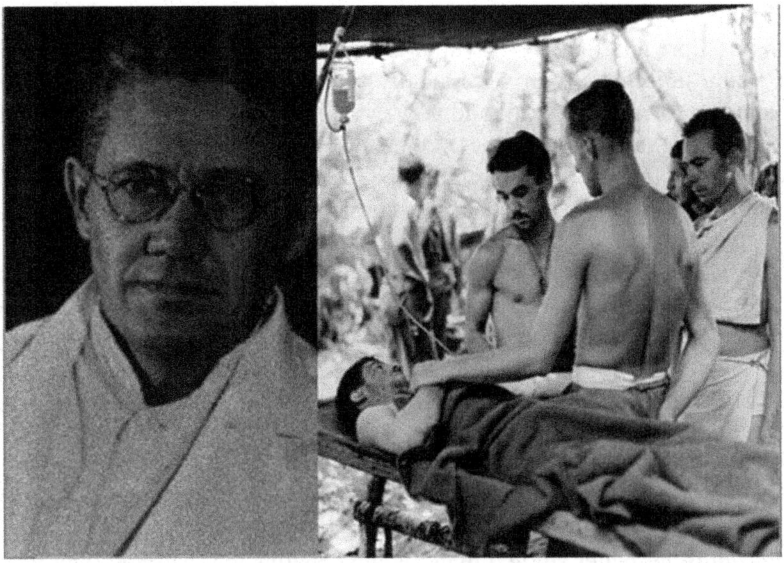

Fig. 2.2 Dr. Henry Knowles Beecher, 1904–1976, Professor Emeritus at the Harvard Medical School, was an anesthesiologist whose observations on psychological effects on pain perception during his World War II service in North Africa led him ultimately to propose what we now know as placebo-controlled trials. Other notable achievements include his groundbreaking 1966 article *Ethics and Clinical Research*, which led to the concept of informed consent and the academic Institutional Review Board system; he also trained Danish anesthesiologist Dr. Bjorn Ibsen, who later pioneered positive-pressure ventilation during a 1952 poliomyelitis outbreak and created the first intensive care unit

manner analogous to local anesthetic action [18]. Fifthly, at a postsynaptic level, endorphins/MOR ligands activate potassium channels on the second-order neuron, leading to hyperpolarization and reduction of transmission [19]. Sixthly, the activity of endorphins/MOR ligands upon both nicotinic and muscarinic acetylcholine receptors within the spinal cord have been shown to contribute significantly to analgesic effects of these compounds [20]. Finally, endorphins/MOR ligands act indirectly on the spinal cord via the aforementioned PAG/RVM descending modulation system.

Opioid receptors exist in the periphery but have not been shown to mediate any meaningful analgesic effects under normal circumstances. In states of local inflammation, however, administration of various opioid receptor ligands (mu, delta, and kappa) have all shown efficacy in reducing inflammation and pain when applied peripherally to hyperalgesic tissue [21]. It is unclear if these data are relevant to physiologic situations and endogenous opioids.

Endomorphins, first described by Zadina in 1997 [22], are powerful and apparently highly selective MOR ligands whose precursor molecule has yet to be identified. Their selectivity for the MOR is 4000 times greater than their affinity for the DOR and 15,000 times greater than their affinity for the KOR [23]. They are known to be more resistant to enzymatic degradation than the other three classes of endogenous opioids and also display vasodilatory activity via activation of nitric oxide upregulation [24]. Synthetic analogs of endomorphins have shown potent analgesic effects with significantly reduced psychomotor retardation and also addictive potential [25, 26] and may evolve as very useful clinical opioids.

First to be identified among the endogenous opioids, but least well studied, are the *enkephalins*, found primarily within the CNS (the name indicates the observation that these substances exist and act primarily within the brain). The proenkephalin molecule is cleaved into two main peptides, met-enkephalin and leu-enkephalin, both of which are rapidly degraded within the bloodstream and various tissues [27, 28]. The enkephalins are considered to be the primary endogenous ligands of the delta-opioid receptor (DOR) [29], although they also possess some mu-opioid receptor activity as well. They are thought to be related to the processing of pain sensation beginning at the level of the dorsal horn and spinal trigeminal nucleus and to limbic modulation of these sensations by the amygdala, hippocampus, and frontal cortex [19]. Due to the relative paucity of our understanding of the DOR system, and the very short half-life of enkephalins, no lasting efforts to harness this family for therapeutic use have been undertaken.

Dynorphins are better studied than the enkephalins, but perhaps even less well understood due to their complex and confusing interactions with various pathways. These powerful compounds have been shown to be regulated in part by the stress response with release being modulated by corticotropin-releasing factor [30]. They are found primarily in the central nervous system (hypothalamus, medulla, pons, midbrain, and spinal cord) and exert their effects primarily through the kappa-opioid receptor (KOR). The name (from the Greek root for "power") indicates the potency of these endogenous ligands; they have been shown to be six to ten times more potent as an analgesic than morphine [31, 32]. However, there is evidence that dynorphins may also be pronociceptive via bradykinin activity stimulation [33]; dynorphin levels within the spinal cord have also been shown to be elevated in chronic pain states [34]. Further complicating their biology (and clinical relevance), dynorphins have been shown to be intricately involved in KOR-mediated dysphoria and the complex neuropsychobiology of addiction [35–37]. The latter has been the major focal area of research on dynorphins and will likely continue to be so as the phenomenon of opioid addiction increases in clinical and public health significance.

Opioid Receptors

Opioid receptors belong to the ubiquitous superfamily of *G-protein-coupled receptors (GPCRs)*, which mediate the known actions of most neurotransmitters and hormones. GPCRs are cell membrane-bound proteins with seven helices arranged spanning the membrane, with three intracellular and three extracellular loops forming a pocket for their ligand(s) to bind (Fig. 2.3). The GPCR is coupled to a separate regulatory protein (the G protein) that binds guanosine diphosphate (GDP) in its

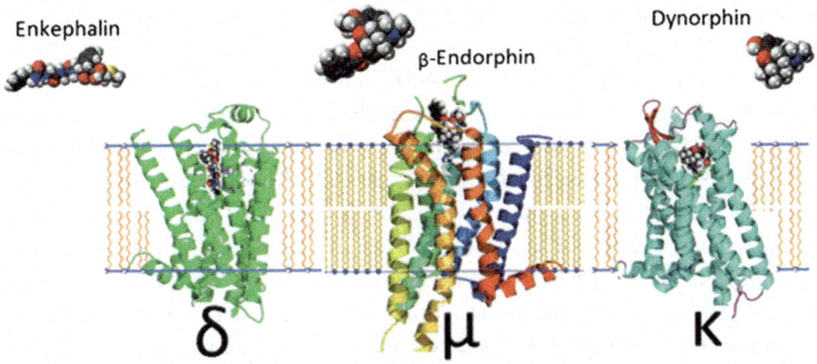

Fig. 2.3 Opioid receptors and their endogenous ligands

resting state. Upon activation by its ligand, the GPCR undergoes a conformational change that causes the G protein to exchange GDP for GTP and undergo dissociation of its component subunits which then effect a number of downstream changes. In the case of opioid receptor activity, some of these effects include inhibition of adenylyl cyclase (which reduces cyclic AMP levels), activation of potassium channels, and inhibition of voltage-gated calcium channels; the net effect of these changes results in hyperpolarization of the cell. In the case of neurons, reduction of neurotransmitter release as well as action potential propagation may result.

One feature of GPCRs that may confer clinically relevant effects is their ability to form oligomers or complexes of multiple receptors, whether homogenous (e.g., MOR-MOR dimer) or heterogenous (e.g., MOR-DOR dimer). Such multimer formation has been proposed as one possible explanation for a variety of unpredictable laboratory and clinical effects, including incomplete cross-tolerance to different therapeutic opioid drugs [38].

The *mu-opioid receptor (MOR)* is the receptor best-studied and most utilized therapeutically. All clinically used opioids today are agonists of the MOR (with varying agonist activities and in some cases antagonist activity at other opioid receptors). Located extensively throughout the central nervous system and also within the peripheral nervous system, gut, and various immune system cells, the MOR is responsible for the majority of therapeutic opioid-related activity (analgesia) as well as several of the more serious and acute adverse effects, such as respiratory depression and constipation/ileus. Mu-receptor subtypes have been proposed by various groups, but have not been accepted as definitive due to very incomplete evidence confounded by multiple alternative explanations (e.g., receptor oligomerization) for the disparity in biologic effects from different ligands [38]. Nonetheless, the mu-1 receptor subtype is suggested to confer analgesia and physical dependence; the mu-2 receptor, euphoria, respiratory depression, ileus, pruritis, miosis, and physical dependence; and the mu-3 receptor, vasodilatation.

The *delta-opioid receptor (DOR)* is currently an area of intense investigation, as its properties may prove to be uniquely useful in modulation of chronic pain and addiction. Located primarily within the cortex and basal ganglia in humans [39], there is a considerable degree of interspecies heterogeneity in terms of peripheral distribution; among primates, DOR seems to be primarily located in small- and medium-sized afferents [40]. As with MOR, subtypes have been proposed, including DOR1 and DOR2. Its natural ligands, as discussed above, are thought to be the enkephalins. Early studies showed somewhat confusing and contradictory effects on CGRP release [41] and substance P release [42]. More recent evidence suggests that complicated interactions between the MOR and DOR (as well as other factors influencing the expression of at least the DOR in various pathologic states) including heteromerization are responsible for the difficulties in assigning clearly defined "effect profiles" for these receptors. Nonetheless, there is some suggestion that DOR agonism may confer superior neuropathic pain control, reduced respiratory depression, constipation, and physical dependence, compared to pure MOR agonism [41, 42]. Alternative roles for DOR agonists including antidepressants and cardiac myocyte ischemic preconditioning agents have also been suggested but have not yet borne fruit clinically [39, 40, 43].

The *kappa-opioid receptor (KOR)* is distributed widely throughout the brain (hypothalamus, periaqueductal gray, and claustrum), substantia gelatinosa, and in peripheral nerves. It is also represented in significant proportion throughout the viscera. Putative subtypes for this receptor have also been proposed. As discussed above, its endogenous ligands include the dynorphins. Other naturally occurring KOR ligands include menthol and the hallucinogen salvia. A disproportionate amount of adverse psychiatric effects seems to be mediated by the KOR (dysphoria/depression, dissociation and hallucinations); however, it has been suggested that this activity may confer a "natural addiction control mechanism." Of clinical interest is the observation that buprenorphine, a partial agonist at the MOR and an antagonist at the KOR that is used primarily in addiction management, seems to possess antidepressant qualities unique to the opioid family. Numerous investigations have demonstrated the superiority of KOR agonists in alleviating pain and discomfort from visceral sources [44]; however, given the high rate of adverse effects, no clinically useful drug has yet been developed.

The *nociceptin/orphanin FQ receptor (NOR)* is a recently discovered opioid receptor "cousin" demonstrating significant interactions with both the classic opioid systems and also a highly diverse array of other physiologic functions. First isolated in 1994, the NOR was initially named opioid receptor-like 1 (ORL1) and shares a little over 50% homology to the "classic" MOR, DOR, and KOR but does not bind any of the known endogenous opioid ligands (other than dynorphin A). Its natural ligand has been independently named nociceptin (reflecting its pronociceptive activities) and orphanin FQ (the most common acronym in the literature, N/OFQ references both titles). As with most things opioid-related, it turns out the N/OFQ system is exceedingly complex, and it is found in tremendous dispersion throughout the CNS, including the cerebral cortex, thalamus, hypothalamus, hippocampus, habenula, amygdala, locus ceruleus, substantia nigra, periaqueductal gray, ventral tegmental area and raphe complex, and both dorsal and ventral horns of the spinal cord; in addition, the system is found throughout the intestinal and other visceral organs and also on many leukocytes [45, 46]. Besides facilitating both pronociception and antinociception (discussed in greater detail below), the widespread activities of this system reflect its ubiquitous distribution and include effects on cognitive functions such as learning and memory; emotional functions related to stress and anxiety; feeding behaviors; respiratory, cardiovascular, and renal function; and immune function [45–48].

Finally, at one time, a proposed *sigma-opioid receptor* was widely accepted (the author remembers memorizing it and its effects, most of which are adverse, in second-year medical school pharmacology class) but has since been shown to be completely structurally unrelated to opioid receptors and is no longer considered to be one.

Opioid-Modulating Systems

As early as the 1980s, it was becoming apparent that endogenous "anti-opioid" systems exist within the CNS. A growing body of evidence supports the hypothesis that the body possesses its own "check and balance" system regulating the pain-modulating effects of endogenous opioids and possibly protecting us against disadvantageous phenomena such as tolerance and dependence.

Adenosine has been studied for decades as an analgesic in its own right and has been shown to undergo opioid-related release in the spinal cord, and the A3 receptor subtype is an area currently undergoing active research for possible therapeutics [49].

The *cholecystokinin (CCK)* system was among the earliest endogenous neuropeptide opioid modifier studied and is generally regarded as an opioid-inhibitory system in addition to its inherent pro-inflammatory action. At the level of both brain and spinal cord, CCK has been shown to both block opioid activity and enhance opioid-induced hyperalgesia [29]. CCK however has been shown to exert both suppressive and potentiating effects upon opioid analgesia that has been proposed to be dependent upon competing actions of subtypes of CCK (CCK-A vs. CCK-B) upon encephalin effects at the MOR vs. the DOR [29]. Differential and possibly dose-dependent effects of CCK on RVM "ON" and "OFF" cells have been invoked to explain differential supraspinal activity [50, 51]. CCK-opioid interactions are exceedingly complex and display responsiveness to stress and anxiety states as well as other endocrine perturbation [52–54].

The *neuropeptide FF (NPFF)* system is another opioid-modulating peptide system with effects that include attenuation not only of anti-nociceptive effects of opioids but also psychological reward [54–57]. This system may play an important role in the iatrogenic phenomenon of opioid-induced hyperalgesia [57].

The *neurokinin-1 receptor (NK1R)* is the main receptor in the tachykinin receptor family, whose main ligand is the neurotransmitter known as *substance P*. While initially thought to be primarily a pain neurotransmitter active primarily within the dorsal horn, it is expressed widely by multiple cell types including neurons, glia, endothelia, fibroblasts and other poeitic cells, and leukocytes as a primary inflammatory mediator and also plays an important role in initiating a number of "constructive" processes as well including hematopoiesis, wound healing, and cell survival [58, 59]. The modulatory effects of NK1R upon opioid activity are not well characterized, but one study showed that activation of NK1R co-localized with MOR in striatal cells prevented MOR endocytosis (which finding was in contradiction to previous studies showing an increase in MOR endocytosis/inactivation) [60].

Perhaps the best-studied of the endogenous opioid-modifying systems is the *N-methyl-D-aspartate (NMDA)* system. The NDMA receptor (NMDAR) is a glutamate (one of the major excitatory neurotransmitters) receptor widely distributed throughout the CNS that is tonically inactivated by the presence of a magnesium ion within its channel. When bound by glutamate (and a co-ligand such as serine or glycine) and when the neuron undergoes depolarization, magnesium then dissociates from the channel, and various cation traffic (primarily calcium influx) results in downstream effects via calcium-sensing proteins and other mediators including G-protein complexes that result in long-term potentiation and other synaptic plasticity events [61, 62]. NMDA activity is increasingly shown to play a role in a number of physiologic events (e.g., learning) and pathophysiologic states (e.g., depression, schizophrenia, autism spectrum disorders, chronic pain states). Of relevance to opioid pharmacology is the fact that since the early 1990s, we have known that NDMA activity results in rapid development of tolerance to opioids and conversely NMDA antagonism prevents or reduces such development of tolerance. One mechanism for NMDA-opioid interactions at least at the level of the periaqueductal gray has recently been shown to be disruption of normal MOR-NMDAR coupling by binding of ligands to either receptor, which activates protein kinase C (PKC) or protein kinase A (PKA) both of which effect tolerance perhaps by internalization of the MOR [63].

The recently discovered *nociceptin/orphanin FQ (N/OFQ)* system demonstrates significant bidirectional modulatory relationships with the classic opioid receptors; depending on species and specific stimulation patterns, ligand dosing, location and chronicity, and a host of other variables, N/OFQ may exert pronociceptive or antinociceptive effects [45–47, 64]. It appears that supraspinal actions may be more complex in terms of pain responses, whereas spinal actions more consistently demonstrate analgesic tendency [46, 47]. Multiple studies have shown heterodimerization of NOR with the classic receptors, adding to the complexity of interactions between these cousins [46]. Furthermore, the pro-inflammatory effects of the NOR system effected by its neuroimmune activities and the stress/anxiety-mediated effects of the NOR system effected by limbic and hypothalamic-pituitary-adrenal axis activities confer additional layers of real-life complexity surrounding NOR modulation.

Activation of the *platelet-derived growth factor receptor type-beta (PDGFR-β)* has been shown in animal models to be activated among other things by MOR activity, and PDGFR-β activity in turn results in opioid tolerance [65]. The mechanism of action is not clear and is furthermore confounded by the fact that PDGFR-β activity inhibits NMDAR [66] which should according to our understanding of that receptor's activity decrease opioid tolerance.

Synergistic effects of *α_2-adrenoreceptor (α_2-AR)* activity with that of opioids have been known for decades and intrathecal administration of clonidine has been commonplace by anesthesiologists for many years. Both α_2-AR and opioid receptors A118G variant (DOR in particular) have been shown to co-localize at the terminus of the primary afferent, and α_2-AR are also abundant on interneurons in the substantia gelatinosa; however, the exact mechanism of this cooperative activity remains unknown. The formation of opioid-adrenoreceptor heteromers has been suggested as one potential explanation [67].

Finally, a fascinating area of research involves the bidirectional relationship of opioids and neuronal support cells (astrocytes, microglia). Long thought to be fairly devoid of any activity other than supporting neurons, our understanding of this dynamic cell population has grown exponentially over the past decade, and we now know that glia are actively involved in neurotransmission, regulating neuronal activity, remodeling synapses, and many other functions. Glia are also very active in modulating the pain response and can function to amplify and perpetuate neuronal signaling by pro-inflammatory means (including cytokines, chemokines, prostaglandins, and other mediators), alter neurotransmitter release and receptor expression, and even actively participate in signaling [68, 69]. Opioid receptors have been demonstrated on glia [49, 69], and activation of these receptors results in inflammatory mediator released/increased pain sensitivity and also opioid tolerance. A distinct innate immune receptor on glia named the *Toll-like receptor 4 (TLR4)* is activated by both stress/inflammatory signals and also by opioids and has been shown to be intricately involved with the development of opioid tolerance, dependence, psychological reward, and also opioid-induced hyperalgesia [68–70].

Overview of Non-analgesic Opioid Effects and Interactions

No twenty-first-century discussion of opioid pharmacology is complete without at least salutatory reference to the vast body of research indicating what appears to be "the most extensive and diverse peptidergic transmission system… widely involved in various pleiotropic functions" [43]. Multiple physiologic processes from the cellular to the organ level are influenced by the opioid system, and while a rigorous discussion of such interactions is well beyond the scope of this book, it bears mention that both endogenous and therapeutic applications of opioids have widespread effects upon the organism as a whole that are just now beginning to be elucidated [43, 69]. Adverse effects of opioids are discussed in a later section.

Opioid Pharmacology

Opioid Pharmacodynamics and Pharmacokinetics

Pharmacodynamics is sometimes defined as "what the drug does to the body" and is concerned with mechanisms of action of drugs and effects produced. Conversely, pharmacokinetics is described as "what the body does to the drug" and is concerned with the processes of absorption, distribution, metabolism, and excretion of drugs.

Simple dose-response curves describing the effects of a drug as invariably correlated with the amount administered or the concentration of the drug are a gross oversimplification increasingly complicated by our expanding understanding of the effects of genetic differences, drug-drug interactions, and dynamic factors such as mutable expression or function of transporters, receptors, and post-receptor mechanisms (e.g., second-messenger systems). Tolerance, for example, discussed in its own subsection below alters pharmacodynamics with almost individual-level variance and is a phenomenon with tremendous clinical impact on opioid therapy.

Beyond the complex issues inherent within the opioid "system" proper, an ever-increasing body of evidence bears witness to the possibly unparalleled diversity of interaction between endogenous or exogenous opioids and their receptors and multiple other physiologic processes from ionic homeostasis, hypoxic/ischemic protection, and cell proliferation at the microscopic level to organ-level alteration of cerebral, respiratory, cardiac, immune, endocrine, and gastroenterologic systems [43, 71]. These interactions are frequently "two-way streets," with complex signaling and reciprocal feedback/control mechanisms that are not fully understood but likely have their basis in dynamic receptor alterations including oligomerization, uncoupling, and endocytosis.

Similarly, the simplicity of basic pharmacokinetic concepts taught for decades (such as zero vs. first-order kinetics, single or two-compartment models) is increasingly challenged by our expanding understanding of phenomena such as pharmacogenetics, epigenetics, drug-drug interactions, induction and inhibition, and other such pharmacodynamic factors that influence metabolism. Disease states also have profound effects on pharmacokinetics (and pharmacodynamics).

It should also be noted that pharmacodynamic and pharmacokinetic principles/processes are occurring simultaneously within the body, and though they are phenomena without innate intelligence, they can be conceptualized as being at odds with each other. The drug "desires" to exert an effect on the body (pharmacodynamics), while the body "desires" to be rid of the drug (pharmacokinetic). For continuity of understanding the biological and biochemical processes involving these molecules from administration to elimination, this discussion will of necessity progress to some extent back and forth from topics within the categories of pharmacodynamics and pharmacokinetics. We will begin our examination of opioid pharmacology with processes that fall under the rubric of pharmacokinetics, such as absorption and distribution. We will then proceed to examination of endogenous opioid ligands and opioid receptors and their pharmacodynamics. Natural opioid-modifying systems will be reviewed next, followed by a brief survey of non-analgesic activities resulting from opioid receptor activation. The pharmacokinetic function of metabolism, and a brief survey of pharmacogenetic factors affecting both opioid pharmacology, and finally a review of the important phenomenon of opioid tolerance will follow before progressing to discussion of individual therapeutic agents. Therapeutic and adverse effects of opioids, evidence-based guidance for use, and alternatives will be discussed in Sect 3.

Absorption and Transport

The vast majority of clinical opioid use is oral, and after ingestion/digestion, the drugs first enter the portal circulation from the intestines via both simple diffusion and also by active transport mechanisms such as the solute carrier (SLC) superfamily of influx transporters, which in conjunction with the ATP-binding cassette (ABC) superfamily of efflux transporters regulates in part net uptake of molecules through the mucosa into the bloodstream [72, 73]. Hepatic uptake is also governed in large part by these transporters. The relatively recent development of controlled-/extended-release technology, which retards the rate of dissolution within the alimentary canal, does not alter any of these fundamental biologic mechanisms.

The drug then undergoes immediate ("first-pass") metabolism as described in more detail below in the pharmacokinetics section—the body is already trying to degrade and eliminate the drug. Parenterally administered drugs of course are not subject to first-pass metabolism but still experience hepatic metabolism every time they circulate through the organ.

In some cases, the drug taken is a relatively ineffective precursor agent that the liver "unwittingly" alters into an active or more potent state. In either case, after running the gauntlet of the liver, the agent (or altered agent) exits the portal circulation and enters the systemic venous circulation for left-heart distribution to the rest of the body.

Distribution is a pharmacokinetic concept that will be explored in slightly more detail below; "macrodistribution" by the cardiovascular system and subsequent "microdistribution" by diffusion and active transport mechanisms into tissues and organs are both encompassed in this phase. Within the latter category, an intermediary system of opioid transporters (the SLC and ABC superfamilies) again exerts either facilitatory or inhibitory effects respectively upon the agent to ferry it across to or restrict its access to the CNS wherein lies the main arena of opioid effects. Continuous active efflux of drugs by ABC superfamily transporters within the vascular luminal endothelium may comprise the major hurdle within the blood-brain barrier for opioids and other psychoactive drugs [74, 75].

Distribution and Metabolism

Distribution of a drug to target organs and receptors, as well as inert tissues such as the muscle, bone, and fat, occurs immediately following entry of the agent to the systemic circulation. Several factors influence the transport and transfer of these molecules, including protein binding and lipophilicity.

Plasma proteins such as albumin and alpha-1 acid glycoprotein (AAG) may bind a drug and prolong its circulation within the bloodstream/retard its uptake by tissues and also retard hepatorenal elimination. The proportion of protein-bound drug varies widely among opioids, from roughly 30% for morphine to 90% for alfentanil (an intravenous opioid). This percentage may be dynamic, however, as competition for plasma protein binding sites, and various metabolic conditions (e.g., hypoalbuminemia or acid-base disturbances) may influence binding. Furthermore, AAG is an acute phase reactant with significantly increased plasma presence during inflammation, which may alter opioid pharmacokinetics.

Lipophilicity is another variable with significant pharmacokinetic effect. As a general rule, the more lipophilic a substance, the more readily it is able to diffuse through cell membranes, which of course are composed of a lipid bilayer. This is particularly important in the context of the blood-brain barrier, where the agent must pass through the endothelial membrane, both apical and basal (all the while undergoing efflux transport back out of the cell into the bloodstream) on its journey to the CNS. There is significant variation in lipophilicity among the opioids, ranging from fairly hydrophilic molecules such as morphine to highly lipophilic molecules such as fentanyl and sufentanil (an intravenous opioid with ten times the potency of fentanyl). Discussions of these characteristics have generally been relegated to the realm of parenteral opioids, as lipophilic distribution considerations significantly impact spinal and epidural administration. However, these issues are not without relevance to the outpatient world as well, as agents with a high degree of lipophilicity (generally presented in pharmacologic textbooks as the octanol: buffer partition coefficient) also store up in adipose tissues, and in obese individuals, this can yield a volume of distribution significantly larger than anticipated. In the case of fentanyl, for example, a significant reservoir of drug can accumulate in the obese individual and wind up contributing to far greater plasma levels than would be expected from a given transdermal dose.

Infrequently discussed in the opioid literature, but commonly taught in pharmacology classes and anesthesiology residency programs is the concept of vessel-rich and vessel-poor compartments, and these theoretical compartments complicate the simple pharmacokinetic concept of half-life [76]. The so-called vessel-rich compartment is comprised of organs and tissues that are highly perfused, such as the brain, heart, lung, liver, and kidney. An intermediately, perfused group is often taught as well, comprising primarily the muscle. Finally, the vessel-poor group consists of the adipose and bone. The apparent reality of this multicompartmental model significantly complicates the simplistic concept of half-life ($t_{½}$), which describes the amount of time required for plasma levels of an agent to fall by 50%, and has been described for first-order kinetics as a constant (with a linear downslope of the logarithm of concentration) for virtually all medications and toxins in classic pharmacology textbooks. In a multicompartmental model, there are multiple half-lives reflecting not only elimination kinetics, but distribution kinetics as well. In the simplest form, $t_{½}\alpha$ refers to distribution half-life and has in general a steeper downslope, at least for agents that readily leave the bloodstream, i.e., are not highly protein-bound nor markedly hydrophilic. In this model, $t_{½}\beta$ refers to elimination half-life and assumes equilibrium between plasma and the compartments.

As a side note, this multicompartmental model has clinical significance also in terms of unanticipated reservoirs. As mentioned previously, fentanyl, due to its very high lipophilicity, will store preferentially in adipose. Adipose is also very poorly perfused, and while it takes a long time for stores to build up in this tissue, the converse is also true; due to very limited blood flow, the rate of egress back into the circulation and out the hepatorenal system is very slow. This phenomenon is perhaps even more well recognized clinically with methadone, which has a lipophilicity roughly an order of magnitude less than fentanyl, but two orders of magnitude greater than morphine.

Again, it should be kept in mind that all of these processes described are not occurring sequentially, but rather simultaneously. Elimination begins with first-pass exposure to the liver for orally administered agents, even before distribution.

In basic terms, the vast majority of pharmacologic compounds (including naturally occurring substances such as opium) despite therapeutic benefit are "considered toxins" by the organism and undergo alteration, degradation, and elimination (as opposed to nutrients and vitamins, etc. which are incorporated into cells and tissues for sustaining and improvement of the organism). After initial alteration by gastric acid and upper gastrointestinal enzymes (in the case of enteral administration), metabolism classically is described as beginning in the liver, where the drug undergoes transformation to render it capable of excretion by the kidneys. Opioids, like many drugs, are for the most part rather hydrophobic, which facilitates their passage into the CNS. Hepatic processes therefore alter the structure of the drug to a more hydrophilic state such that glomerular filtration and excretion can occur. As described above, oral medications undergo immediate hepatic "first-pass metabolism" upon absorption from the intestines; for parenterally administered medications (e.g., sublingual, transdermal, intravenous) "first-pass metabolism" does not apply; nonetheless, the circulating drug burden must still eventually and repetitively pass through the liver and will eventually undergo transformation by these same processes.

These hepatic processes are classified into so-called Phase 1 and Phase 2 metabolism. Both are catalyzed by enzymes, and Phase 1 is generally facilitated by the *cytochrome P450* family which will be discussed in greater detail below. In this phase, one of these "CYP" enzymes acts to modify the structure of the drug by a variety of means, such as oxidation (the most common reaction) but also by reduction, hydrolysis, and cyclization/decyclization reactions. Phase 2 is facilitated by enzymes such as *uridine diphosphate glucuronosyltransferase (UGT)* and consists of the addition of another hydrophilic moiety such as glucuronate (or sulfate, glutathione, glycine, or sulfate). The addition of these large anionic groups renders the molecule more polar as well as larger, with resultant reduction in both diffusion and active transport across cell membranes. The conjugated molecule is also much more readily excreted as discussed above.

Phase 1 metabolism, especially that performed by CYP3A4, has been shown to be highly subject to both induction (increased activity of the enzyme resulting from exposure to certain substrates) and inhibition (decreased enzymatic activity from other substrates). The CYP3A4 enzyme is thought to have at least 40 alleles and is responsible for over 50% of all drug metabolisms. CYP3A4 is responsible for the primary metabolism of fentanyl and oxycodone and is also involved in the metabolism of tramadol and methadone [77]. Many drugs or other chemicals (e.g., bergamottin in grapefruit juice) can induce or inhibit CYP3A4 activity, yielding significant unpredictability in metabolism. Tables showing known inducers and inhibitors of CYP3A4 are ubiquitous and as such are not reproduced here; commonly used inducers include many statins, anticonvulsants, and antiretroviral agents. Commonly used inhibitors include estrogens, cimetidine, amiodarone and quinidine, many calcium channel blockers, many antibiotics, many of the antidepressants, and most of the antiretrovirals. In addition, as so many drugs are metabolized by this pathway, it is conceivable that polypharmacy may effect competition for this enzyme.

Exceptions to this basic pattern exist; for example, remifentanil, an intravenous opioid commonly used in operative anesthesia, is degraded by enzymes within the bloodstream itself (RBC esterase) and as such has an extremely short half-life. Intravenous, subarachnoid and epidural, and peripheral parenteral administration of opioids is not discussed within this volume.

Pharmacogenetics

While technically falling under host factors and therefore more applicable to the last section of this book, the effect of pharmacogenetic variance on opioid therapy will be covered in this basic science section for continuity of understanding the drugs. Pharmacogenetic factors are likely one of the major factors conferring much of the interpersonal variability seen with both therapeutic effects and misuse/abuse of opioids and can affect both pharmacodynamics and pharmacokinetics (Table 2.1).

Table 2.1 Pharmacodynamic and pharmacokinetic polymorphisms affecting opioid therapy

Enzyme/receptor	Variants	Effects
COMT (catechol-*O*-methyltransferase)	Val158Met variant	Decreased catecholamine metabolism – Increased pain perception – Reduced opioid effectiveness – Multiple other psychiatric disorders
ORM1 (mu-opioid receptor)	A118G variant	– Increased pain perception – Reduced opioid effectiveness
CYP2B6	Reduced activity	Reduced S-methadone metabolism with increased risk of torsades de pointe
CYP2D6	"Poor metabolizer"	Decreased plasma levels/efficacy of prodrugs (e.g., codeine, hydrocodone) Reduced metabolism of tramadol, oxycodone, methadone
	"Ultrarapid metabolizer"	Increased plasma levels/efficacy of prodrugs (e.g., codeine, hydrocodone) Increased metabolism of tramadol, oxycodone, methadone
UGT2B7	Reduced activity	Reduced metabolism/increased plasma levels of morphine (hydromorphone? oxymorphone?)

Among pharmacodynamic polymorphisms, only two major genes have been studied extensively for their contribution to differences in pain perception/experience and opioid response: the *catechol-O-methyltransferase (COMT)* gene and the *mu-opioid receptor (OPRM1)* gene.

COMT is an enzyme that metabolizes catecholamines (dopamine, norepinephrine, epinephrine) and thus reduces sympathetic activity. Several studies have shown that alterations of this enzyme (the most well studied of which is the Val158Met allelic variant which involves substitution of methionine for valine at position 158 of the enzyme, resulting in reduced catabolism) are associated with significant increases in pain perception and reductions in opioid responsiveness [78, 79]. Recent analyses have suggested that the Val158Met variant of COMT may only confer clinically significant alterations in chronic pain related to musculoskeletal complaints and specifically fibromyalgia and other chronic widespread pain conditions [80, 81]. However, it must be kept in mind that COMT activity is exceedingly broad, with complex effects on cognition and executive function, emotional processing, and sense of well-being, and has been implicated in the pathophysiology of depression, bipolar mood disorder, anxiety, posttraumatic stress disorder, schizophrenia, and various substance use disorders and addiction.

The OPRM1 gene manifests over 3000 known polymorphisms, and the most well studied is the A118G variant which involves a substitution of guanine for adenosine in the coding region on chromosome 6. This mutation has been shown to result in highly variable mu-receptor biochemistry among various ligands and across species with no consistent pattern yet identified [82, 83]. Clinical observations have been similarly confusing with several studies and meta-analyses suggesting that the A118G variant is associated with increased pain perception/reported pain scores and increased opioid requirements [83, 84], while others show no significant association [79, 85, 86]. Of note, the meta-analyses favoring a clinical effect focus on the postoperative period [83, 84].

Pharmacogenetics affecting pharmacokinetics shows more consistency in effects and have been well characterized especially in regard to the CYP450 system. As mentioned previously, the majority of drugs including opioids undergo Phase 1 metabolism by this hepatic family, and alterations herein result in significant effects upon activation of prodrugs and inactivation of drugs. Commercially available assays for several enzymes within this family (especially CYP2D6, CYP2C19, and CYP2B6) are beginning to show some utility in guiding pharmacotherapeutic choices for a number of psychoactive drugs including opioids, benzodiazepines, and antidepressants, and the narrow therapeutic window of many of these substances coupled with increased access to the assays may eventually render pharmacogenetic testing standard of care.

The *CYP3A4* enzyme is thought to have at least 40 allelic variants and is responsible for over 50% of all drug metabolisms. CYP3A4 is responsible for the primary metabolism of fentanyl and oxycodone and is also involved in the metabolism of tramadol and methadone [77]. The effects of polymorphisms at this locus have not been well characterized; alterations (e.g., CYP3A4*1G, a common variant in Asians) have been reported but have not shown any consistency in clinical effect

[84]. Of much more significance are the effects of drug-drug interactions involving induction or inhibition of this enzyme as discussed above in the section on pharmacokinetics.

The *CYP2D6* enzyme is primarily responsible for the metabolism of codeine and hydrocodone and partially responsible for the metabolism of tramadol, oxycodone, and methadone. CYP2D6 is responsible for the metabolism of far fewer drugs overall and thus is less subject to induction and inhibition by other substances. CYP2D6 however has over 100 known allelic variants [84], and this heterogeneity has shown much more significant clinical effects than has CYP3A4s. Four phenotypic categories resulting from these variances have been proposed: poor metabolizers (the result of homozygous nonfunctional alleles), intermediate metabolizers, extensive metabolizers, and ultrarapid metabolizers (the result of multiple functional allelic copies or promoter mutations) [78]. Intermediate and extensive metabolizers have not been shown to exhibit significant variability in clinical effect and may be considered baseline or normal subjects. Poor CYP2D6 metabolizers will show increased plasma levels and prolonged effects (both of which may confer toxicity) of drugs that rely primarily on this pathway for degradation; conversely, they will show decreased plasma levels and effects of prodrugs such as codeine and hydrocodone that rely on transformation by the cytochrome enzyme to a more active and potent form (e.g., codeine to morphine, hydrocodone to hydromorphone). Conversely, ultrarapid CYP2D6 metabolizers will show reduced plasma levels and shorter duration of action of active drugs and greatly increased plasma levels of active metabolites of prodrugs that may confer significant toxicity. A tragic and well-reported incident involving the death of a neonate due to maternal ultrarapid CYP2D6 activity occurred in April 2005; postmortem analysis revealed that the infant's plasma morphine levels were sevenfold higher than morphine levels in infants prescribed morphine, due to maternal breast milk morphine levels that were one to two orders of magnitude higher than that normally seen [1]. The US Food and Drug Administration subsequently issued a warning highlighting the dangers of postpartum codeine prescriptions in 2007; the same caution must of course apply to any opioid or toxic substances metabolized through the CYP2D6 pathway. CYP2D6 polymorphisms have not shown consistent clinical effects with regard to tramadol nor oxycodone [84]; however, it should be noted that this enzyme converts oxycodone to oxymorphone.

The *CYP2B6* enzyme is one of many that metabolize methadone; however, it is the main enzyme that degrades the S-enantiomer of methadone [87], which is the isomer conferring that agent's *N*-methyl D-aspartate (NMDA) blockade and also the isomer associated with QT interval prolongation [88]. Individuals deficient in CYP2B6 activity are thus at higher risk for torsades de pointe and may warrant more frequent/intensive ECG monitoring and lower doses.

The *UGT2B7* enzyme is the predominant mediator of Phase 2 metabolism of morphine, which does not undergo substantial Phase 1 metabolism. It also conjugates glucuronide to hydromorphone and oxymorphone. Allelic variants of this enzyme have been demonstrated among various populations [78, 79] and decreased activity results in increased plasma levels of morphine, as would be expected.

Tolerance

Many drugs used clinically demonstrate a phenomenon of inducing tolerance with repeated use; while our understanding of underlying mechanisms is far from complete, drug tolerance is conceptualized as occurring largely due either to increased metabolism and elimination of the drug (so-called pharmacokinetic tolerance) or due to a decreased response to the drug at its site of action (so-called pharmacodynamic tolerance).

Pharmacokinetic tolerance is thought to occur primarily due to upregulation of degradative function in the liver, with "induction" (increased activity) of cytochrome P450 enzymes. Many drugs induce their own metabolism, and the more of a substance the organism is exposed to, the more actively it works to eliminate the substance.

The mechanisms underlying pharmacodynamic tolerance are more complex and are not fully understood and involve a number of alterations at the level of the receptor, its downstream effects, and also other modulatory systems. Early observations of alterations in both second messenger function (such as hyperactivity of the adenylyl cyclase system) and in transmembrane ion flux and polarization were followed by discoveries that other pathways (most notably the NMDA system) are very involved in the development or prevention of opioid tolerance [89] More recent advances in the understanding of G-protein-coupled receptor signal attenuation across the family indicate that the initial step in the development of desensitization involves phosphorylation of the receptor (by G-protein receptor kinases) that serves to prepare the activated receptor for binding by proteins called arrestins which then initiate the process of receptor endocytosis. The endocytosed receptors are held within the cell until a recycling process of cell membrane reinsertion occurs [90]. Receptor oligomerization is currently being invoked to explain a number of phenomena involving the complex and still mysterious details underlying the opioid system, and some investigators have proposed that MOR-DOR heteromerization in particular may occur in the context of chronic ligand exposure with resultant functional alteration [91].

A mechanistically different process contributing to the "diminishing returns" with chronic opioid use is an actual upregulation in pain sensitivity known as opioid-induced hyperalgesia (OIH) which is discussed in more detail in Chap. 3. As alluded to briefly in the endogenous opioid-modulation section above, native processes involved in the "check and balance" system related to opioid analgesia are likely involved in OIH. In addition, however, compensatory upregulation of non-opioid-influenced nociceptive pathways in the CNS could be responsible (in part) for both OIH and tolerance [92]. Teleologically, both phenomena perhaps represent a common means for preserving the ability of the organism to detect threats (by means of nociception).

Finally, it should be mentioned that although the situation is almost certainly the exception rather than the rule, a decrease in therapeutic efficacy of long-term opioid use may be the result of progressive "organic" pathology. Cancer grows and spreads, and autoimmune inflammatory conditions progressively destroy more tissue. However, our understanding of the interactions between nociception and endogenous modulation of pain is expanding as discussed above in limited detail, and there is growing evidence that in the absence of modifying factors such as concurrent neuropsychological pathology (including but not limited to maladaptive neural plasticity) or OIH, even in states of aggressive tissue pathology the body (and mind) may well be capable of significantly more innate pain management than we generally give it credit for. Nonetheless, it is incumbent upon the physician to remain ever vigilant for the spread of disease within the patient, whether from the condition being treated (e.g., metastasis) or the treatment itself—such as occult bowel pathology from opioid-induced ileus/obstruction, pathologic fracture owing to opioid-induced endocrinopathy, or OIH.

Summary

The physician's safe, ethical, and effective prescription of opioids (conceptualized as the agent in classic epidemiologic paradigm) is predicated upon a thorough understanding not only of the drug class itself, which is explored in greater detail in the next chapter, but also of the biologic systems wherein/upon which they act.

Opioids are produced by the body and act as part of a comprehensive homeostatic self-preservation effort geared toward the well-being of the organism. The most salient aspect of this system is acute pain relief, but within seconds modulating and counter-regulatory effects are initiated to balance pain relief with perception of danger thus facilitating help. Different endogenous opioids exist, with primary affinity for different opioid receptors, which exert different effects toward this overall goal.

Therapeutic (exogenous) opioids exist within nature as well (e.g., opiates) and have been modified and copied pharmaceutically to harness the potent analgesic qualities of this system. Unlike the endogenous system, however, the only limitation upon exogenous opioid exposure is volitional (or imposed) discretion on the part of the consumer, and in a situation of excess exposure—whether by quantity or chronicity—both tolerance and adverse effects reduce analgesic efficacy and tip the balance of risk:benefit away from the positive. The body is prepared to some extent to reduce these potential threats by eliminating the agent metabolically. Genetic factors play an increasingly appreciated role in varying efficiency of this process from individual to individual.

Again, to date no therapeutic opioid compound (nor any known analgesic) is without limiting adverse effects which are discussed in greater detail in Chap. 3. Reducing the "virulence" of these agents must involve some degree of attenuation of not only morbid or lethal complications but also euphoria-inducing and addictive qualities, and these efforts will be reviewed in Chap. 4.

References

1. Koren G, Cairns J, Chitayat D. Pharmacogenetics of morphine poisoning in a breastfed neonate of a codeine-prescribed mother. Lancet. 2006;368:704.
2. Salzet M, Vieau D, Day R. Crosstalk between nervous and immune systems through the animal kingdom: focus on opioids. Trends Neurosci. 2000;23:550–5.
3. Krude H, Biebermann H, Luck W, Horn R, Brabant G, Grüters A. Severe early-onset obesity, adrenal insufficiency and red hair pigmentation caused by POMC mutations in humans. Nat Genet. 1988;19:155–7.
4. Liem EB, Lin CM, Suleman MI, Doufas AG, Gregg RG, Veauthier JM, et al. Anesthetic requirement is increased in redheads. Anesthesiology. 2004;101:279–83.
5. Liem EB, Joiner TV, Tsueda K, Sessler DI. Increased sensitivity to thermal pain and reduced subcutaneous lidocaine efficacy in redheads. Anesthesiology. 2005;102:509–14.
6. Mogil JS, Ritchie J, Smith SB, Strasburg K, Kaplan L, Wallace MR, et al. Melanocortin-1 receptor gene variants affect pain and mu-opioid analgesia in mice and humans. J Med Genet. 2005;42:583–7.
7. Fields HL, Bry J, Hentall I, Zorman G. The activity of neurons in the rostral medulla of the rat during withdrawal from noxious heat. J Neurosci. 1983;3:2545–52.
8. Fields HL, Malick A, Burstein R. Dorsal horn projection targets of ON and OFF cells in the rostral ventromedial medulla. J Neurophysiol. 1995;74:1742–59.
9. Heinricher MM, Tavares I, Leith JL, Lumb BM. Descending control of nociception: specificity, recruitment and plasticity. Brain Res Rev. 2009;60:214–25.
10. Levine JD, Gordon NC. Influence of the method of drug administration on analgesic response. Nature. 1984;312:755–6.
11. Fields HL. Pain modulation: expectation, opioid analgesia and virtual pain. Prog Brain Res. 2000;122:245–53.
12. Eippert F, Bingel U, Schoell ED, Yacubian J, Klinger R, Lorenz J, et al. Activation of the opioidergic descending pain control system underlies placebo analgesia. Neuron. 2009;63:533–43.
13. Heinke B, Gingl E, Sandkühler J. Multiple targets of μ-opioid receptor-mediated presynaptic inhibition at primary afferent Aδ- and C-fibers. Neuroscience. 2011;31:1313–22.
14. Takasusuki T, Yaksh TL. Regulation of spinal substance p release by intrathecal calcium channel blockade. Anesthesiology. 2011;115:153–64.
15. Kumamoto E, Mizuta K, Fujita T. Opioid actions in primary afferent fibers-involvement in analgesia and anesthesia. Pharmaceuticals. 2011;4:343–65.
16. Cesselin F, Benoliel JJ, Bourgoin S, et al. Spinal mechanisms of opioid analgesia. In: Stein C, editor. Opioids in pain control: basic and clinical aspects. Cambridge: Cambridge University Press; 1999. p. 70–95.
17. Baillie LD, Schmidhammer H, Mulligan SJ. Peripheral mu-opioid receptor mediated inhibition of calcium signaling and action potential-evoked calcium fluorescent transients in primary afferent CGRP nociceptive terminals. Neuropharmacology. 2015;93:267–73.
18. Smith HS. Optimizing pharmacologic outcomes: individualization of therapy. In: Smith HS, editor. Opioid therapy in the twenty-first century. New York: Oxford University Press; 2013. p. 135–44.
19. Yaksh TL, Wallace MS. Opioids, analgesia, and pain management. In: Brunton L, editor. Goodman and Gilman's pharmacologic basis of therapeutics. New York: McGraw–Hill; 2011. p. 481–525.
20. Chen SR, Pan HL. Spinal endogenous acetylcholine contributes to the analgesic effect of systemic morphine in rats. Anesthesiology. 2001;95:525–30.
21. Sehgal N, Smith HS, Manchikanti L. Peripherally acting opioids and clinical implications for pain control. Pain Physician. 2011;14:249–58.
22. Zadina JE, Hackler L, Ge LJ, Kastin AJ. A potent and selective endogenous agonist for the mu-opiate receptor. Nature. 1997;386:499–502.

23. McConalogue K, Grady EF, Minnis J, Balestra B, Tonini M, Brecha NC, et al. Activation and internalization of the mu-opioid receptor by the newly discovered endogenous agonists, endomorphin-1 and endomorphin 2. Neuroscience. 1999;90:1051–9.
24. Sarić A, Balog T, Sobocanec S, Marotti T. Endomorphin 1 activates nitric oxide synthase 2 activity and downregulates nitric oxide synthase 2 mRNA expression. Neuroscience. 2007;144:1454–61.
25. Varamini P, Blanchfield JT, Toth I. Endomorphin derivatives with improved pharmacological properties. Curr Med Chem. 2013;20:2741–58.
26. Zadina JE, Nilges MR, Morgenweck J, Zhang X, Hackler L, Fasold MB. Endomorphin analog analgesics with reduced abuse liability, respiratory depression, motor impairment, tolerance, and glial activation relative to morphine. Neuropharmacology. 2016;105:215–27.
27. Dupont A, Cusan L, Garon M. Extremely rapid degradation of [3H] methionine-enkephalin by various rat tissues in vivo and in vitro. Life Sci. 1977;21:907–14.
28. Milloy D. Enkephalins and endorphins: the endogenous opiates. AANA J. 1982;50:569–73.
29. Roques BP, Noble F, Fournie-Zaluski MC. Endogenous opioid peptides and analgesia. In: Stein C, editor. Opioids in pain control: basic and clinical aspects. Cambridge: Cambridge University Press; 1999. p. 21–45.
30. Land BB, Bruchas MR, Lemos JC, Xu M, Melief EJ, Chavkin C. The dysphoric component of stress is encoded by activation of the dynorphin κ-opioid system. J Neurosci. 2008;28:407–14.
31. Goldstein A, Tachibana S, Lowney LI, Hunkapiller M, Hood L. Dynorphin-(1-13), an extraordinarily potent opioid peptide. Proc Natl Acad Sci U S A. 1979;76:6666–70.
32. Han JS, Xie CW. Dynorphin: potent analgesic effect in spinal cord of the rat. Sci Sin, Ser B, Chem Biol Agric Med Earth Sci. 1984;27:169–77.
33. Lai J, Luo MC, Chen Q, Ma S, Gardell LR, Ossipov MH, et al. Dynorphin a activates bradykinin receptors to maintain neuropathic pain. Nat Neurosci. 2006;9(12):1534–40.
34. Podvin S, Yaksh T, Hook V. The emerging role of spinal dynorphin in chronic pain: a therapeutic perspective. Annu Rev. Pharmacol Toxicol. 2016;56:511–33.
35. Butelman ER, Yuferov V, Kreek MJ. κ-opioid receptor/dynorphin system: genetic and pharmacotherapeutic implications for addiction. Trends Neurosci. 2012;35:587–96.
36. Tejeda HA, Shippenberg TS, Henriksson R. The dynorphin/κ-opioid receptor system and its role in psychiatric disorders. Cell Mol Life Sci. 2012;69:857–96.
37. Wee S, Koob GF. The role of the dynorphin-kappa opioid system in the reinforcing effects of drugs of abuse. Psychopharmacology. 2010;210:121–35.
38. Dietis N, Rowbotham DJ, Lambert DG. Opioid receptor subtypes: fact or artifact? Br J Anaesth. 2011;107:8–18.
39. Peppin JF, Raffa RB. Delta opioid agonists: a concise update on potential therapeutic applications. J Clin Pharm Ther. 2015;40:155–66.
40. Gendron L, Mittal N, Beaudry H, Walwyn W. Recent advances on the delta-opioid receptor: from trafficking to function. Brit J Pharmacol. 2015;172:403–19.
41. Beaudry H, Dubois D, Gendron L. Activation of spinal mu- and delta-opioid receptors potently inhibits substance P release induced by peripheral noxious stimuli. J Neurosci. 2011;31:13068–77.
42. Quock RM, Burkey TH, Varga E, Hosohata Y, Hosohata K, Cowell SM, et al. The delta-opioid receptor: molecular pharmacology, signal transduction, and the determination of drug efficacy. Pharmacol Rev. 1999;51:503–32.
43. Xia Y, editor. Neural function of the delta-opioid receptor. New York: Springer; 2015.
44. Arendt-Nielsen L, Olesen AE, Staahl C, Menzaghi F, Kell S, Wong GY, et al. Analgesic efficacy of peripheral kappa-opioid receptor agonist CR665 compared to oxycodone in a multi-modal, multi-tissue experimental human pain model: selective effect on visceral pain. Anesthesiology. 2009;111:616–24.
45. Schroder W, Lambert DG, Koch T. Functional plasticity of the N/OFQ-NOP receptor system determines analgesic properties of NOP receptor agonists. Br J Pharmacol. 2014;171:3777–800.

46. Donica CL, Awwad HO, Thakker DR, Standifer KM. Cellular mechanisms of nociceptin/orphanin FQ (N/OFQ) peptide (NOP) receptor regulation and heterologous regulation by N/OFQ. Mol Pharmacol. 2013;83:907–18.
47. Mallimo EM, Kusnecov AW. The role of orphanin FQ/nociceptin in neuroplasticity: relationship to stress, anxiety and neuroinflammation. Front Cell Neurosci. 2013;7:1–18.
48. Bodera P, Stankiewicz W, Kocik J. Interactions of orphanin FQ/Nociceptin (OFQ/N) system with immune system factors and hypothalamic-pituitary-adrenal (HPA) axis. Pharmacol Rep. 2014;66:288–91.
49. Trang T, Al-Hasani R, Salvemini D, Salter MW, Gutstein H, Cahill CM. Pain and poppies: the good, the bad and the ugly of opioid analgesics. J Neurosci. 2015;35:13879–88.
50. Heinricher MM, McGaraughty S, Tortorici V. Circuitry underlying antiopioid actions of cholecystokinin within the rostral ventromedial medulla. J Neurophysiol. 2001;85:280–6.
51. Heinricher MM, Neubert MJ. Neural basis for the hyperalgesic action of cholecystokinin in the rostral ventromedial medulla. J Neurophysiol. 2004;92:1982–9.
52. Hebb AL, Poulin JF, Roach SP, Zacharko RM, Drolet G. Cholecystokinin and endogenous opioid peptides: interactive influence on pain, cognition and emotion. Prog Neuropscyhopharmacol Biol Psychiatry. 2005;29:1225–38.
53. Lovick TA. Pro-nociceptive action of cholecystokinin in the periaqueductal grey: a role in neuropathic and anxiety-induced hyperalgesic states. Neurosci Biobehav Rev. 2008;32:852–62.
54. Bowers ME, Choi DC, Ressler KJ. Neuropeptide regulation of fear and anxiety: implications of cholecystokinin, endogenous opioids, and neuropeptide Y. Physiol Behav. 2012;107:699–710.
55. Mollereau C, Roumy M, Zajac JM. Opioid-modulating peptides: mechanisms of action. Curr Top Med Chem. 2005;5:341–55.
56. Mouledous L, Mollereau C, Zajac JM. Opioid-modulating properties of the neuropeptide FF system. Biofactors. 2010;36:423–9.
57. Elhabazi K, Trigo JM, Mollereau C, Moulédous L, Zajac JM, Bihel F, et al. Involvement of neuropeptide FF receptors in neuroadaptive responses to acute and chronic opiate treatments. Br J Pharmacol. 2012;165:424–35.
58. O'Connor TM, O'Connel J, O'Brien DI. The role of substance P in inflammatory disease. J Cell Physiol. 2004;201:167–80.
59. Garcia-Recio S, Gascon P. Biological and pharmacological aspects of the NK1-receptor. Biomed Res Int. 2015;2015:495704. doi:10.1155/2015/495704.
60. Yu YJ, Arttamangkul S, Evans CJ, Williams JT, von Zastrow M. Neurokinin 1 receptors regulate morphine-induced endocytosis and desensitization of mu-opioid receptors in CNS neurons. J Neurosci. 2009;29:222–33.
61. Fan X, Jin WY, Wang YT. The NDMA receptor complex: a multifunctional machine at the glutaminergic synapse. Front Cell Neurosci. 2014;8:1–9.
62. Vyklicky V, Korinek M, Smejkalova T. Structure, function, and pharmacology of NMDA receptor channels. Physiol Res. 2014;63(Suppl. 1):S191–203.
63. Rodriguez-Munoz MR, Sanchez-Blazquez P, Vicente-Sanchez A, Berrocoso E, Garzón J. The mu-opioid receptor and the NMDA receptor associate in PAG neurons: implications in pain control. Neuropsychopharmacology. 2012;37:338–49.
64. Toll L, Bruchas MR, Calo G, Cox BM, Zaveri NT. Nociceptin/orphanin FQ receptor structure, signaling, ligands, functions, and interactions with opioid systems. Pharmacol Rev. 2016;68:419–57.
65. Wang Y, Barker K, Shi S. Blockade of PDGFR-β activation eliminates morphine analgesic tolerance. Nat Med. 2012;18:385–7.
66. Valenzuela CF, Xiong Z, MacDonald JF, Weiner JL, Frazier CJ, Dunwiddie TV, et al. Platelet-derived growth factor induces a long-term inhibition of N-methyl-D aspartate receptor function. J Biol Chem. 1996;271:16151–9.

67. Chabot-Dore AJ, Schuster DJ, Stone LS, Wilcox GL. Analgesic synergy between opioid and α2-adrenoreceptors. Brit J Pharm. 2015;172:388–402.
68. Watkins LR, Hutchinson MR, Rice KC, Maier SF. The "toll" of opioid-induced glial activation: improving the clinical efficacy of opioids by targeting glia. Trends Pharmacol Sci. 2009;30:581–91.
69. Hutchinson MR, Shavit Y, Grace PM. Exploring the neuroimmunopharmacology of opioids: an integrative review of mechanisms of central immune signaling and their implications for opioid analgesia. Pharmacol Rev. 2011;63:772–810.
70. Hutchinson MR, Bland ST, Johnson KW. Opioid-induced glial activation: mechanisms of activation and implications for opioid analgesia, dependence, and reward. Sci World J. 2007;7:98–111.
71. Feng Y, He X, Yang Y, Chao D, Lazarus LH, Xia Y. Current research on opioid receptor function. Curr Drug Targets. 2012;13:230–46.
72. Klaassen C, Aleksunes L. Xenobiotic, bile acid, and cholesterol transporters: function and regulation. Pharmacol Rev. 2010;62:1–96.
73. König J, Müller F, Fromm M. Transporters and drug-drug interactions: important determinants of drug disposition and effects. Pharmacol Rev. 2013;65:944–66.
74. Shen S, Zhang W. ABC transporters and drug efflux at the blood-brain barrier. Rev Neurosci. 2010;21:29–53.
75. Tournier N, Declèves X, Saubaméa B. Opioid transport by ATP-binding cassette transporters at the blood-brain barrier: implications for neuropsychopharmacology. Curr Pharm Des. 2011;17:2829–42.
76. Buxton ILO, Benet LZ. Pharmacokinetics: the dynamics of drug absorption, distribution, metabolism, and elimination. In: Brunton L, editor. Goodman and Gilman's pharmacologic basis of therapeutics. New York: McGraw Hill; 2011. p. 17–39.
77. Smith HS. Opioid metabolism. Mayo Clin Proc. 2009;84:613–24.
78. Smith H. Variations in opioid responsiveness. Pain Physician. 2008;11:237–48.
79. Sadhasivam S, Chidambaran V. Pharmacogenomics of opioids and perioperative pain management. Pharmacogenomics. 2012;13:1719–40.
80. Kambur O, Männistö PT. Catechol-O-methyltransferase and pain. Int Rev. Neurobiol. 2010;95:227–79.
81. Tammimäki A, Männistö PT. Catechol-O-methyltransferase gene polymorphism and chronic human pain: a systematic review and meta-analysis. Pharmacogenet Genomics. 2012;22:673–91.
82. Kroslak T, LaForge KS, Gianotte RJ, Ho A, Nielsen DA, Kreek MJ. The single nucelotide polymorphism A118G alters functional properties of the human mu opioid receptor. J Neurochem. 2007;103:77–87.
83. Hwang IC, Park JY, Myung SK, Ahn HY, Fukuda K, Liao Q. OPRM1 A118G gene variant and postoperative opioid requirement: a systematic review and meta-analysis. Anesthesiology. 2014;121:825–34.
84. Ren ZY, Xu XQ, Bao YP, He J, Shi L, Deng JH, et al. The impact of genetic variation on sensitivity to opioid analgesics in patients with postoperative pain: a systematic review and meta-analysis. Pain Physician. 2015;18:131–52.
85. Walter C, Lotsch J. Meta-analysis of the relevance of the OPRM1 118A > G genetic variant for pain treatment. Pain. 2009;146:270–5.
86. Vuilleumier PH, Stamer UM, Landau R. Pharmacogenomic considerations in opioid analgesia. Pharmacogenom Personal Med. 2012;5:73–87.
87. Dobrinas M, Crettol S, Oneda B. Contribution of CYP2B6 alleles in explaining extreme (S)-methadone plasma levels: a CYP2B6 gene resequencing study. Pharmacogenet Genomics. 2013;23:84–93.
88. Eap CB, Crettol S, Rougier JS, Schläpfer J, Sintra Grilo L, Déglon JJ, et al. Stereoselective block of hERG channel by (S)-methadone and QT interval prolongation in CYP2B6 slow metabolizers. Clin Pharmacol Ther. 2007;81:719–28.

89. Cox BM. Mechanisms of tolerance. In: Stein C, editor. Opioids in pain control: basic and clinical aspects. Cambridge: Cambridge University Press; 1999. p. 70–95.
90. Williams JT, Ingram SL, Henderson G. Regulation of mu-opioid receptors: desensitization, phosphorylation, internalization, and tolerance. Pharmacol Rev. 2013;65:223–54.
91. Pasternak GW, Pan YX. Mix and match: heterodimers and opioid tolerance. Neuron. 2011;69:6–8.
92. Goldberg JS. Chronic opioid therapy and opioid tolerance: a new hypothesis. Pain Res Treat. 2013;2013:407504. doi:10.1155/2013/407504.

Chapter 3
Understanding the Agent, Part II: Adverse Effects

A 40-year-old female traveling to her methadone clinic developed nausea, vomiting, and tremulousness and presented to the ED where she was noted initially to be in ventricular bigeminy. Past medical history was positive for hypertension, for which she took 100 mg of metoprolol daily. She had no history of other cardiovascular diseases. The only other reported medication was 135 mg of methadone administered daily at a local methadone clinic for the management of an addiction to heroin. On physical examination, the patient was a well-developed and well-nourished woman who was initially alert and lucid, with hyperdynamic vital signs. She exhibited multiple runs of polymorphic ventricular tachycardia consistent with torsades de pointes. Shortly after arrival she had a prolonged episode associated with a loss of consciousness. There was no palpable pulse. The patient was defibrillated at 120 J (biphasic) and converted to sinus rhythm. She was treated with 2 g intravenous magnesium sulfate infused over 10 min. The rhythm initially stabilized; however, 2 min later a second prolonged run of torsades commenced. A loading dose of lidocaine was given, accompanied by a 2 mg/min infusion. Ten mEq of potassium chloride were infused over 1 h. After the lidocaine drip was initiated, the patient experienced no further dysrhythmias. A post-conversion ECG was remarkable for a QTc interval of 577 ms.

The patient was admitted to the intensive care unit. The dosage of methadone was reduced to 60 mg per day, and metoprolol was discontinued. A repeat ECG the following day showed reduction of the QTc interval to 485 ms. The patient had an internal cardioverter-defibrillator implanted 3 days after initial presentation and was discharged in stable condition [1].

H.B. McAnally, *Opioid Dependence*, DOI 10.1007/978-3-319-47497-7_3

As Dr. Scott Fishman points out in his excellent handbook *Responsible Opioid Prescribing* [2], "Opioids are neither inherently 'good' nor inherently 'bad.'" As with virtually any tool in the therapeutic armamentarium, they have beneficial and harmful effects. And as with any decision in clinical medicine, their use—whether short term or long term—must be grounded in a full understanding of the drug class and the current evidence for both benefit (examined in detail in Chap. 7) and risk.

The previous chapter initiated our examination of opioids with a presentation of the organism's endogenous opioid system including ligands, receptors, and opioid-modulating systems as fundamental to understanding opioids in general. Basic pharmacologic principles including the relatively new field of pharmacogenetics completed this introduction to the agent. We now move on to examine the *virulence* of the agent, so to speak. Adverse effects (AEs) and tolerance to opioids' analgesic effects (which often tip the risk-benefit ratio in favor of the former by encouraging increasing use) are almost universal with use of the class. AE ranges from annoying (pruritis, nausea) to life-threatening (addiction, respiratory depression, cardiac dysrhythmias), and these more significant outcomes of course (when reported) comprise the descriptive statistics that underlie the epidemic. Adverse effects are discussed by physiologic system.

Opioid Adverse Effects

Psychiatric

The distinction between psychiatric and neurologic (or endocrine) may be in many cases artificial; in this section we are focusing on effects that are historically considered to have some significant "nonorganic" component, e.g., mood.

While relatively rare, *delusional phenomena* and *hallucinations* with opioid use have been reported for centuries. Case reports and anecdotal experience are ubiquitous for these complications, but no good-quality research at either basic-science level (likely impossible due to in vitro or species limitations in assessing outcomes) or the clinical level exists. Historically morphine has been associated with a higher rate of delusional phenomena than other opioids, but this may mirror its greater relative use in the past, prior to the development of newer agents. There is some speculation that its metabolites morphine-6-glucuronide and, more so, morphine-3-glucuronide are responsible for the bulk of these symptoms [3]. Delusions and psychotic reactions are more frequently reported in the palliative care population, many of whom have metabolism limiting end-stage organ disease, which lends some additional plausibility to this hypothesis. It also emphasizes the point however that a number of potential physiologic alterations irrespective of opioid use per se may be responsible for these symptoms in this population. Meperidine and methadone have also seen a disproportionate case reporting of hallucinatory/delusional phenomena. Mechanistically it appears that kappa-receptor (KOR) agonism is responsible for the majority of opioid-induced delusions and psychosis [4, 5]. Alternative support for this hypothesis was shown in a case series of schizophrenics whose psychosis was successfully treated with buprenorphine, which is a KOR antagonist [6].

The incidence and prevalence of *depressive disorders* in general are difficult to estimate, as they rely on self-report for the most part and lack easily measured and objective variables. Nonetheless, it is well-accepted that an increased frequency of depressive disorders is common with opioid use and also with chronic pain; attempts to tease out the independent contributions of both conditions to depression have been challenging to say the least. Disproportionately high rates of baseline depression have been reported among patients suffering with chronic pain, and underlying mood disorders including depression frequently drive patients to seek opioid and other CNS-depressant pharmacotherapy. A high-powered study however recently examined the question of correlation between chronic opioid use and new onset depression, i.e., not present at the outset of treatment [7]. This very large retrospective analysis included over 100,000 patients in three separate environments (the Veterans' Administration, an academic medical center, and a managed care system), and the data were stratified by treatment duration (≤30 days, 31–90 days, and >90 days) and daily dose (≤50 morphine equivalent dose or "MED," 51–100 MED, and ≥100 MED.) All three groups showed duration-dependent incidence of new onset depression ranging from 8.4–11.6% in the ≤30 days group and 14.4–19.3% in the ≥90 days group. In the VA sample, the MED was strongly correlated with increased incidence of depression as well, ranging from 11.9% in the ≤50 MED group to 20.1% in the ≥100 MED group. The authors reported similar findings of dose-dependent increasing depression risk in a previous study [8].

Opioid-induced depression has also been mechanistically attributed largely to kappa-opioid receptor (KOR) agonism [9]. Again, interestingly buprenorphine (a KOR antagonist) has been shown to confer significant antidepressant activity [10, 11], and delta-opioid receptor (DOR) agonism is also associated with clinically measurable antidepressant effect [9, 12]. It should be noted again that in vitro and species limitations render bench research into opioid effects on depression difficult to interpret at best, and as such our understanding of the effects of opioids on mood are limited to observational clinical studies which are fraught with confounding by both pre-existing/comorbid psychiatric disorders and also pain.

While infrequently considered an adverse effect, *euphoria* is very common with opioid use, and we consider it an AE in theory and practice, as it is clearly associated with the development of both psychological dependence and addiction. These conditions are lately conceptualized as belonging to a continuum of opioid use disorder (OUD) and comprise psychopathology in their own right. OUD is surveyed briefly below, while its complex (and only partially understood) biology and pharmacology will be discussed in greater detail in Sect. 4 of this book. Briefly, however, euphoria from opioids is thought to be mediated via the mu-opioid receptor (MOR) and current understanding of addiction biology links psychological dependence upon all addictive substances to dopaminergic activity within the limbic structures including the ventral tegmental area, medial forebrain bundle, and nucleus accumbens [13]. However, it is also known that most drugs of abuse (including alcohol) release not only dopamine but also opioid peptides into the ventral striatum [14, 15], and dopaminergic activity may not be essential for opioid addiction as dopamine receptor blockade does not prevent heroin self-administration in animal models [14].

Descriptive statistics for opioid abuse and dependence rely on self-report, which likely underestimates the true frequency of the condition. Definitions furthermore are murky, with terms such as "misuse," "abuse," "dependence," and "addiction" used loosely throughout the literature without consensus. *Misuse* is an action with somewhat imprecise definition in the literature; the National Institute on Drug Abuse (NIDA) defines misuse as "taking a medication in a manner or dose other than prescribed [17]." Misuse may represent a single event or repetitive episodes of prescription noncompliance or illicit drug use; it may be accidental or very self-limited. NIDA historically differentiated *abuse* from misuse by an intentional component underlying abuse. More recently, their definition has consolidated both terms together under the rubric of abuse with the definition being "the use of a medication without a prescription, in a way other than as prescribed, or for the experience or feelings elicited [18]." The fourth edition of the *Diagnostic and Statistical Manual of Mental Disorders* (DSM-4) conceptualized "abuse as a mild or early phase and *dependence* as the more severe manifestation [16]." The two categories were based upon the number of criteria met over a 12-month period, with some differences in the criteria: abuse criteria all included recurrent use as the main indicator, whereas dependence criteria included a broader array of both physiologic variables (tolerance and withdrawal) and behavioral variables (desire/unsuccessful attempts to quit, effort expended in pursuit, etc.) *Addiction* is a term deliberately avoided by the American Psychiatric Association (and the World Health Organization) yet commonly used in the scientific community (e.g., NIDA) to describe "compulsive drug seeking despite negative consequences."

The trend is currently toward abandoning the specificity of categorical variables for the sensitivity of a continuum, and the DSM-5 has recently described a spectrum of *opioid use disorder (OUD)* that "includes signs and symptoms that reflect compulsive, prolonged self-administration of opioid substances that are used for no legitimate medical purpose or, if another medical condition is present that requires opioid treatment, that are used in doses greatly in excess of the amount needed for that medical condition [16]." Diagnostic criteria are listed in Table 3.1. There are four main "symptom clusters" within the current substance use disorder framework including:

- Impairment of control
- Social problems
- Risky use
- Physical effects (tolerance, withdrawal)

In practice (as well as in evaluating the literature), it may be useful to remember that in common parlance misuse and abuse describe actions, whereas dependence and addiction represent conditions or states.

Table 3.1 Opioid use disorder criteria: Diagnostic and statistical manual of mental disorders, fifth edition [16]

A problematic pattern of opioid use leading to clinically significant impairment or distress, as manifested by at least two of the following, occurring within a 12-month period:
1. Opioids are often taken in larger amounts or over a longer period than was intended
2. There is a persistent desire or unsuccessful efforts to cut down or control opioid use
3. A great deal of time is spent in activities necessary to obtain the opioid, use the opioid, or recover from its effects
4. Craving or a strong desire or urge to use opioids
5. Recurrent opioid use resulting in a failure to fulfill major role obligations at work, school, or home
6. Continued opioid use despite having persistent or recurrent social or interpersonal problems caused or exacerbated by the effects of opioids
7. Important social, occupational, or recreational activities are given up or reduced because of opioid use
8. Recurrent opioid use in situations in which it is physically hazardous
9. Continued opioid use despite knowledge of having a persistent or recurrent physical or psychological problem that is likely to have been caused or exacerbated by the substance
10. Tolerance, as defined by either of the following:
(a) A need for markedly increased amounts of opioids to achieve intoxication or desired effect
(b) A markedly diminished effect with continued use of the same amount of an opioidNote: This criterion is not considered to be met for those taking opioids solely under appropriate medical supervision
11. Withdrawal, as manifested by either of the following:
(a) The characteristic opioid withdrawal syndrome (refer to criteria A and B of the criteria set for opioid withdrawal)
(b) Opioids (or a closely related substance) are taken to relieve or avoid withdrawal symptomsNote: This criterion is not considered to be met for those individuals taking opioids solely under appropriate medical supervision

The United Nations Office on Drugs and Crime estimated that in 2012 between 26 and 36 million people globally abuse opioids [19]. The Substance Abuse and Mental Health Services Administration reports that in 2014 nearly 2 million people in the United States met criteria for prescription OUD, with another 0.6 million addicted to heroin; this translates roughly into a prevalence of 0.8% [20]. The TROUP study examined diagnoses for 45,000 patients from a Medicaid population and a research database comprising patients from five commercial plans from 2000 to 2005; the investigators reported a prevalence of diagnosed opioid abuse dependence of approximately 3% in each population [21], not markedly dissimilar to the federally reported statistics. A recent controversial review by Vowles et al. [22] however reported a prevalence of opioid "misuse" (using prescription opioids in a manner other than prescribed) ranging between 21 and 29% and a prevalence of addition ranging between 8 and 12%. Other data from the chronic pain population support a prevalence of abuse/dependence on the same order of magnitude, ranging from 3 to 26% [21, 23, 24].

As far as incidence, a large review of 67 studies performed by Fishbain et al. in 2008 concluded that only 3.27% (with a range from 0 to 45%) of patients became addicted to opioids over a variable time period of exposure, and again the authors admit that the definition/diagnostic criteria in the literature reviewed were hopelessly vague [25]. They also reported an 11.5% (range from 0 to 44.6%) incidence of aberrant drug-related behavior (ADRB) from the data, which outcome consisted of qualitative variables such as aggressively demanding more opioids, unsanctioned dose escalation, etc. They posit that the true incidence of OUD with exposure to chronic opioids lies somewhere between these two numbers.

Besides contributing to lost quality of life and productivity, OUD also amplifies the risks of other "organic" morbidity and mortality from opioids and their use. The compulsion to procure and use opioids despite significant risks to the individual's well-being increases exposure to/incidence of direct risks such as respiratory depression and bowel obstruction and also to indirect risks such as contracting infectious diseases from injection or sexual transmission and injury or death from violence or mishap.

Neurologic

Sedation is extremely common with opioid use and ranges from mild drowsiness to outright obtundation/coma. Estimating incidence and prevalence is virtually impossible due to the lack of standardized outcome definition, variable patient awareness/report, frequent co-administration of sedatives in patients using opioids, and also rather rapid adaptation to this AE in the majority of individuals. Electroencephalography has shown that the administration of increasing doses of opioids can render depression of consciousness to the point of delta wave predominant sleep/anesthesia without achieving full-blown burst suppression as seen with the sedative hypnotics or general anesthetics [26]. Mu-opioid receptor (MOR) agonism is thought to underlie the depressant effects of opioids upon consciousness [27] and probably occurs through a number of mechanisms including suppression of hypocretin/orexin release from the hypothalamus [28], direct reduction of forebrain acetylcholine [29], and alteration of norepinephrine activity at the locus coeruleus [30, 31].

The effects of opioids upon sleep are difficult to assess and confounded by underlying pain in many cases and also by the common co-administration of other CNS depressants in the relevant patient population. Most clinical sleep studies are also performed outside the patient's normal environment which introduces other potentially interfering variables. However, some research indicates that opioid use inhibits both rapid eye movement and non-rapid eye movement sleep patterns [32]. Obstructive sleep apnea is discussed below but bears mention here as another contributor to sleep disturbance. Regardless of the underlying etiology, sleep deprivation may also contribute to apparent sedation.

Delirium may result from the effects of opioids or active metabolites upon the consciousness [33, 34]; in clinical situations this is very difficult to tease out from potential co-administration of other CNS depressants, and underlying neurocognitive disorders. A broad differential diagnosis for delirium should always be considered under any circumstance as metabolic, infectious, endocrine and other system pathology are ubiquitous and may be easily overlooked.

Neuroexcitation leading to *myoclonus* and *seizures* has been reported, most notoriously with meperidine (pethidine) in the context of renal insufficiency but also with virtually all of the commonly used agents [34]. In vitro work suggests that these actions are MOR and KOR related without any contribution from the DOR [26]. Mechanisms are likely multifactorial but may involve excitation of hippocampal pyramidal neurons by GABA inhibition [35].

Opioid-induced hyperalgesia (OIH) has been observed for nearly 150 years [36] and has been somewhat contentious, as it appears for all intents and purposes to manifest symptoms congruent with both tolerance (analgesic inefficacy of current dosing) and also withdrawal (generalized misery.) A key difference observed frequently in clinical practice however is a generalized increase in disproportionate pain (hyperalgesia) or pain experienced from normally non-painful stimuli (allodynia) with OIH; tolerance does not in itself confer increased pain nor a greater distribution thereof. An example from my practice is presented at the beginning of Chap. 10 as a case study. Virtually all opioids have been implicated in the development of OIH; however, certain drugs seem anecdotally to confer a greater incidence of the condition. Postanesthetic care unit and intensive care unit nurses frequently complain of inability to adequately control pain in patients whose anesthetics included the ultra-short-acting intravenous opioid remifentanil. Interventional pain physicians who perform a significant amount of minor mechanical insults to patients on chronic opioid therapy frequently note a disproportionate association with oxycodone use and exaggerated pain perception/behaviors in response to blood pressure cuff inflation or local anesthetic skin wheal placement with a fine needle.

Extended duration of opioid exposure does not seem to be requisite for the development of OIH. Angst and Clark's systematic review of the phenomenon [37] examined nine human case reports/series and 75 rodent studies and noted that OIH responses persisted up to 10 days following a single exposure. They also reference a particularly enlightening study by Celerier [38] that demonstrated that after apparent resolution of OIH, animals challenged with a single dose of either opioid agonist or antagonist demonstrated immediate and increased OIH symptomatology, suggesting not only prolonged sensitization to OIH but also conceptually the development of a new allostatic pain threshold with both pronociceptive and antinociceptive activities in a tenuous and heightened balance.

Mechanistically, OIH appears to be a complex process involving activities of the NMDA, Neurokinin-1, Neuropeptide FF, serotonin, spinal dynorphin, and possibly TRPV1 systems [36, 39]. Alterations of opioid receptor structure and function seem intuitively (and experimentally) to be essential for development and propagation of the condition; in addition, alteration of rostral ventral medullary neuron "ON" and OFF" cell balance (see Chap. 2) likely plays a role [36].

Treatment approaches to OIH include rotation of agent (discussed briefly in Chap. 8) and more rationally in the author's mind, cessation of opioid therapy. Many examples of chronic pain abatement with opioid cessation support this approach. It is no small task to convince patients to desist from seeking more of the agent they believe to be alleviating their suffering, but in clear-cut cases of OIH, we see nearly universal improvement in symptoms for those who endure the detoxification process. Low-dose naltrexone therapy, increasingly used in the treatment of some central sensitization disorders such as fibromyalgia may provide an answer to OIH as well; theoretically the homeostatic recruitment of increased endogenous opioid release by very low intermittent exposure to an antagonist underlies this practice. NMDA antagonists may also provide some therapeutic benefit.

Inhibition of adaptive neural plasticity may be one of the most insidious effects of chronic opioid therapy and from both an individual and public health perspective may be one of the more devastating legacies of our recent 20-year national experiment in attempting to treat chronic pain with chronic opioids. A tremendous accumulation of evidence suggests that many chronic pain states, especially neuropathic pain or those involving central sensitization (but extending even to chronic low back pain [40–42], now a ubiquitous complaint in this nation), may be the result of maladaptive changes in cortical and limbic system synaptic patterns and even neuronal viability. Proposed mechanisms for this pathologic/maladaptive "re-wiring" of pain pathways include multifactorial long-term potentiation in both the dorsal horn and also higher central structures including the thalamus, limbic structures, and cortex [43–45]. Beyond supportive basic and clinical research, the teleologic argument that short-term pain is essential for survival and danger avoidance but long-term pain is pathologic and without any advantage to the organism is a sound one.

Under normal circumstances brain-derived neurotropic factor (BDNF) and other mediators act throughout the brain to facilitate learning and adaptive neuroplasticity. Chronic pain itself can inhibit these changes as does depression, but (exogenous) opioids have also been shown to play a role in inhibiting BDNF activity and other mechanisms of adaptive plasticity at the level of both the brain and spinal cord [46–49]. It is entirely conceivable that the chronic pain epidemic is the scion of the opioid epidemic.

Respiratory

Respiratory depression is the best-appreciated and most-feared complication of opioid use and statistically the AE responsible for the lion's share of opioid-related mortality. Incidence/prevalence data on respiratory depression in the outpatient setting is of course impossible to collect, and only extreme events are captured via vital statistics. The inpatient arena however has provided some insight into occurrence of opioid-related respiratory depression in hospitalized patients. A recent review reported an overall incidence of significant respiratory depression among patients treated with opioids at slightly less than 0.5%; outcome definitions among the studies reviewed however were highly variable and included different cutoff values for bradypnea or otherwise comprised vague terminology such as "respiratory depression" or "ventilatory depression." [50]. A slightly older review of nearly 20,000 inpatients pooled from 165 studies provided summed respiratory depression incidence data stratified by the following outcome variables: 0.3% required naloxone resuscitation, 1.1% exhibited "hypoventilation," 3.3% exhibited "hypercarbia," and 17% exhibited "oxygen desaturation" [51].

Increases in arterial pCO_2 (resulting from either increased production of CO_2 or decreased ventilation) cause corresponding decreases in pH. Under normal circumstances, central chemoreceptors located primarily in the brainstem but also the medulla, and to a far lesser degree, peripheral chemoreceptors located primarily in the carotid and aortic bodies sense acidosis and respond by increasing both diaphragmatic and accessory muscle activity [52]. Similarly, carotid body chemoreceptors normally respond to hypoxemia with consequential ventilatory increases as well. Opioids acting primarily on the mu-opioid receptor (MOR) [53] cause dose-dependent suppression of the ventilatory responses to both hypercapnia and hypoxemia [54], with decreases in both respiratory rate and to a much lesser degree tidal volume. (In fact it is very common to see compensatory increases in tidal volume with heavily narcotized but spontaneously breathing patients in the operating room or postanesthesia care unit.)

Fortunately, adaptation to opioid-induced respiratory depression is relatively efficient, with the majority of patients on short- or long-term opioid therapy escaping an opioid-induced apneic death by rapid development of tolerance to the mechanisms discussed above [27]. Conversely, it is not uncommon to see rapid "sensitization" to the respiratory depressant effects of opioids in the acute care setting at least, when sudden and effective analgesia removes the competing nociceptive stimulus to breathe. The parturient who has been "loaded up" with systemic opioids prior to initiation of labor epidural analgesia or the postoperative patient with substantial residual plasma opioid levels from the operating room who then receives a supplemental regional anesthetic in the recovery room for intractable pain is frequently seen to become acutely hypopneic or even apneic and desaturate.

In any circumstance, respiratory depression and in severe cases apnea remain a significant threat in any situation involving opioid use, and this issue comprises the central and paramount risk assumed by the patient and practitioner with every prescription and use of the drug. Underlying respiratory pathology from airway obstruction to pulmonary disease (e.g., COPD or interstitial lung disease) heightens these risks, as does concomitant CNS depressant use; a large percentage of opioid overdose death victims are positive for benzodiazepine, alcohol, and other sedatives [55, 56].

Regardless of the validity of observations and clinical lore indicating that substantial tolerance develops to the overall respiratory depressant effects of opioids, a high prevalence of *sleep-disordered breathing (SDB)* is associated with opioid use and may reflect sleeping decrement in hypoxic (rather than hypercarbic) ventilatory response [57]. Central apnea (CSA) occurs via mechanisms described above, with decreased ventilatory response to both hypercarbia and hypoxemia. Obstructive apnea (OSA) occurs when the upper airway is occluded, primarily due to the tongue collapsing against the posterior pharynx, and it is well established that opioids depress genioglossal tone. More recently it has been shown that opioids also decrease laryngeal aperture [58]. The rates of severe SDB (with an apnea-hypopnea index ≥15) in the general US populace are likely underestimated but have been reported on the order of 10%; the figure increases to 26% with relaxation of the criteria to include AHI ≥ 5 [59]. By comparison, Webster et al. showed a SDB (AHI prevalence ≥5) of 75% in a cohort of 140 patients on chronic opioid therapy [60]; the authors reported a similar figure (85%) in another study published the following year [61]. Walker et al. compared opioid users vs. nonusers and found no significant difference in the rate of OSA but a sixfold higher incidence of CSA in the former group [57], with dose-dependent increases in AHI. Coupled with the alarming increases in both obesity and sedative prescriptions in this country, opioid-associated SDB demands a dramatic rethinking of recent opioid prescribing practices as well as heightened vigilance in screening for OSA.

Other than histamine-induced *bronchospasm* (reportedly occurring primarily if not exclusively in individuals with some underlying degree of reactive airways), direct pulmonary pathology such as obstructive bronchial/bronchiolar disease has not been reported. Infrequently these days restrictive pathology is observed in the operative arena primarily from high-dose fentanyl use causing *rigid chest syndrome*. This phenomenon may be prevalent and unappreciated in the illicit drug community, with similarly high plasma levels of opioids occurring via intravenous injection.

Cardiovascular

Opioids in general are thought to be fairly benign from a cardiovascular system standpoint and have long enjoyed therapeutic use in treating ischemic cardiac disease and the symptoms of congestive heart failure. The author remembers as a student learning the mnemonic "MONA [morphine/oxygen/nitroglycerin/aspirin] greets all patients at the door" as a time-honored empiric treatment protocol for suspected coronary syndrome. Sympatholysis and reduction of pulmonary venous pressures from opioid agonism have been known and utilized for decades to treat both symptoms and underlying pathology of both CAD and CHF. More recently, evidence linking delta-opioid receptor (DOR) agonism with cardiac myocyte ischemic preconditioning is growing [62, 63] and may lead to novel cardioprotective strategies.

However, there are also well-known AEs of opioids upon the cardiovascular system. *Bradycardia* is commonly seen due to both direct sympatholytic and also provagal effects. While frequently utilized clinically for cardioprotection, *sympatholysis* and/or vagal stimulation from opioids may also result in catastrophic circulatory failure in patients who are severely hypovolemic or suffering from significant left ventricular dysfunction that are "living on sympathetic drive." Any anesthesiologist (even in training) has seen profound hemodynamic collapse in trauma or cardiac patients with even the "gentlest cardiac induction" which traditionally consists largely if not even exclusively of intravenous opioid administration. Much less frequently *sympathomimetic* or *anticholinergic effects* may result from opioid use, and meperidine (pethidine) has long been known to confer atropine-like hemodynamic changes including *tachycardia.* Several agents (most notably levorphanol, tramadol, and tapentadol) also possess intrinsic norepinephrine reuptake inhibitory properties that increase sympathetic tone.

While opioids are generally thought to be either rhythm-neutral or antiarrhythmic [26], dangerous electrophysiologic alterations are receiving increasing attention with opioid use, most notably QT interval prolongation with methadone and possibly buprenorphine [64] (although most studies refute these findings) and oxycodone [65]. Fatal cardiac rhythm disturbances such as torsades de pointes are now well-recognized risks of therapy with methadone.

Preload and *afterload* can be affected in a number of ways by opioids including volume alteration from renal and neuroendocrine (hypothalamic-pituitary-adrenal) effects and also via indirect vascular pathology from *histamine release*, leading in extreme cases to significant hypotension and distributive shock.

Decreased cardiac output from sympatholytic effects upon rate and afterload is well known; however, another mechanism may include direct *cardiac myocyte depression* [26, 66, 67], resulting from perturbation of sodium and calcium flux in both in vitro and in vivo models. However, there is also evidence of direct inotropic effects of opioids in other experimental settings [26]; these contradictory findings as well as the complex interactions of opioids with the autonomic system and neuroendocrine system (e.g., cytokine profile alterations) render the net effect of opioids on cardiac contractility still mysterious.

Endocrine

Evidence is accumulating that opioid use profoundly alters normal endocrine balance, with effects on many hormonal systems. The most well recognized and perhaps clinically relevant is opioid-induced *hypogonadism*. Opioids inhibit gonadotropin-releasing hormone (GnRH) secretion from the hypothalamus [68, 69] which results in reduction of anterior pituitary secretion of luteinizing hormone (LH) and to a much lesser degree follicle-stimulating hormone (FSH) which in turn reduce gonadal production of sex hormones (testosterone and estradiol) and also gamete production. In men, besides sexual effects, increased adiposity, decreased muscle mass and maintenance/repair, reduced energy and exercise tolerance, and decreased bone mineral density to the point of osteoporosis may occur [70]. Increased inflammation and reductions in pain tolerance due to hypogonadism have been reported as well. Opioid-related bone mineral density loss has not been as well characterized in women; however, infertility, amenorrhea, night sweats and hot flashes, fatigue, poor exercise tolerance, and decreased healing have all been demonstrated in women undergoing chronic opioid therapy [69–71]. The prevalence of hypogonadism in the opioid-using population has been reported consistently at around 90% [68, 69] versus a population baseline of 40% or less. These effects may begin within hours to days of opioid administration and do not require long-term exposure [69]. Screening for hypogonadism and testosterone supplementation in hypogonadal male patients on chronic opioid therapy has been recommended but is not currently widespread.

The effects of opioid use on the hypothalamic-pituitary-adrenal (HPA) axis are only partially understood; the interactions between native opioid ligand-receptor systems and the HPA and indeed the entire homeostatic neuroimmunoendocrine milieu are tremendously complex and affected by a host of both physical and psychological events, not least of which are the confounding effects of pain, stress, and anxiety. Several case reports and series document at least relative *adrenal insufficiency* in patients exposed to chronic opioids; the incidence is estimated at up to 10% [68]. Decreased glucocorticoid release from the adrenals may be due to direct primary action upon the zona fasciculata but is thought to be mainly due to a secondary effect upon pituitary release of ACTH, possibly via decreased sensitivity to hypothalamic CRH. Measurements of CRH, ACTH, and cortisol however are subject to tremendous variability under normal circumstances due to diurnal variation and other factors, and the presence of pain and stress may complicate serologic measurements to the point of unreliability. Recently dehydroepiandrosterone sulfate (DHEAS) levels have been demonstrated to be a more sensitive and perhaps more robust marker for adrenal insufficiency and seem to be reduced in patients on opioid therapy, particularly females [69, 72].

Prolactin levels are increased in human males receiving chronic opioid therapy; this is thought to occur via opioid-induced release of tonic dopaminergic inhibition from the arcuate nucleus acting upon the pituitary [35]. Such effects have not been conclusively seen in premenopausal women and may reflect a "buffering" effect of estrogen [68].

Growth hormone (GH) levels are usually increased by acute opioid use; however, chronic effects are poorly characterized. It has been theorized that the acute effects are due to release of previously synthesized and stored GH and that chronic exposure may result in deficiency of synthesis [68].

Conflicting evidence exists in the literature regarding the effects of opioid use upon thyroid function [68, 73], and as of yet no reliable conclusions can be drawn.

Neurohypophysial (posterior pituitary) hormones are also affected by opioid use. *Antidiuretic hormone (ADH)/vasopressin* secretion appears to be decreased by opioid use [68]; however, some studies indicate opioid-induced increases in ADH. It must be kept in mind that ADH release is a highly dynamic phenomenon influenced by volume and osmolar status and direct renal (angiotensin) and intestinal (cholecystokinin) regulation; ADH also exhibits complex bidirectional interactions with other endocrine systems such as the HPA axis. *Oxytocin* levels appear to be decreased by opioid use during both labor and the postpartum period but not prior [68].

Immunologic

Immunosuppressive effects of opioids have been recognized for over 500 years [74]; recent advances in our understanding of the role of the endogenous opioid system as part of the neuroimmunoendocrine system as a whole reveal a highly complex interaction between native opioid peptides and the immune system

[75–77]. A review of the current state of our understanding of *opioid immunomodulation (OIM)* is beyond the scope of this work, and the reader is encouraged to investigate the literature; however, the following observations bear mentioning here:

- The MOR appears to be the most important mediator as MOR-knockout mice models display no OIM [74].
- The nociceptin/orphanin-FQ (N/OFQ) system has been shown to have pro-inflammatory effects and may exert suppression of cytokine and chemokine activity [74, 78]. The clinical relevance of this has been shown in ICU populations, especially those suffering from sepsis; whether exogenous opioid use effects OIM through some alteration of this pathway remains to be seen.
- Central effects may comprise the majority of clinically relevant opioid immunomodulation as opioids that do not cross the blood-brain barrier seem to exert less pronounced effects [74].
- The HPA system's activity is known to be affected by opioids in a complex manner (see above); it exerts profound enhancing or suppressive effects upon immune system function subject to many other variables.
- Altered sympathetic nervous system (SNS) outflow may negatively affect natural killer cell activity and lymphocyte proliferation [76, 79]. It must be remembered that SNS and HPA activity are closely intertwined.
- Opioids may exert peripheral effects upon immunocytes via the Toll-like receptor 4 (TLR4) [74, 76]. The presence of classic opioid receptors (MOR in particular) on immunocytes has been recently challenged by intensive mRNA assaying; NOR mRNA however was detected [74].
- The role of astrocytes and microglia in central immunomodulation is an area of intensive research currently, and the effects of opioids upon these cells have recently been thoroughly reviewed [77].

The most relevant clinical arena in which to consider the immunomodulatory effects of opioids is undoubtedly oncology, where severe pain is common and known to suppress immune function and accelerate tumor growth and metastasis in animal models. Al-Hashimi et al. [74] recently performed a systematic literature review of the effect of exogenous opioids on immune function in the cancer population and found highly variable data on leukocyte counts, cytokine activity, killer cell activity, etc. They caution against drawing any conclusions in the absence of any demonstrated effects on clinical outcomes. The immunosuppressed population in pain may well experience increased immunocompetence from good analgesia; opioids are likely not the optimal vehicle but are often the only option in most situations worldwide and in this country.

Gastroenterologic

Nausea and vomiting are highly prevalent AE of opioids and have been reported with every agent used therapeutically (or illicitly.) Nausea occurs in roughly one third of patients treated with opioids and is thought to result from a combination of effects at the medullary chemoreceptor trigger zone, inhibition of gut motility, and also vestibular stimulation [80]. All three opioid receptor types are involved and their contributions vary by site and other factors not well elucidated. With continued use, most patients report a decrease in or resolution of nausea and vomiting, but in some cases, it is persistent.

Opioid-induced bowel dysfunction (OIBD) ranges from mild constipation to life-threatening paralytic ileus. Relaxation of fundal musculature combined with contraction of antral and duodenal muscle delays gastric emptying. Ileus results from intestinal MOR-mediated alteration/inhibition of normal contractile patterns [81] and in mild form contributes to constipation. It may be so severe, however (more likely in conjunction with postoperative ileus), that potentially fatal complications, e.g., abdominal compartment syndrome, may occur [82]. *Opioid-induced constipation (OIC)* occurs in between 15 and >50% of patients on chronic opioid therapy [27] and, unlike most adverse (and therapeutic) effects, does not seem to diminish over time. In addition to the ileus described above, mechanisms include MOR-mediated increased fluid absorption and decreased enterocyte secretion and increased sphincter tone. OIC like any constipation can predispose to nausea and vomiting, hemorrhoids, prolapse and in severe cases bowel obstruction and perforation. Prophylaxis with stool softeners such as docusate has long been standard operating procedure and should be included with any opioid prescription along with instructions for plentiful hydration. Osmotic agents such as polyethylene glycol are another reasonable routine recommendation; we frequently recommend magnesium in doses of 500–750 mg/day and titrating upward to effect, as this agent is also an adjunctive analgesic (NMDA blocker) and membrane stabilizer conferring some benefit in neuropathic pain. More aggressive treatment with stimulant laxatives or enemas may be obviated in the future with the advent of newer pharmacologic agents such as peripherally acting MOR antagonists whose activity is essentially confined to gastrointestinal MOR (e.g., methylnaltrexone, naloxegol, alvimopan). Lubiprostone (which exerts its effect by activating chloride channels, achieving a net effect similar to the action of cholera toxin) has recently been marketed for the treatment of OIC; methadone however seems to inhibit its effect [83]. Unlike most of the adverse effects of the drug class, tolerance to OIBD does not seem to develop.

Cholangiographic and manometric studies have confirmed *sphincter of Oddi spasm* with opioid use; this complication has particular relevance for the treatment of pain from biliary colic and pancreatitis. Anecdotal evidence in the 1980s and 1990s favored meperidine (pethidine) compared to morphine (which seems to confer the greatest degree of spasm), but a review of the literature concluded that there is no clinical superiority with any particular opioid agent and the risks of meperidine outweigh the benefits [84].

Urologic

Urinary retention occurs not infrequently in patients on opioid therapy; the rate has been estimated at around 10% [85] but has been reported as high as 18.1% in post-operative patients [86] where surveillance and monitoring (i.e., Foley urometrics) are prevalent. The pathophysiology is thought to be due to a MOR and possibly DOR-mediated combination of inhibition of the spinobulbospinal voiding reflex, decreased detrusor activity, and increased sphincter tone. As with OIBD, peripheral MOR antagonists appear to ameliorate these symptoms.

Dermatologic

Pruritis is a common adverse effect of opioid therapy, with an incidence estimated between 2 and 10% [87]. Neuraxial (epidural or intrathecal) administration seems to be associated with a higher incidence (up to 80% [88]) and may suggest a primarily central mechanism as opposed to a peripheral histaminergic response. The inefficacy of antihistamine therapy on this condition and reasonable success with low-dose antagonist therapy (naloxone or naltrexone) support a specific opioid receptor-mediated pathway.

Literature Review of Adverse Effects

The findings of several recent systematic reviews examining the incidence of various adverse effects from opioids are summarized below and in Table 3.2.

Kalso et al. (2004) reviewed 15 randomized controlled trials (RCTs) comparing opioid therapy for chronic non-cancer pain to placebo [90]. Data from 1445 patients were analyzed showing an 80% rate of report of at least one adverse effect in the opioid group vs. 56% in the placebo group. Rates for specific AEs were reported by treatment group and are presented in the table.

Furlan et al. (2006) performed a meta-analysis of 41 RCTs of opioid use in chronic non-cancer pain; 30 of these were placebo-controlled [91]. Altogether data from 6019 patients were analyzed, and data on adverse effects were presented in terms of risk differences, without raw numbers/rates presented. Risk differences for specific AEs that showed statistically significant differences between treatment groups are presented in the table.

Trescot et al. (2008) reviewed a number of studies examining opioid effectiveness and AE and render a unique presentation of AE stratified by specific drug [92]. These data are presented in the table.

Papaleontiou et al. (2010) performed a systematic review and meta-analysis of 31 RCTs and 12 observational studies comparing opioids to placebo or non-opioid

Table 3.2 Systematic reviews of adverse effects of opioids vs. placebo

Study	Adverse effect	Rate in cases	Rate in controls	Other analyses
Kalso et al. [89]	Constipation	41%	11%	
	Nausea	32%	12%	
	Somnolence	29%	10%	
	Dizziness	20%	7%	
	Vomiting	15%	3%	
	Pruritis	15%	7%	
Furlan et al. [90]				Risk difference in opioid vs. placebo (95%CI)
	Constipation			16% (10–22%)
	Nausea			15% (11–19%)
	Somnolence			9% (5–13%)
	Dizziness			8% (5–12%)
	Vomiting			5% (2–7%)
	Dermatologic sxs			4% (1–6%)
Trescot et al. [91]				Drug AE prevalence
				Morphine nausea 37%
				Fentanyl nausea 31%
				Constipation 4.6–23.1%
				Somnolence 18%
				Methadone nausea/vomiting 23.6%
				Sedation 18.5%
				Pruritis/rash 13%
				Constipation 11.7%
				Oxycodone constipation 15%
				Nausea 12%
				Somnolence 8%
				Vomiting 7%
				Depression 2%
Papaleontiou et al. [92]	Constipation	30%		
	Nausea	28%		
	Dizziness	22%		
	Somnolence	21%		
Furlan et al. [93]	Nausea	28%	9%	EERW opioid vs. placebo data[a]
	Constipation	26%	7%	Nausea 16% 8%
				Constipation 15% 3%
				Somnolence 10% 5%
	Somnolence	24%	7%	Dizziness 10% 5%
	Dizziness	18%	5%	Dermatologic sxs 5% 2%
	Dermatologic sxs	15%	2%	
	Vomiting	15%	3%	
	Dry mouth	12%	6%	

(continued)

Table 3.2 (continued)

Study	Adverse effect	Rate in cases	Rate in controls	Other analyses
McNicol et al. [94]	Constipation	34%	9%	
	Somnolence	29%	14%	
	Nausea	27%	9%	
	Dizziness	22%	8%	
	Vomiting	12%	4%	
Chou et al. [96]				Odds ratios for opioid vs. none groups
				"Serious" overdose 8.4
				"Any" overdose 5.2
				Myocardial infarction 2.66
				Fracture 1.27

[a]*EERW* enriched enrollment randomized withdrawal trials

analgesics in chronic non-cancer pain, with 10,545 patients total [93]. Inclusion criteria included an age equal to or greater than 60 years old (mean age 64.) Rates for specific AEs were reported for the opioid group and are presented in the table.

Furlan et al. in 2011 updated their earlier analysis with 21 additional studies for a total of 62 RCTs comparing opioids vs. placebo or other drug for chronic non-cancer pain in 11,927 patients [94]. The purpose of this subsequent investigation was to evaluate whether enriched enrollment randomized withdrawal trials (EERW, a type of RCT in which potential participants receive the study drug on a trial basis prior to randomization into the actual study) provided improved data quality by augmenting the pool with participants with improved tolerance. An *a priori* assumption of this design is that AE will be underrepresented, as potential participants who cannot tolerate the drug will not enroll. In this analysis, the rate of AE was substantially higher in traditional RCTs than in the EERW trials, and the data are presented in the table.

McNicol et al. (2013) reviewed 31 RCTs (n = 1237 patients) comparing opioids vs. placebo specifically for neuropathic pain [95]; rates for specific AEs were reported for the opioid vs. placebo groups and are presented in the table.

Reinecke et al. (2015) performed a meta-analysis of 46 RCTs (n = 10,742 patients) evaluating treatment methodologies in chronic non-cancer pain [96]; 24 of these RCTs evaluated pharmacologic interventions involving both opioid and non-opioid drugs compared to placebo (the remainder evaluated physical and psychological therapy modalities.) Data on AE, which included in descending order of frequency nausea, constipation, somnolence, dizziness, and vomiting, were reported only in the aggregate, and the authors state that the incidence was "10–20% higher in opioid than placebo groups."

Chou et al. (2015) in a study funded by the Agency for Healthcare Research and Quality reviewed 39 studies including RCTs and observational studies that compared opioid therapy for at least 3 months vs. other modalities including placebo

[97]. No studies reported on long-term (greater than 12 months) efficacy in terms of pain relief, functional improvement, etc.; however AE was evaluated for greater than 12 months in 19 studies, and these data are presented in a non-pooled manner; those which are amenable to tabular representation are shown below (see Table 3.2).

Finally, an unprecedented prospective study involving the entire state of North Carolina in 2010 was carried out using prescription drug monitoring program data [98]. Subjects receiving an opioid prescription in 2010 (n = 2,182,374 patients) as well as the remainder of the state's population (totaling almost 9.5 million individuals) were followed forward for 1 year, and mortality data related to opioid use was examined. There were 629 total prescription opioid-related deaths (478 of which had a valid prescription and 151 apparently were using prescription opioids illicitly, i.e., via diversion.) There was a strong correlation between dose and mortality without any specific "inflection point" noted. Concurrent alcohol use was identified in only 12% of opioid deaths; however, benzodiazepine use was identified in over 60% of opioid decedents. (The authors draw attention to the fact that the overall general prescription rate for benzodiazepines is on the order of 5% nationwide.) The mortality rate was tenfold higher in patients receiving prescriptions for both opioids and benzodiazepines compared to those receiving prescriptions for opioids alone.

Summary

Opioids are powerful and yet seemingly capricious agents with a historically unparalleled ability to efficiently relieve pain coupled with a myriad of adverse effects ranging from trivial to life-threatening. They also display near-universal but relatively unpredictable loss of efficacy in the context of chronic use. Such tolerance is a major factor in amplifying the incidence and severity of adverse effects as patients often consume (sanctioned or unsanctioned) increasing quantities of opioids in an attempt to either relieve pain or withdrawal symptoms or simply for recreational purposes.

References

1. Pimentel L, Mayo D. Chronic methadone therapy complicated by torsades de pointes: a case report. J Emerg Med. 2008;34:287–90.
2. Fishman SM. Responsible opioid prescribing–a clinician's guide. 2nd ed. Washington, D.C.: Waterford Life Sciences; 2014.
3. Chowdhury MM, Board R. Morphine-induced hallucinations - resolution with switching to oxycodone: a case report and review of the literature. Cases J. 2009;2:9391.
4. White KL, Roth BL. Psychotomimetic effects of kappa opioid receptor agonists. Biol Psychiatry. 2012;72:797–8.
5. Dogra S, Yadav PN. Biased agonism at kappa opioid receptors: implication in pain and mood disorders. Eur J Pharmacol. 2015;763(Pt B):184–90.

6. Schmauss C, Yassouridis A, Emrich HM. Antipsychotic effect of buprenorphine in schizophrenia. Am J Psychiatry. 1987;144:1340–2.
7. Scherrer JF, Salas J, Copeland LA, Stock EM, Ahmedani BK, Sullivan MD, et al. Prescription opioid duration, dose, and increased risk of depression in 3 large patient populations. Ann Fam Med. 2016;14:54–62.
8. Scherrer JF, Salas J, Lustman PJ, Burge S, Schneider FD, Residency Research Network of Texas (RRNeT) Investigators. Change in opioid dose and change in depression in a longitudinal primary care patient cohort. Pain. 2015;156:348–55.
9. Lutz PE, Kieffer BL. Opioid receptors: distinct roles in mood disorders. Trends Neurosci. 2013;36:195–206.
10. Bodkin JA, Zornberg GL, Lukas SE. Buprenorphine treatment of refractory depression. J Clin Psychopharmacol. 1995;15:49–57.
11. Machado-Vieira R, Zarate CA Jr. Proof of concept trials in bipolar disorder and major depressive disorder: a translational perspective in the search for improved treatments. Depress Anxiety. 2011;28:267–81.
12. Peppin JF, Raffa RB. Delta opioid agonists: a concise update on potential therapeutic applications. J Clin Pharm Ther. 2015;40(2):155–66.
13. Gardner E. Introduction: addiction and brain reward and anti-reward pathways. Adv Psychosom Med. 2011;30:22–60.
14. Chartoff EH, Connery HS. It's MORe exciting than mu: crosstalk between mu opioid receptors and glutamatergic transmission in the mesolimbic dopamine system. Front Pharmacol. 2014;5:116.
15. Koob GF. The dark side of emotion: the addiction perspective. Eur J Pharmacol. 2015;753:73–87.
16. American Psychiatric Association. Diagnostic and statistical manual of mental disorders. 5th ed. Washington, D.C.: American Psychiatric Association; 2013.
17. National Institute on Drug Abuse. Misuse of prescription drugs. 2017. https://www.drugabuse.gov/publications/research-reports/misuseprescription-drugs/summary. Accessed 18 Aug 2017
18. National Institute on Drug Abuse. NIDA research report series–prescription drug abuse. 2014. Available from: https://www.drugabuse.gov/publications/research-reports/prescription-drugs/what-prescription-drug-abuse.
19. UNODC, World drug report 2012. http://www.unodc.org/unodc/en/data-and-analysis/WDR-2012.html.
20. Substance Abuse and Mental Health Services Administration, Center for Behavioral Health Statistics and Quality. Behavioral health trends in the United States: results from the 2014 national survey on drug use and health. Rockville, MD: Substance Abuse and Mental Health Services Administration; 2015.
21. Edlund MJ, Martin BC, Fan MY, Devries A, Braden JB, Sullivan MD. Risks for opioid abuse and dependence among recipients of chronic opioid therapy: results from the TROUP study. Drug Alcohol Depend. 2010;112:90–8.
22. Vowles KE, McEntee ML, Julnes PS, Frohe T, Ney JP, van der Goes DN. Rates of opioid misuse, abuse, and addiction in chronic pain: a systematic review and data synthesis. Pain. 2015;156:569–76.
23. Sehgal N, Manchikanti L, Smith HS. Prescription opioid abuse in chronic pain: a review of opioid abuse predictors and strategies to curb opioid abuse. Pain Physician. 2012;15:ES67–92.
24. Palmer R, Carrel D, Cronkite D, Saunders K, Gross D, Masters E, et al. The prevalence and characteristics of patients with indicators of opioid abuse within an integrated group practice. J Pain. 2014;15(Supplement):S25.
25. Fishbain DA, Cole B, Lewis J, Rosomoff HL, Rosomoff RS. What percentage of chronic nonmalignant pain patients exposed to chronic opioid analgesic therapy develop abuse/addiction and/or aberrant drug-related behaviors? A structured evidence-based review. Pain Med. 2008;9:444–59.
26. Fukuda K. Opioid analgesics. In: Miller R, editor. Miller's anesthesia. Philadelphia: Saunders; 2014. p. 864–914.

27. Smith HS, McCleane G, Thompson G. Optimizing pharmacologic outcomes: assessing and managing opioid side effects. In: Smith HS, editor. Opioid therapy in the 21st century. Oxford: Oxford University Press; 2013. p. 79–103.
28. Li Y, van den Pol AN. Mu-opioid receptor-mediated depression of the hypothalamic hypocretin/orexin arousal system. J Neurosci. 2008;28:2814–9.
29. Osman NI, Baghdoyan HA, Lydic R. Morphine inhibits acetylcholine release in rat prefrontal cortex when delivered systemically or by microdialysis to basal forebrain. Anesthesiology. 2005;103:779–87.
30. Bagetta G, De Sarro GB, Sakurada S. Different profile of electrocortical power spectrum changes after micro-infusion into the locus coeruleus of selective agonists at various opioid receptor subtypes in rats. Br J Pharmacol. 1990;101:655–61.
31. Van Bockstaele EJ, Valentino RJ. Neuropeptide regulation of the locus coeruleus and opiate-induced plasticity of stress responses. Adv Pharmacol. 2013;68:405–20.
32. Cheatle MD, Webster LR. Opioid therapy and sleep disorders: risks and mitigation strategies. Pain Med. 2015;16:S22–6.
33. Dhingra L, Ahmed E, Shin J, Scharaga E, Magun M. Cognitive effects and sedation. Pain Med. 2015;16:S37–43.
34. McNicol E, Horowicz-Mehler N, Fisk RA. Management of opioid side effects in cancer-related and chronic noncancer pain: a systematic review. J Pain. 2003;4:231–56.
35. Yaksh TL, Wallace MS. Opioids, analgesia, and pain management. In: Brunton L, editor. Goodman and Gilman's pharmacologic basis of therapeutics. New York: McGraw-Hill; 2011. p. 481–525.
36. Lee MD, Silverman S, Hansen H, Patel VB, Manchikanti L. A comprehensive review of opioid-induced hyperalgesia. Pain Physician. 2011;14:145–61.
37. Angst MS, Clark JD. Opioid-induced hyperalgesia: a qualitative systematic review. Anesthesiology. 2006;104:570–87.
38. Celerier E, Laulin JP, Corcuff JB, Le Moal M, Simonnet G. Progressive enhancement of delayed hyperalgesia induced by repeated heroin administration: a sensitization process. J Neurosci. 2001;21:4074–80.
39. Chen L, Mao J. Optimizing pharmacologic outcomes: opioid-induced hyperalgesia. In: Smith HS, editor. Opioid therapy in the 21st century. Oxford: Oxford University Press; 2013. p. 105–19.
40. Apkarian AV, Sosa Y, Sonty S, Levy RM, Harden RN, Parrish TB, et al. Chronic back pain is associated with decreased prefrontal and thalamic gray matter density. J Neurosci. 2004;24:10410–5.
41. Siddall PJ, Stanwell P, Woodhouse A, Somorjai RL, Dolenko B, Nikulin A, et al. Magnetic resonance spectroscopy detects biochemical changes in the brain associated with chronic low back pain: a preliminary report. Anesth Analg. 2006;102:1164–8.
42. Ivo R, Nicklas A, Dargel J. Brain structural and psychometric alterations in chronic low back pain. Eur Spine J. 2013;22:1958–64.
43. Zhuo M. Long-term potentiation in the anterior cingulate cortex and chronic pain. Phil Trans Royal Soc B. 2014;369:20130146.
44. Price TJ, Inyang KE. Commonalities between pain and memory mechanisms and their meaning for understanding chronic pain. Prog Mol Biol Transl Sci. 2015;131:409–34.
45. Doan L, Manders T, Wang J. Neuroplasticity underlying the comorbidity of pain and depression. Neural Plast. 2015;2015:504691.
46. Beltrán-Campos V, Silva-Vera M, García-Campos ML, Diaz-Cintra S. Effects of morphine on brain plasticity. Neurologia. 2015;30:176–80.
47. Kandasamy R, Price TJ. The pharmacology of nociceptor priming. Handb Exp Pharmacol. 2015;227:15–37.
48. Sahbaie P, Liang DY, Shi WY. Epigenetic regulation of spinal cord gene expression contributes to enhanced postoperative pain and analgesic tolerance subsequent to continuous opioid exposure. Mol Pain. 2016;12:1–11.

49. Mao J, Mayer DJ. Spinal cord neuroplasticity following repeated opioid exposure and its relation to pathological pain. Ann N Y Acad Sci. 2001;933:175–84.
50. Dahan A, Aarts L, Smith TW. Incidence, reversal, and prevention of opioid-induced respiratory depression. Anesthesiology. 2010;112:226–38.
51. Cashman JN, Dolin SJ. Respiratory and haemodynamic effects of acute postoperative pain management: evidence from published data. Br J Anaesth. 2004;93:212–23.
52. West JB. Respiratory physiology: the essentials. 9th ed. Baltimore, MD: Lippincott Williams and Wilkins; 2012.
53. Dahan A, Sarton E, Teppema L, Olievier C, Nieuwenhuijs D, Matthes HW, et al. Anesthetic potency and influence of morphine and sevoflurane on respiration in mu-opioid receptor knockout mice. Anesthesiology. 2001;94(5):824–32.
54. Pattinson KTS. Opioids and the control of respiration. Br J Anesth. 2008;100:747–58.
55. Jann M, Kennedy WK, Lopez G. Benzodiazepines: a major component in unintentional prescription drug overdoses with opioid analgesics. J Pharm Pract. 2014;27:5–16.
56. Jones CM, Paulozzi LJ, Mack KA. Alcohol involvement in opioid pain reliever and benzodiazepine drug abuse–related emergency department visits and drug-related deaths — United States, 2010. MMWR. 2014;63(40):881–5.
57. Walker JM, Farney RJ, Rhondeau SM, Boyle KM, Valentine K, Cloward TV, et al. Chronic opioid use is a risk factor for the development of central sleep apnea and ataxic breathing. J Clin Sleep Med. 2007;3:455–61.
58. Mulier JP. Perioperative opioids aggravate obstructive breathing in sleep apnea syndrome: mechanisms and alternative anesthesia strategies. Curr Opin Anaesthesiol. 2016;29:129–33.
59. Peppard PE, Young T, Barnet JH, Palta M, Hagen EW, Hla KM. Increased prevalence of sleep-disordered breathing in adults. Am J Epidemiol. 2013;177:1006–14.
60. Webster LR, Choi Y, Desai H. Sleep-disordered breathing and chronic opioid therapy. Pain Med. 2008;9:425–32.
61. Mogri M, Desai H, Webster L, Grant BJ, Mador MJ. Hypoxemia in patients on chronic opiate therapy with and without sleep apnea. Sleep Breath. 2009;13:49–57.
62. Feng Y, He X, Yang Y, Chao D, Lazarus LH, Xia Y. Current research on opioid receptor function. Curr Drug Targets. 2012;13:230–46.
63. Xia Y, editor. Neural function of the delta-opioid receptor. Basel: Springer International Publishing; 2015.
64. Fareed A, Patil D, Scheinberg K, Blackinton Gale R, Vayalapalli S, Casarella J, et al. Comparison of QTc interval prolongation for patients in methadone versus buprenorphine maintenance treatment: a 5-year follow-up. J Addict Dis. 2013;32:244–51.
65. Fanoe S, Jensen GB, Sjogren P, Korsgaard MP, Grunnet M. Oxycodone is associated with dose-dependent QTc prolongation in patients and low-affinity binding of hERG activity in vitro. Br J Clin Pharmacol. 2009;67:172–9.
66. Ventura C, Spurgeon H, Lakatta EG, Guarnieri C, Capogrossi MC. Kappa and delta opioid receptor stimulation affects cardiac myocyte function and Ca2+ release from an intracellular pool in myocytes and neurons. Circ Res. 1992;70:66–81.
67. Fry CH, Henry J. The mode of action of several opioids on cardiac muscle. Exp Physiol. 1997;82:261–72.
68. Vuong C, Van Uum SHM, O'Dell LE, Lutfy K, Friedman TC. The effects of opioids and opioid analogs on animal and human endocrine systems. Endocr Rev. 2010;31:98–132.
69. Gudin JA, Laitman A, Nalamachu S. Opioid related endocrinopathy. Pain Med. 2015;16:S9–15.
70. De Maddalena C, Bellini M, Berra M. Opioid-induced hypogonadism: why and how to treat it. Pain Physician. 2012;15:ES111–8.
71. Elliott JA, Horton E, Fibuch EE. The endocrine effects of long-term oral opioid therapy: a case report and review of the literature. J Opioid Manag. 2011;7:145–54.
72. Rhodin A, Stridsberg M, Gordh T. Opioid endocrinopathy: a clinical problem in patients with chronic pain and long-term opioid treatment. Clin J Pain. 2010;26:374–80.

73. Gozashti MH, Mohammadzadeh E, Divsalar K, Shokoohi M. The effect of opium addiction on thyroid function tests. J Diabetes Metab Disorders. 2014;13:5–10.
74. Al-Hashimi M, Scott SW, Thompson JP, Lambert DG. Opioids and immune modulation: more questions than answers. Br J Anaesth. 2013;111:80–8.
75. Pomorska DK, Gach K, Janecka A. Immunomodulatory effects of endogenous and synthetic peptides activating opioid receptors. Mini-Rev Med Chem. 2014;14:1148–55.
76. Boland JW, McWilliams K, Ahmedzai SH, Pockley AG. Effects of opioids on immunologic parameters that are relevant to anti-tumour immune potential in patients with cancer: a systematic literature review. Br J Cancer. 2014;111:866–73.
77. Hutchinson MR, Shavit Y, Grace PM, Rice KC, Maier SF, Watkins LR. Exploring the neuroimmunopharmacology of opioids: an integrative review of mechanisms of central immune signaling and their implications for opioid analgesia. Pharmacol Rev. 2011;63:772–810.
78. Bodera P, Stankiewicz W, Kocik J. Interactions of orphanin FQ/nociceptin (OFQ/N) system with immune system factors and hypothalamic-pituitary-adrenal (HPA) axis. Pharmacol Rep. 2014;66:288–91.
79. Hall DM, Suo JL, Weber RJ. Opioid mediated effects on the immune system: sympathetic nervous system involvement. J Neuroimmunol. 1998;83:29–35.
80. Porreca F, Ossipov MH. Nausea and vomiting side effects with opioid analgesics during treatment of chronic pain: mechanisms, implications, and management options. Pain Med. 2009;10:654–62.
81. Poulsen JL, Brock C, Olesen AE, Nilsson M, Drewes AM. Evolving paradigms in the treatment of opioid-induced bowel dysfunction. Therap Advan Gastroenterol. 2015;8:360–72.
82. Van Noord BA, Roffey P, Thangathurai D. Abdominal compartment syndrome following opioid-induced postoperative ileus. J Clin Anesth. 2013;25:146–9.
83. Cuppoletti J, Chakrabarti J, Tewari K, Malinowska DH. Methadone but not morphine inhibits lubiprostone-stimulated cl^- currents in T84 intestinal cells and recombinant human ClC-2, but not CFTR cl^- currents. Cell Biochem Biophys. 2013;66:53–63.
84. Thompson DR. Narcotic analgesic effects on the sphincter of Oddi: a review of the data and therapeutic implications in treating pancreatitis. Am J Gastroenterol. 2001;96:1266–72.
85. Verhamme KM, Sturkenboom MC, Stricker BH. Drug-induced urinary retention: incidence, management and prevention. Drug Saf. 2008;31:373–88.
86. Benyamin R, Trescot AM, Datta S, Buenaventura R, Adlaka R, Sehgal N, et al. Opioid complications and side effects. Pain Physician. 2008;11(2 Suppl):S105–20.
87. Cherny N, Ripamonti C, Pereira J, Davis C, Fallon M, McQuay H, et al. Strategies to manage the adverse effects of oral morphine: an evidence-based report. J Clin Oncol. 2001;19:2542–54.
88. Kumar K, Singh SI. Neuraxial opioid-induced pruritus: an update. J Anaesthesiol Clin Pharmacol. 2013;29:303–7.
89. Kalso E, Edwards J, Moore R, McQuay HJ. Opioids in chronic non-cancer pain: systematic review of efficacy and safety. Pain. 2004;112:372–80.
90. Furlan AD, Sandoval JA, Mailis-Gagnon A, Tunks E. Opioids for chronic non—cancer pain: a meta—analysis of effectiveness and side effects. Can Med Assoc J. 2006;174:1589–94.
91. Trescot AM, Glaser SE, Hansen H, Benyamin R, Patel S, Manchikanti L. Effectiveness of opioids in the treatment of chronic non-cancer pain. Pain Physician. 2008;11:S181–200.
92. Papaleontiou M, Henderson CR, Turner BJ, Moore AA, Olkhovskaya Y, Amanfo L, et al. Outcomes associated with opioid use in the treatment of chronic non-cancer pain among older adults: a systematic review and meta-analysis. J Am Geriatr Soc. 2010;58:1353–69.
93. Furlan A, Chaparro LE, Irvin E, Mailis-Gagnon A. A comparison between enriched and non-enriched enrollment randomized withdrawal trials of opioids for chronic noncancer pain. Pain Res Manag. 2011;16:337–51.
94. McNicol ED, Midbari A, Eisenberg E. Opioids for neuropathic pain. Cochrane Reviews. 2013; doi:10.1002/14651858.CD006146.pub2.
95. Reinecke H, Weber C, Lange K, Simon M, Stein C, Sorgatz H. Analgesic efficacy of opioids in chronic pain: recent meta-analysis. Br J Pharmacol. 2015;172:324–33.

96. Chou R, Turner JA, Devine EB, Hansen RN, Sullivan SD, Blazina I, et al. The effectiveness and risks of long-term opioid therapy for chronic pain: a systematic review for a national institutes of health pathways to prevention workshop. Ann Intern Med. 2015;162:276–86.
97. Dasgupta N, Funk MJ, Proescholdbell S, Hirsch A, Ribisl KM, Marshall S. Cohort study of the impact of high-dose opioid analgesics on overdose mortality. Pain Med. 2016;17:85–98.
98. Dasgupta N, Funk MJ, Proescholdbell S, Hirsch A, Ribisl KM, Marshall S. Cohort study of the impact of high-dose opioid analgesics on overdose mortality. Pain Med. 2016;17(1):85–98.

Chapter 4
Understanding the Agent, Part III: Specific Drugs

A 24-year-old right hand-dominant male presents to your practice with a complaint of right upper extremity pain that he describes as "burning, throbbing, and electric-like." The pain began 2 years ago immediately following a work-related injury where his arm was caught in a cable and hyperextended. He underwent a rotator cuff repair shortly after the incident, without any improvement in his symptoms nor function, and states that ever since, he has had worsening of both pain and function. He reports that light touch, water, or even wind is exquisitely painful to the limb, and he describes intermittent color changes and swelling from the elbow and distal to that. The limb constantly feels cold to him. He requests "Percocet" which he has been prescribed ever since his operation. He states that 2 months after the operation his orthopedic surgeon prescribed him tramadol, but he sustained a generalized tonic-clonic seizure and fractured three ribs as a result of the seizure. He did some Internet research and learned that there is an interaction between tramadol and bupropion, which he has been using for the past 4 years. After bringing this to the attention of his surgeon, he was referred to a pain management clinic where he has been treated by a series of stellate ganglion blocks and oxycodone combination products. He is a smoker but denies alcohol consumption. He is disabled and not working presently. Family history is noncontributory. Review of systems is positive for insomnia, anxiety, and depression.

On exam he is well-developed, well-nourished, alert, and oriented x4. VS: T97.3, HR 88, BP 142/95, RR 18. Pupils are 3 mm. The RUE shows a livedo reticularis erythematous pattern and is mildly edematous with a shiny and waxy appearance, and the hand has some flexion contractures of all digits. There is obvious atrophy of the limb compared to the LUE. He guards the limb, and there is hyperalgesia to palpation and passive ROM. It feels cold to the touch compared to the LUE.

H.B. McAnally, *Opioid Dependence*, DOI 10.1007/978-3-319-47497-7_4

Currently Available (Outpatient) Prescription Opioids

Opioids are generally classified either according to chemical structure or by pharmacokinetic properties, i.e., duration of action. Currently available outpatient prescription opioids in the United States are arranged in this chapter alphabetically for ease of reference. Excluded from this list are:

- Agents that are no longer available, such as propoxyphene
- Mixed agonist/antagonists, such as butorphanol, nalbuphine, and pentazocine
- Strictly intravenous agents, such as alfentanil and remifentanil
- Illicit agents, such as heroin and kratom

Before proceeding to individual agents, however, some basic definitions should be clarified. *Opioids* are molecules that act upon opioid receptors as described above and may include natural substances such as opiates, semisynthetic derivatives, or fully synthetic compounds. *Opiates* are plant alkaloids found in the opium poppy (*Papaver somniferum*). *Partial agonists* are substances that exert submaximal effect at a receptor compared to one that exerts full effect. *Mixed agonist/antagonists* exert agonist effects at some receptors and antagonist effects at others; this is generally due to differing activity at receptor subtypes.

Buprenorphine

Buprenorphine is a synthetic thebaine derivative, developed in 1969, with introduction into clinical practice in the 1970s in injectable form and in the 1980s in a sublingual formulation. Bioavailability is very poor orally due to high hepatic first-pass metabolism. Due to high lipophilicity, however, it is suitable for sublingual administration, and this has become the preferred route of administration clinically. Sublingual bioavailability is on the range of 50% [1]. Time to onset of effect is on the order of 10 min. It is highly (96%) protein bound.

Buprenorphine is a partial agonist at the MOR and an antagonist at both the KOR and DOR. It displays unique tenacity for the MOR, with a dissociation constant many orders of magnitude higher than most other opioids [1, 2], which confers both an extended duration of action and also the unique ability to "block" other opioid agonists from occupying the MOR, an attractive feature in terms of addictionology but one with problematic features in the acute care arena; both of these issues are discussed later. The potency of buprenorphine is rather contested in the literature; conservative estimates place it at 15–20 times the potency of morphine, whereas in some studies, it appears to be closer to 70 times more potent than morphine.

Buprenorphine undergoes both hepatic Phase I metabolism by CYP3A4 to norbuprenorphine and also direct Phase II glucuronidation. Norbuprenorphine is an active metabolite with roughly 20% efficacy of buprenorphine and also undergoes glucuronidation. The elimination of buprenorphine is primarily fecal, with 10–30%

of the dose excreted renally (as conjugated compounds.) Renal dosing does not appear to be necessary [3]. The half-life of buprenorphine is very long, with estimates as high as 37 h [2]. This is in part due to its long MOR association but also a very long proposed biophase equilibration time [4], which is a theoretical/modeled parameter explaining differences in concentration and effect between plasma and site of effect (in this case the central nervous system.)

Buprenorphine is formulated for both transdermal and sublingual administration, as noted above, and is supplied currently as a monoproduct transdermal system, as a monoproduct tablet, and as a combination (with naloxone) tablet and also film. The transdermal system is FDA approved for the treatment of chronic pain, whereas the sublingual formulations, while increasingly used off-label for chronic pain treatment, are FDA approved for the treatment of opioid dependence. The complex issues surrounding this indication are discussed at greater length in subsequent chapters.

If chronic opioid therapy is being considered, many features of buprenorphine render it an attractive choice. It displays ceiling effects of both therapeutic and also adverse effects (especially respiratory depression), little or no need for renal dosing, and overall a very good safety profile. Buprenorphine does not affect respiratory rate; there is some evidence in animal models suggesting reduction in tidal volume attributable to the glucuronidated metabolite [5], but from a respiratory depression standpoint, it remains the safest of all opioids currently available. Early reports suggested a possible association between buprenorphine use and QT interval prolongation, but several recent investigations seem to have laid these concerns to rest, and at present, routine ECG monitoring is not recommended for buprenorphine therapy as it is for methadone [5–7]. Despite widespread and increasing prevalence of use (and abuse) discussed in greater detail below, mortality associated with the drug is extremely low; a postmortem analysis of drug overdose-related deaths in New York City during a 5-month period in 2013 showed buprenorphine metabolites in only 2% of decedents, and all overdose victims had multiple CNS depressants present in serum [8]. Only three deaths attributable to buprenorphine were reported by the American Association of Poison Control Centers in 2011 (http://www.deadiversion.usdoj.gov/drug_chem_info/buprenorphine.pdf). Concurrent benzodiazepine use is thought to be responsible for most fatalities where buprenorphine is involved.

From a psychiatric standpoint, opioid use is associated with a high risk of depression and possibly suicidality; buprenorphine is uniquely antidepressant, likely owing to its KOR antagonism, and in fact many psychiatrists have called for expanded FDA treatment indications to include refractory depression. In addition, given the high prevalence of comorbid opioid use disorder among chronic pain patients, buprenorphine's unique ability to render other opioids basically ineffective is an attractive feature deserving of consideration.

Buprenorphine may not confer typical chronic opioid-induced hyperalgesia states; experimental data in both animals and humans indicate significant antihyperalgesic effects [5, 9]; these may however be dose-dependent and of clinical relevance only at high doses [10]. Antagonism at KOR, DOR, and N/OFQR has all been invoked as potential mechanisms underlying this phenomenon. Buprenorphine displays the most potent sodium channel blockade of any opioid agonist and in fact is classified as a strong local anesthetic [11]; this mechanism may partially explain the apparent antihyperalgesia conferred by this agent.

There is currently an unfortunate paucity of high-quality evidence in the literature for the use of buprenorphine for treating chronic pain; the vast majority of investigations pertain to its efficacy in treating opioid dependence. One recent systematic review of buprenorphine for chronic pain examined 12 studies and reported that all studies reported that sublingual buprenorphine demonstrated some effectiveness for analgesia in chronic pain patients; however, the evidence was deemed low quality and insufficient to draw any conclusions from [12]. A Cochrane review of buprenorphine for use in treating neuropathic pain found no studies of sufficient quality to analyze. A recent Cochrane review of buprenorphine in cancer pain examined 19 studies ($n = 1421$ patients) and found that of 11 studies comparing buprenorphine to an alternate (non-placebo) therapeutic regimen, five studies showed superiority, three showed no difference, and three showed inferiority [13]. Further high-quality investigation is warranted into the question of efficacy of buprenorphine treatment in chronic pain, especially neuropathic pain, as the only current FDA-approved vehicle is the transdermal system which is very expensive and not covered by many payers; accumulation of evidence demonstrating superior risk-benefit ratio of buprenorphine compared to other options may convince more payers to include sublingual vehicles to their formulary for treating refractory chronic pain.

One potentially problematic issue with buprenorphine use has to do with its MOR tenacity/virtual blockade of other opioids in the context of acute care. In situations of trauma or other emergent operations, a patient on buprenorphine may not experience analgesia from other opioids administered. This issue may be circumvented in many cases by regional anesthesia (e.g., spinal/epidural blockade or peripheral nerve blockade.) In the case of elective surgery, it is wise to wean off of buprenorphine ahead of time to allow for unhindered access to the MOR.

By far the majority of buprenorphine use in this country and worldwide is for the maintenance and treatment of opioid dependence. The US federal law (discussed in greater detail in Chap. 8) allows for any physician with a DATA 2000 waiver ("X-number") addendum to their DEA registration to prescribe buprenorphine for this purpose. Office-based opioid treatment (OBOT) is a term that has become synonymous with buprenorphine, as no other opioid agonist is allowed to be used solely for the treatment of opioid use disorder outside of federally sanctioned opioid treatment programs (OTPs) which rely primarily on methadone. Combination buprenorphine-naloxone products are preferred for OBOT as they have been shown repeatedly to suffer less abuse than the buprenorphine monoproduct. The use of the monoproduct is actively discouraged by current guidelines/standard of care (e.g., the Substance Abuse Mental Health Services Administration Consensus Panel on Buprenorphine) [14] as well as the Drug Enforcement Agency, except in the case of pregnancy. Methadone has historically been used for the treatment of opioid use disorder in pregnancy; however, a recent prospective, double-blinded randomized trial (the "MOTHER" study—Maternal Opioid Treatment: Human Experimental Research) showed that infants born to mothers maintained on buprenorphine required significantly less morphine (by an order of magnitude), had a significantly shorter hospital stay (by a week), and had a significantly shorter duration of treatment for neonatal abstinence syndrome (4.1 days vs. 9.9 days) compared to infants whose mothers were maintained on methadone [15].

Buprenorphine therapy has been shown to be highly effective in meeting its goals of reducing illicit opioid abuse and improving retention in substance abuse treatment. OBOT has also been shown to decrease high-risk sexual behaviors and to reduce emergency department utilization and overall opioid-related mortality [16–21].

Although far less prone to abuse than other opioids, buprenorphine is subject to abuse. In some countries (e.g., Malaysia, Finland), high rates of abuse have been seen, arguably related to the lack of other widely available opioid options. In the United States, buprenorphine products generally rank as the least abused or misused opioid among those studied [22]; nonetheless, the products may be tampered with and injected, insufflated, etc. The formulation of the combination naloxone products came about in order to discourage such abuse, as the bioavailability of naloxone is relatively low when the product is used appropriately (sublingually) but much higher with intravenous use, and studies bear out that abusers prefer the monoproduct over the combination buprenorphine-naloxone formulations [23, 24].

Diversion of buprenorphine is a more significant issue; from 2002 to 2008, the retail distribution of buprenorphine increased more than 7000-fold from 107 grams to 800,317 grams. Between 2009 and 2014 the 26 Health's National Prescription Audit Plus Retail database showed a 144% increase in the number of buprenorphine prescriptions filled [25]. This tremendous increase in availability certainly facilitates greater distribution, and during this period buprenorphine items reported to the National Forensic Laboratory Information System (NFLIS) also increased more than 250-fold from 13 items to 5627 items [26]. As with abuse, diversion favors the monoproduct; data from several programs show a diversion rate for monoproduct tablets averaging 6.4 times the rate of that of the combination film [24]. Furthermore, each individually packaged combination film product in the United States contains a unique ten-digit ID number and QR code that can be scanned at any point in the chain of medication distribution which may be used to help in diversion investigation.

Many addictionologists and other interested parties however maintain that from a public health standpoint, buprenorphine diversion may represent a boon in disguise, as it may be expanding (unsupervised) treatment with an agent that has been shown to be highly effective and extraordinarily low risk, and thus providing net benefit in terms of reducing opioid misuse morbidity and mortality (Table 4.1).

Codeine

Codeine is one of the three main phenanthrene alkaloids contained in opium (morphine and thebaine being the other two). Structurally, codeine is a morphine molecule with an extra methyl group attached and in itself possesses relatively weak

Table 4.1 Comparison of currently available (outpatient) opioids

Drug	Potency relative to morphine (p.o.)	Receptor activities	Metabolism	Active metabolites	Unique issues
Tramadol	0.1 × MSO_4	MOR agonist SNRI	CYP2D6; renal excretion	*O*-desmethyltramadol	Seizures, serotonin syndrome may occur with antidepressant co-Rx
Codeine	0.1 × MSO_4	MOR agonist	UGT2B7 > CYP2D6; renal excretion	Morphine	CYP2D6 ultrarapid metabolizers experience elevated MSO_4
Meperidine (Pethidine)	0.1 × MSO_4	MOR agonist	CYP3A4/2B6; renal excretion	Normeperidine	Normeperidine accumulation causes seizures in renal failure; seizures, serotonin syndrome may occur with antidepressant co-Rx
Tapentadol	0.15 × MSO_4	MOR agonist NRI	UGT2B7/1A9; renal excretion	–	–
Hydrocodone	0.8 × MSO_4	MOR agonist	CYP3A4/2D6, also non-P450; renal excretion	Hydromorphone	–
Morphine	1 × MSO_4	MOR agonist	UGT2B7; renal excretion	M-6-glucuronide	M6G more potent than parent MSO_4 and accumulates in renal failure

Methadone	1 - ? × MSO_4	MOR agonist	CYP3A4/2B6/2C19; biliary excretion	–	Very long half-life; QTc prolongation
Oxycodone	2 × MSO_4	MOR agonist KOR agonist	CYP3A4/2D6; renal excretion	Oxymorphone	Anecdotally most addictive, most hyperalgesia-inducing p.o.opioid
Oxymorphone	3–5 × MSO_4	MOR agonist	UGT2B7	?	–
Hydromorphone	5 × MSO_4	MOR agonist	UGT2B7; renal excretion	–	–
Buprenorphine	15–75 × MSO_4	MOR agonist KOR antagonist	CYP3A4, UGT2B7; biliary excretion	Norbuprenorphine	Tenacity for MOR “blocks” other opioids
Fentanyl	80 × MSO_4	MOR agonist	CYP3A4; renal excretion	–	–

efficacy in terms of opioid agonism unless demethylated by the CYP2D6 system into morphine. Codeine itself and its primary metabolite codeine-6-glucuronide (C6G) have only a fraction of the potency of morphine but given their quantitative preponderance may confer (especially C6G) the majority of the drug's analgesia [27, 28]. Codeine has a fairly high oral bioavailability with around 90% absorption. It is relatively unbound by plasma proteins (7–25% binding) with an average volume of distribution between 3 and 6 L/kg (http://www.drugbank.ca/drugs/DB00318). Codeine binds to and exerts its known effects via the MOR and is not reported to interact significantly with either the DOR or KOR. Its potency is generally thought to be between 10 and 15% that of morphine.

O-methylation to morphine via CYP2D6 comprises a relatively small fraction of its disposition; its primary metabolism is (Phase II) glucuronidation to codeine-6-glucuronide. Its half-life is generally reported to be 2–3 h. Hepatic impairment has not been reported to be a significant issue in terms of dose adjustment, but it should be kept in mind that due to its prodrug nature, therapeutic efficacy will be markedly reduced. Codeine is 90% renally excreted, and as such, dosing adjustment should be made in cases of renal impairment [29, 30], especially considering that morphine is its most potent metabolite.

Codeine (as well as other opioids, most notably hydrocodone) has been used for decades as an antitussive; several different pathways affected by various triggers including mechanical and chemical (e.g., bradykinin) stimuli are involved, and some of these have been shown to be very responsive to opioids, while others have not [30].

Codeine is reported to be the most commonly used opioid therapeutically throughout the world; in the United States it ranks #4. It is available primarily as a combination analgesic with acetaminophen in this country in three different strengths (15 mg, 30 mg, and 60 mg codeine with acetaminophen 300 mg) and also exists in pure form as an antitussive syrup. Other more obscure forms exist but are rarely used and not generally available. Between 2009 and 2014 the 26 Health's National Prescription Audit Plus Retail database showed a 9% decrease in the number of codeine prescriptions filled [25]; with the reclassification of hydrocodone to a Schedule II drug however, it is expected that codeine products will enjoy a renaissance of prescription as the drug remains Schedule III presently, meaning that prescriptions for codeine may be telephoned or FAXed in rather than requiring a hard copy prescription.

Fentanyl

Fentanyl is a synthetic phenylpiperidine derivative and the only one of its class (including alfentanil, remifentanil, and sufentanil) to have any use in the outpatient arena. All are highly potent opioids that exist primarily as intravenous preparations; however, fentanyl is available and used primarily as a transdermal preparation and to a lesser extent as a transmucosal (buccal or nasal) preparation. Fentanyl is highly protein bound (80–85%) with a volume of distribution between 3 and 8 L/kg (http://www.drugbank.ca/drugs/DB00813). Due to its significant lipophilicity and potency, it is suitable for transdermal delivery, and it diffuses readily into the epidermis where it forms a depot for slower release into the dermis and circulation. Despite individual variability owing to skin thickness and keratinization, absorption is fairly predictable with the drug achieving therapeutic levels generally within 12–16 h of application [31]. Bioavailability of the transdermal system is reported as 92% (http://www.drugbank.ca/drugs/DB00813). Fentanyl "patches" are designed for 72 h use and are most commonly prescribed as such. Individual and environmental factors (e.g., increased ambient or skin temperatures) may result in altered absorption kinetics.

Transmucosal forms are prescribed almost exclusively for "breakthrough pain" in terminal cancer situations and comprise the most rapid parenteral delivery option at present. Roughly one-fourth of a transmucosal dose enters the circulation almost immediately due to sublingual absorption with the remaining three-fourths swallowed and subjected to hepatic first-pass metabolism, with roughly 25% of the enteral portion escaping to enter the circulation [32]. Onset of analgesia is generally within 15 min and lasts roughly an hour.

Fentanyl is an extremely potent (estimated at 80 times the potency of morphine) agonist at the MOR. Effects at the DOR and KOR have not been well characterized. It is metabolized almost exclusively through the CYP3A4 pathway and undergoes dealkylation to norfentanyl, which is held to be an inactive molecule. Hepatic impairment and probably more importantly CYP3A4 inhibition (which is very common given the vast amount of drugs that are metabolized via this enzyme) certainly warrant caution; due to its potency and almost exclusively renal elimination, dose adjustment is recommended once the GFR drops below 50 mL/min [30]. While more of an issue with intravenous infusions, the lipophilicity of the drug alters normal kinetics substantially and may result in significantly underestimated depot reservoirs in the obese.

Two transdermal forms currently exist; the original delivery system contains an actual liquid reservoir contained within the backing and adhesive layer, while the newer "matrix" formulation contains the drug within the adhesive layer. Both formulations are subject to abuse; the reservoir may be accessed for noncontrolled applications, and the matrix formulation may be cut and applied transmucosally. Recent "lacing" of heroin with fentanyl has resulted in an increased number of deaths from heroin use and has gained considerable media coverage over the past couple years. Between 2009 and 2014 the 26 Health's National Prescription Audit Plus Retail database showed only a 5% increase in the number of fentanyl prescriptions filled [25]; however, there was a two- to tenfold increase (varying by geographic region of the country) in fentanyl items submitted to forensic laboratories during this time period.

Hydrocodone

Hydrocodone is a semisynthetic phenanthrene opioid derived from codeine. It is well absorbed from the gastrointestinal tract, with greater than 50% bioavailability. In blood, 20–50% of hydrocodone is bound to protein; the volume of distribution is not known (http://www.drugbank.ca/drugs/DB00956). Time to onset of analgesia is generally reported as being within half an hour. It acts primarily on the MOR, with some affinity for the DOR. Potency data for hydrocodone are conflicting and confusing; this may be in part to the extensive metabolism and numerous active metabolites, with pharmacogenetic variance conferring marked individual variability in effect. Most textbooks and equianalgesic conversion tables report the potency of hydrocodone to be between 0.6 and 1.0 times that of morphine.

Hydrocodone undergoes metabolism by CYP2D6 to hydromorphone, a much more potent opioid. CYP3A4 metabolism renders norhydrocodone, a molecule generally held to be inactive but may have some analgesic effects [33]; other metabolites include dihydrocodeine, which is an active molecule and available by prescription, and nordihydrocodeine, the CYP3A4 metabolite of dihydrocodeine. Forty percent of hydrocodone metabolism is reported to occur independently of the cytochrome P450 pathway [34]. While strong recommendations regarding hepatic and renal dosing of hydrocodone are not generally touted, given hydromorphone's potency (and significant hepatic metabolism) dose adjustment should be considered in terms of metabolic organ dysfunction.

Hydrocodone has been available in the United States almost exclusively as a combination product with acetaminophen (or ibuprofen); more recently pure mono-product hydrocodone formulated as an extended-release/long-acting drug has been made available. Hydrocodone was reclassified from a Schedule III to a Schedule II drug in October 2014, making it slightly more onerous for prescribers. Despite a downturn in prescription in 2014 (−1% between 2009 and 2014) [25], hydrocodone products are the most prescribed opioid in the United States, with more than 125 million prescriptions written that year; to put it in global perspective, this country is responsible for approximately 99% of the world's hydrocodone consumption (http://www.deadiversion.usdoj.gov/drug_chem_info/hydrocodone.pdf#search=hydrocodone). Not surprisingly, hydrocodone products are the most commonly diverted opioid in this nation [35].

Hydromorphone

Hydromorphone is a potent semisynthetic hydrogenated ketone derivative of morphine. Its absorption and bioavailability (13–50%) [36] are relatively low; it also has relatively low protein binding (20%) (http://www.drugbank.ca/drugs/DB00327). It is slightly more lipophilic than morphine and together with low protein binding has a slightly greater volume of distribution at 4.1 L/kg [37]. Time to onset of analgesia following an oral dose is reported to be roughly 30 minutes. It is a strong MOR agonist, generally held to be five times more potent than morphine.

Hydromorphone is metabolized almost exclusively by Phase II glucuronidation to hydromorphone-3-glucuronide which is held to be inactive from an analgesic standpoint but may accumulate in renal impairment and cause neuroexcitatory toxicity (similar to the well-known effects of normeperidine in renal failure). For this reason, hepatic dosing seems prudent and renal dosing is recommended [30].

Hydromorphone is available on an outpatient basis in various immediate-release strengths, and an extended-release once-a-day formulation has been available now for over a decade. Between 2009 and 2014 the 26 Health's National Prescription Audit Plus Retail database showed a 45% increase in the number of hydromorphone prescriptions filled [25]; NFLIS data showed a significant (twofold) increase in hydromorphone products submitted to forensic laboratories from 2011 to 2013 in the South.

Levorphanol

Rarely used, levorphanol (the levo-enantiomer to dextromethorphan) is a long-acting synthetic phenanthrene with very diverse activity. Its bioavailability is roughly 70%, and it is approximately 40% protein bound with a volume of distribution between 10 and 13 L/kg (http://www.drugbank.ca/drugs/DB00854). Time to peak effect is roughly 1 h. While a potent agonist at the MOR, levorphanol also avidly binds the DOR and KOR (which is responsible for much of its limiting psychomimetic effects, although it also has anticholinergic properties) [38] and is also an NMDA antagonist and furthermore a serotonin/norepinephrine reuptake inhibitor. This complement of activities renders it a theoretically attractive alternative agent in the treatment of refractory chronic pain states, especially neuropathic pain [39]. It is reportedly four to eight times more potent as agonist than morphine at the MOR.

It is metabolized via hepatic glucuronidation to levorphanol-3-glucuronide, an active metabolite that is excreted by the kidney and as such should be renally dosed. Its half-life is reported to be between 11 and 30 h [37, 40].

Levorphanol possesses many of the qualities of methadone (long half-life, NMDA blockade), but unlike the latter it is not known to prolong the QTc interval. Nonetheless, its widespread use and acceptance have been limited by relative lack of availability and high cost and significant constellation of neuropsychiatric adverse effects (thought to be due primarily to anticholinergic effects).

Meperidine

Meperidine (pethidine in the U.K. and elsewhere) is a synthetic phenylpiperidine and the first fully synthetic opioid. It has largely fallen out of favor in the United States but remains one of the more commonly used opioids elsewhere. It has oral bioavailability similar to that of morphine (50–60%) and is relatively protein bound

(60–80%) (http://www.drugbank.ca/drugs/DB00454). Its volume of distribution is reported to be 2.6 L/kg, almost equal to morphine's. Peak plasma concentrations are reported to occur within 1–2 h of oral administration.

Meperidine is a relatively weak MOR agonist with roughly one-tenth the potency of morphine. It is a relatively strong KOR agonist, and this may account for some of its well-known dysphoric and even hallucinogenic effects in certain individuals. Meperidine is hydrolyzed by hepatic carboxylesterase to an inactive metabolite known as meperidinic acid (pethidinic acid) and also undergoes Phase I demethylation to normeperidine (norpethidine) via the CYP3A4 and CYP2B6 pathways. Both of these metabolites are further glucuronidated for renal excretion. Due to the significant neuroexcitatory toxicity of normeperidine, meperidine is contraindicated in renal impairment due to buildup. Avoiding it in hepatic impairment is prudent as well, and many have called for a moratorium on its use in chronic pain altogether [41, 42].

Meperidine also has serotonin reuptake inhibition properties. A well-known interaction between meperidine and monoamine oxidase inhibitors (MAOI) has been described for decades; concurrent use may result in an agitated neurotoxic state that may be fatal. More recently we have learned that this likely represents a serotonin syndrome with liability well beyond meperidine and the MAOI class; phenylpiperidines in general are serotonin reuptake inhibitors, and most antidepressants are as well, and the combination of these two classes is contraindicated.

Meperidine possesses anticholinergic activity and confers tachycardia and mydriasis unique among opioids. Anecdotally (and possibly owing to its anticholinergic activity), meperidine reportedly confers reduced visceral tone and intraluminal pressures; there is conflicting evidence however in vivo for this activity. It has also been the best studied of the opioids historically in terms of sodium channel blockade and has found utility for this local anesthetic-like activity in regional anesthesia; it is unlikely that there is much clinical significance for this phenomenon with oral dosing.

Meperidine is falling out of favor in this country as indicated above; between 2009 and 2014 the 26 Health's National Prescription Audit Plus Retail database showed a 49% decrease in the number of meperidine prescriptions filled [25].

Methadone

Methadone is a structurally unique synthetic opioid of the diphenylheptane class, unique in many ways. The least expensive of the opioids and the one with the widest range of therapeutic uses historically, it is also the most lethal; a 2012 CDC report of opioid fatality surveillance in 13 states showed that while comprising less than 2% of all opioid prescriptions in 2009, methadone had by far the highest mortality, responsible for nearly 40% of the single-drug deaths in this sample [43].

Methadone has a highly variable oral bioavailability ranging from 36 to 100% (http://www.drugbank.ca/drugs/DB00333). It is highly protein bound (primarily to alpha-1 acid glycoprotein) but is relatively lipophilic with a volume of distribution reported between 1 and 8 L/kg. Time to onset of analgesia ranges between 30 and 90 minutes. Like most organic chemicals, methadone exhibits chirality, and its enantiomers have been well-studied. R-methadone (the levo-isomer) is a full MOR agonist with relatively weak DOR and KOR affinity, whereas S-methadone (the dextro-isomer) is an NMDA antagonist and also possesses some serotonin/norepinephrine reuptake inhibitory activity [44]. The reported potency of methadone varies widely from roughly equipotent to morphine to upward of ten times that; many sources make vague statements about dynamically increasing potency correlating with accumulation; given what we know of overall receptor sensitization, the likelihood of actual MOR agonism increase over time is unlikely. Methadone's joint NMDA antagonism is thought to confer some reduction in the development of opioid tolerance. One thing is clear: methadone is unpredictable. It also appears that the pharmacokinetic parameters of methadone do not parallel its analgesic duration which is reported to be between 4 and 8 h [44, 45].

Metabolism of methadone is primarily via Phase I reactions catalyzed by multiple cytochrome P450 enzymes, with CYP3A4 providing the majority of its conversion to the inactive metabolite 2-ethylidene-1,5-dimethyl-3,3-diphenylpyrrolidine (EDDP). The different enantiomers undergo other enzyme-specific metabolisms as well; CYP2C19 preferentially metabolizes R-methadone, while CYP2B6 preferentially metabolizes S-methadone [46]. The half-life of methadone is generally reported in the range of 15–55 h [45] but may be as high as 150 hours; such variability is perhaps due to multicompartmental model kinetics as the drug undergoes extensive tissue sequestration as evidenced by animal and human forensic studies. Elimination is largely biliary/fecal [44] which reduces the need for dose adjustment in renal impairment.

Methadone has been associated with prolongation of the QT interval, and ventricular dysrhythmias (e.g., torsade de pointes) may be responsible for a number of deaths from its use. The *S*-enantiomer has been shown to block the human ether-a-go-go (hERG) voltage-gated calcium channel in cardiac myocytes which is involved in repolarization [47]. Methadone also seems to confer what may be a disproportionate degree of central apnea [48].

The efficacy of methadone in treating chronic non-cancer pain was recently investigated in a Cochrane review; only two randomized controlled trials and one non-randomized study, with 181 total subjects, were included in the analysis. The authors state that no conclusions can be made on the basis of the limited data available [49]. Similar uncertainty has been reported by previous reviewers on the basis of lack of data.

Far more literature exists related to the use of methadone in the treatment of opioid dependence; numerous studies support the efficacy of "methadone maintenance therapy (MMT)" in reducing illicit opioid use, improving substance abuse treatment retention, reducing high-risk behaviors such as intravenous drug use and reducing conversion to HIV seropositivity, and reducing criminal activity and incarceration [49–53]. Decreased illicit drug use and improved treatment retention appear to be dose-dependent when comparing daily doses less than 60 mg to doses between 60 and 100 mg [54–56]. Duration of MMT however is the strongest predictor of reduction in heroin use as evidenced by the Drug Abuse Reporting Program (DARP) in the 1980s and the Treatment Outcome Perspective Study (TOPS) in the 1990s. Both demonstrated about a 40% reduction in illicit opioid use at the end of 1 year after methadone maintenance treatment [57, 58].

From a prescription opioid mortality standpoint, however, methadone represents the most dangerous opioid in terms of case fatality, and its use (and associated mortality) increased significantly over the past two decades (peaking in the late 2000s), associated with increased use for pain management rather than MMT. Prescriptions for methadone increased nearly sevenfold from 1998 to 2006, with mortality very nearly paralleling that, with a 5.5-fold increase from 1999 to 2009 [43]. Between 2009 and 2014 the 26 Health's National Prescription Audit Plus Retail database showed a 7% decrease in the number of methadone prescriptions filled [25]. The case fatality rate involving methadone seems to have stabilized and even decreased slightly since 2007; nonetheless, in 2010, methadone accounted for 31.4% of all opioid-related deaths (and 39.8% of all single-opioid-related deaths) in 13 states submitting medical examiner data to the Drug Abuse Warning Network (DAWN.) Methadone represented only 4.5% and 18.5% of the opioids distributed by state.

Morphine

Morphine is the prototypical therapeutic opioid, well represented in classical literature and popular media as a wartime boon, and remains the standard by which all others are judged; this is reflected by equianalgesic tables comparing all opioid to a "standard" 30 mg oral dose of morphine, and more recently the concept of morphine equivalent daily dose (MEDD) which is discussed later in the book. It is also the starting point for synthesis of most of the commercially available semisynthetic opioids, and approximately 70% or so is used in the creation of hydrocodone, hydromorphone, oxycodone, oxymorphone, and others [59]. It is a phenanthrene opiate, one of the three main alkaloids of *P. somniferum*, and the most potent of the three. The oral absorption of morphine is relatively poor, with a bioavailability of approximately 30%. It is between 30 and 40% protein bound, is relatively hydrophilic (among opioids) with an octanol-water coefficient of one, and has a volume of distribution between 1 and 6 L/kg (http://www.drugbank.ca/drugs/DB00295). Time to peak analgesia following an oral dose is reported to be roughly 1 h. Morphine is an effective MOR agonist and also displays lesser affinity for the DOR and KOR.

The metabolism of morphine is held to be primarily via Phase II glucuronidation. The principal metabolite, morphine-6-glucuronide (M6G), is active and is in fact a more potent agonist than the parent compound. Other metabolites including morphine-3-glucuronide are largely devoid of analgesic activity but may confer adverse effects. It is thought that in chronic use, buildup of M6G confers most of the analgesia from morphine [41]. Elimination is largely renal, with less than 10%

biliary/fecal excretion. As such, renal impairment can lead to toxic buildup of M6G, and dose adjustment (or avoidance of the agent altogether) is necessary.

Morphine is available for outpatient use as both immediate-release preparations and various extended-release formulations as well. A novel combination of extended-release morphine with embedded naltrexone was introduced last decade in hopes of reducing abuse but was withdrawn from the market in 2011 due to safety concerns raised by the FDA; it was reintroduced in a newer formulation in 2015 and is discussed in greater detail in Chap. 5.

Morphine is well tolerated overall as evidenced by its long-standing reign as the primary parenteral analgesic in the inpatient arena. Like all opioids it has an adverse effect profile (which comprises the subject matter of Chap. 3), but it may confer a higher incidence of nausea/vomiting and pruritis than some of the newer semisynthetic and synthetic opioids. The latter is likely due to disproportionate histamine release from this agent, and in the anesthesia community, it has been common practice to avoid the use of morphine in severe asthmatics for the past half century, for fear of precipitating severe bronchoconstriction. Newer data question this practice [60]. Another long-standing acute care practice, namely, the administration of morphine for the treatment of acute pulmonary edema, has been called into question recently as well [61, 62]. For decades, morphine-related reduction in pulmonary venous pressures has been noted experimentally and clinically in the setting of pulmonary edema, and as noted in the previous chapter, the use of morphine for suspected acute coronary pain or congestive heart failure in the emergency setting has been the standard practice. The availability of newer and more selective vasodilators without the adverse effects of opioids may replace the routine use of morphine in these situations.

Between 2009 and 2014 the 26 Health's National Prescription Audit Plus Retail database showed a 33% increase in the number of morphine prescriptions filled [25].

Oxycodone

Oxycodone is a semisynthetic derivative of thebaine, one of *P. somniferum*'s three opiate alkaloids. It is relatively well absorbed with oral bioavailability of 60–87% (http://www.drugbank.ca/drugs/DB00497). It is roughly 50% protein bound, with a volume of distribution of 2.6 L/kg. Time to onset of analgesia following an oral dose is reported to be roughly 30 minutes. It is a strong MOR agonist, generally held to be roughly twice as potent as morphine; this fact is underappreciated by most patients and clinicians, and the latter may be due in part to the historic classification of oxycodone as a "weak opioid" in many algorithmic treatment guidelines, e.g., the WHO analgesic ladder. It also binds the KOR with greater affinity than most therapeutic opioids [63], and the relative contributions of KOR to MOR agonism to oxycodone's therapeutic and adverse effects have been debated in the literature for over a decade. Regardless of the degree of relative receptor specificity, KOR agonism confers both potential benefit and an increased constellation of adverse effects, discussed in greater detail below.

Oxycodone undergoes extensive hepatic P450 metabolism, yielding numerous metabolites all of which confer some MOR and KOR agonism also. CYP3A4 demethylates oxycodone to noroxycodone, a weak MOR agonist, which represents roughly 80% of the circulating oxycodone metabolites following an oral dose. CYP2D6 demethylates oxycodone to oxymorphone, which comprises roughly 10% of oxycodone metabolites [64]. It also catalyzes the demethylation of noroxycodone to noroxymorphone. Given the potency of oxymorphone, CYP2D6 polymorphisms would be expected to confer significant variability of both therapeutic and adverse effects, and a recent investigation showed significantly increased incidence of both of these effects in individuals with ultrarapid metabolizer status for this enzyme [64]. Its primary excretion is via the kidney (greater than 80%), and as such the dosage should be adjusted in situations of renal insufficiency. Oxycodone is available in a variety of oral formulations. It exists as a single immediate-release product, a combination product with acetaminophen or salicylate, and various extended-release formulations. The history of ER/LA oxycodone is troubled and in the opinion of many authorities not only parallels but may have been responsible in large part for the early years of the current opioid epidemic. This viewpoint along with data supporting it is discussed in greater detail in subsequent chapters, especially the next one.

Oxycodone has been reported in several studies to confer superior analgesia for visceral pain compared to other opioids, and this is thought to be due to peripheral activity at the KOR [65] . Large recent reviews have shown no superiority for oxycodone compared to other opioids in terms of analgesic efficacy in cancer pain as a whole [66, 67]; nonetheless, this author tends to be more receptive to oxycodone use in palliative situations, especially those involving visceral malignancy due to the possibility of improved KOR-mediated peripheral analgesia and anecdotally reported superiority in terms of reduced fatigue/improved energy. A recent systematic review and meta-analysis suggest that oxycodone may confer less drowsiness than other opioids [68]. Oxycodone has been shown in one small study (n = 24 subjects) to confer superior suppression of allodynia [69]. These results however must be interpreted in light of the very small number of participants and the hitherto substantial evidence of no increased benefit from oxycodone compared to other agents in treating neuropathic pain [70]. Furthermore, anecdotal report and experience shared among many interventional pain physicians favor a disproportionate degree of hyperalgesia associated with oxycodone use.

Oxycodone has enjoyed tremendous popularity in the United States in particular; in 2007 this nation consumed 51.6 tons of oxycodone, representing 82% of global consumption that year [71]. Dispensation of this drug has increased significantly over the past two decades, with milligrams of oxycodone representing both the greatest volume (by mg) of opioids purchased by US pharmacies and the opioid with the largest increase (287%) in purchasing from 2000 to 2010 [72]. Between 2009 and 2014 the 26 Health's National Prescription Audit Plus Retail database showed a 21% increase in the number of oxycodone prescriptions filled [25], with nearly 60 million prescriptions dispensed. Concurrently with the increased availability to the public, it has become one of the most widely recreationally used drugs in America. The National Survey on Drug Use and Health (NSDUH) indicated that 16.0 million people, aged 12 and older in the United States, reported using oxycodone products nonmedically in their lifetime in 2012 [73]. While no methodology currently exists to accurately measure the euphoria-producing and addictive nature of a substance and interpersonal variability for psychological effects and vulnerability ("drug of choice") is a universally observed phenomenon, many patients and prescribers report that oxycodone confers a markedly higher degree of psychological dependence compared to other opioids. Several studies comparing "likability" of various opioids have been performed over the past decade, and oxycodone appears to be the most desired/craved drug in the class [74, 75] owing to a greater degree of positive psychoactive reward and a lower adverse effect profile. Oxycodone is reported as being the drug of choice for almost 80% of nonmedical prescription opioid abusers based on a wide sample [76]. There are also ample data showing that oxycodone products are overall the most abused prescription opioids in the United States [77] although other data [78] rank it second to hydrocodone products (which are more widely prescribed in this country). Canada has experienced significant problems with the drug as well, and in February 2012 Ontario became the first province to remove ER/LA oxycodone from its public benefit program after intense public scrutiny into the problem of oxycodone dependence; the First Nations communities of Ontario reported OxyContin abuse rates as high as 80% [79]. According to the US Drug Enforcement Agency, oxycodone has been the most frequently encountered pharmaceutical drug by law enforcement officers since 2009 (http://www.deadiversion.usdoj.gov/drug_chem_info/oxycodone/oxycodone.pdf#search=oxycodone). Not surprisingly, diversion rates of oxycodone are second only to hydrocodone products [35], again, probably relegated to this place due to the greater number of hydrocodone prescriptions written in this country.

Finally, the prescriber should be aware that ER/LA oxycodone has been implicated as the prescription drug most likely to confer risk of transition to intravenous opioid abuse [80–83]. From the onset of the OxyContin abuse trend in Appalachia in the late 1990s, as opioid-abusing individuals have sought means to increase their psychoactive reward in the face of increasing tolerance, they have discovered and utilized a variety of means to circumvent extended-release and even abuse-deterrent properties to deliver a potent oxycodone dose immediately by insufflation, smoking, or injection.

Given the higher incidence in our experience for adverse effects including opioid-induced hyperalgesia, as well as the extraordinary potential for abuse, addiction, and diversion as well as transition to intravenous use, it is our practice to avoid oxycodone for chronic non-cancer pain scenarios. A recent emergency department initiative in the Seattle area has implemented a similar practice pattern [84].

Oxymorphone

Oxymorphone is a potent semisynthetic thebaine derivative like oxycodone and is one of oxycodone's natural metabolites (via the CYP2D6 pathway.) Although well absorbed from the gut, it undergoes extensive first-pass metabolism, and thus its oral bioavailability is on the order of 10% [85]. The volume of distribution of oxymorphone is 3 L/kg (similar to morphine) with protein binding of about 10%. It is poorly protein bound (10%) and has a volume of distribution of oxymorphone. Time to onset of analgesia following an oral dose is reported to be roughly 30 minutes. It is a strong MOR agonist, generally held to be three to five times more potent than morphine [86].

Oxymorphone primarily undergoes Phase II glucuronidation and only 2% is excreted unchanged by the kidney. Its main metabolite is oxymorphone-3-glucuronide; the analgesic efficacy/opioid receptor affinity of this molecule is unknown currently. Oxymorphone is currently available as a monoproduct in both immediate- and extended-release formulations. Between 2009 and 2014 the 26 Health's National Prescription Audit Plus Retail database showed a 69% increase in the number of oxymorphone prescriptions filled [25].

In our practice we have found utility for oxymorphone primarily in transitioning people away from oxycodone, which we have particular aversion to. As oxymorphone is a metabolite of oxycodone, it is rather doubtful that any adverse reactions or "allergies" could occur.

Tapentadol

Tapentadol is a new synthetic opioid of the phenylpropylamine class, sharing structural and mechanistic qualities with tramadol (discussed below) which is more familiar to most clinicians. It has oral bioavailability of roughly 30%, similar to that of morphine (http://www.drugbank.ca/drugs/DB06204). It is approximately 20% protein bound. Onset of analgesia is roughly 30 min after consumption. Tapentadol is a weak MOR agonist, with 18-fold less affinity for the receptor than morphine. Its potency relative to morphine however is commonly reported to be on the order of 1:3–1:7, which reflects significant analgesic benefit conferred by its norepinephrine reuptake inhibition (NRI) properties. Tapentadol undergoes minor hepatic Phase I metabolism (via CYP2C19 and CYP2D6) but possesses no active metabolites (http://www.drugbank.ca/drugs/DB06204) [87], and the majority of its metabolism is via Phase II glucuronidation, with roughly 97% of the oral dose excreted renally as the glucuronidated form. Its half-life is reported to be between 4 and 24 h (http://www.drugbank.ca/drugs/DB06204) [88].

Tapentadol has been available in this country since 2009 as an immediate-release preparation, and in 2011 an extended-release form was made available; the latter shortly thereafter gained FDA approval for the treatment of refractory diabetic neuropathic pain.

Tapentadol's efficacy in treating neuropathic pain in particular has been examined, and it appears to be a uniquely effective agent within the class for treating neuropathic pain [88, 89] in particular, owing to its NRI activity. It has been reported to confer significantly fewer adverse effects than most opioids [88, 90]. In addition, its abuse potential has been reported to be significantly lower than that of most other opioids in clinical use as assessed by various surveillance methods including substance abuse treatment center data, emergency department and toxicology data, law enforcement data, and surveillance of Internet discussions [91–93]. Whether this represents unfamiliarity with and lesser availability of a new drug remains to be seen.

Tramadol

Tramadol is a synthetic piperidine analog of codeine. It has high oral bioavailability approaching 95% [94]. It is approximately 20% protein bound. The onset of analgesia is roughly 60 min after consumption. Tramadol is a very weak MOR agonist, with affinity reported at 6000 times less than that of morphine [87]. Its potency relative to morphine however is commonly reported to be on the order of 1:10, which reflects significant analgesic benefit conferred by its serotonin and norepinephrine reuptake inhibition (SNRI) properties. Tramadol exists as a racemic mixture, with the R or (+) isomer inhibiting serotonin reuptake and the S or (−) isomer inhibiting norepinephrine reuptake [94]. Limited evidence suggests that there may be a weak component of NMDA blockade inherent to tramadol [95], but these results have not been widely replicated in either in vitro or in vivo models.

Tramadol undergoes extensive (greater than 60%) hepatic Phase I metabolism with CYP2D6 responsible for the generation of an active metabolite (O-desmethyltramadol, denoted M1) which has 200-fold greater affinity for the MOR than the parent compound and six times the reported potency. Polymorphisms of this enzyme have been shown to confer clinically relevant variability in the efficacy of tramadol [96], and case reports exist of severe respiratory depression in ultrarapid metabolizers. CYP3A4 and CYP2B6 generate *N*-desmethyltramadol which is largely devoid of activity. The metabolites are excreted primarily by the kidneys. Tramadol exists as both immediate-release and extended-release formulations in this country.

Tramadol shows improved efficacy in neuropathic pain models compared to pure nociceptive models [97], and this is likely due to the combination SNRI effect. A Cochrane review performed in 2006 and updated in 2008 found strong evidence for good efficacy of tramadol in neuropathic pain [98].

Tramadol (along with other agents in the phenylpiperidine class) has been well-documented to cause both seizures and serotonin syndrome when co-administered with pro-serotonergic agents, and the author is aware of a handful of cases within his community. Pre-existing seizure disorders or head injury may be a contraindication to tramadol even in the absence of antidepressant therapy, as seizures may result in part also from the DOR agonist activity of O-desmethyltramadol [99].

Table 4.2 Opioid prescriptions filled in the United States, 2009 and 2014 [25]

Drug	Prescriptions in 2009	Prescriptions in 2014	% change from 2009 to 2014	% of total opioid prescriptions in 2014
Hydrocodone	126.9 million	125.3 million	−1.2%	42.8%
Oxycodone	49 million	59.5 million	+21%	20.3%
Tramadol	26.1 million	46.2 million	+77%	15.8%
Codeine	26.5 million	24.1 million	−9%	8.2%
Buprenorphine	4.7 million	11.5 million	+144%	3.9%
Morphine	7.7 million	10.3 million	+33%	3.5%
Fentanyl	6.4 million	6.7 million	+5%	2.3%
Hydromorphone	2.6 million	3.8 million	+45%	1.3%
Methadone	3.9 million	3.6 million	−7%	1.2%
Oxymorphone	0.7 million	1.2 million	+69%	0.4%
Meperidine	0.7 million	0.4 million	−49%	0.1%

While typical opioid withdrawal symptoms are generally less pronounced with tramadol, there seems to be an increased incidence of atypical withdrawal symptoms (e.g., mental status changes, significant anxiety/agitation and paranoia, hallucinations and unusual sensory experiences including paresthesias and formication) [100] that may be referable to cessation of the SNRI activity.

Tramadol has been thought to have low abuse liability for the past two decades since its release; however, a recent report by the World Health Organization warns of increased misuse and abuse in Africa and Western Asia [101]. In the United States, the drug was reclassified to a Schedule IV substance by the FDA in August 2014, reflecting concerns about abuse. Anecdotally, an increased incidence of both prescription and suspected diversion has been reported at least within our community; whether that represents increased interest in the drug as a result of tighter regulation is conjecture but interesting to consider. Between 2009 and 2014 the 26 Health's National Prescription Audit Plus Retail database showed a 77% increase in the number of tramadol prescriptions filled [25] (Table 4.2).

Summary

Multiple agents with widely varying potencies, metabolic/elimination pathways, durations of action, adverse effect profiles, and abuse and diversion liability exist. The knowledge of different profiles for somatic and psychiatric adverse effects, propensity to confer hyperalgesia, and risk of abuse and diversion is incumbent upon any provider who writes opioid prescriptions. While the generalist certainly does not need to be expert in all of the agents available, the growing scope of the problem of opioid abuse in this country necessitates some familiarity with all of the commonly used agents, regardless of specialty. The old injunction to "know a few agents really well" is certainly reasonable; however, staying abreast of the current knowledge base is essential when prescribing potentially lethal agents and those that can otherwise ruin a life; perhaps no drug (at least in the opioid class) exemplifies the risk of poorly informed/indiscriminate prescription than oxycodone.

References

1. Bai SA, Xiang Q, Finn A. Evaluation of the pharmacokinetics of single- and multiple-dose buprenorphine buccal film in healthy volunteers. Clin Ther. 2016;38:358–69.
2. Yassen A, Olofsen E, van Dorp E, Sarton E, Teppema L, Danhof M, et al. Mechanism-based pharmacokinetic-pharmacodynamic modelling of the reversal of buprenorphine-induced respiratory depression by naloxone: a study in healthy volunteers. Clin Pharmacokinet. 2007;46:965–80.
3. Böger RH. Renal impairment: a challenge for opioid treatment? The role of buprenorphine. Palliat Med. 2006;20(Suppl 1):s17–23.
4. Yassen A, Olofsen E, Romberg R, Sarton E, Danhof M, Dahan A. Mechanism-based pharmacokinetic-pharmacodynamic modeling of the antinociceptive effect of buprenorphine in healthy volunteers. Anesthesiology. 2006;104:1232–42.
5. Khanna IK, Pillarisetti S. Buprenorphine - an attractive opioid with underutilized potential in treatment of chronic pain. J Pain Res. 2015;8:859–70.
6. Fareed A, Patil D, Scheinberg K, Blackinton Gale R, Vayalapalli S, Casarella J, et al. Comparison of QTc interval prolongation for patients in methadone versus buprenorphine maintenance treatment: a 5-year follow-up. J Addict Dis. 2013;32:244–51.
7. Anchersen K, Clausen T, Gossop M, Hansteen V, Waal H. Prevalence and clinical relevance of corrected QT interval prolongation during methadone and buprenorphine treatment: a mortality assessment study. Addiction. 2009;104:993–9.
8. Paone D, Tuazon E, Stajic M, Sampson B, Allen B, Mantha S, et al. Buprenorphine infrequently found in fatal overdose in New York City. Drug Alcohol Depend. 2015;155:298–301.
9. Koppert W, Ihmsen H, Korber N, Wehrfritz A, Sittl R, Schmelz M, et al. Different profiles of buprenorphine- induced analgesia and antihyperalgesia in a human pain model. Pain. 2005;118:15–22.
10. Ravn P, Secher EL, Skram U, Therkildsen T, Christrup LL, Werner MU. Morphine- and buprenorphine-induced analgesia and antihyperalgesia in a human inflammatory pain model: a double-blind, randomized, placebo-controlled, five-arm crossover study. J Pain Res. 2013;6:23–38.
11. Leffler A, Frank G, Kistner K, Niedermirtl F, Koppert W, Reeh PW, et al. Local anesthetic-like inhibition of voltage-gated Na(+) channels by the partial mu-opioid receptor agonist buprenorphine. Anesthesiology. 2012;116:1335–46.
12. Cote J, Montgomery L. Sublingual buprenorphine as an analgesic in chronic pain: a systematic review. Pain Med. 2014;15:1171–8.
13. Schmidt-Hansen M, Bromham N, Taubert M, Arnold S, Hilgart JS. Buprenorphine for treating cancer pain. Cochrane Database Syst Rev. 2015;3:CD009596. doi:10.1002/14651858.CD009596.pub4.
14. United States Substance Abuse, Mental Health Services Administration. Treatment improvement protocol 40 (TIP 40): clinical guidelines for the use of buprenorphine in the treatment of opioid addiction. Rockville (MD): Substance Abuse and Mental Health Services Administration (US); 2004. p. 169.
15. Jones HE, Kaltenbach K, Heil SH, Stine SM, Coyle MG, Arria AM, et al. Neonatal abstinence syndrome after methadone or buprenorphine exposure. N Engl J Med. 2010;363:2320–233.
16. Fiellin DA, O'Connor PG. Clinical practice. Office-based treatment of opioid-dependent patients. NEJM. 2002;347:817–23.

17. Amass L, Ling W, Freese TE, Reiber C, Annon JJ, Cohen AJ, et al. Bringing buprenorphine-naloxone detoxification to community treatment providers: the NIDA clinical trials network field experience. Am J Addict. 2004;13:S42–66.
18. Maremmani I, Pani PP, Pacini M, Perugi G. Substance use and quality of life over 12 months among buprenorphine maintenance-treated and methadone maintenance-treated heroin-addicted patients. J Subst Abus Treat. 2007;33:91–8.
19. Mattick RP, Kimber J, Breen C, Davoli M. Buprenorphine maintenance versus placebo or methadone maintenance for opioid dependence. Cochrane Database Syst Rev. 2008;2008:CD002207.
20. Sullivan LE, Moore BA, Chawarski MC, Pantalon MV, Barry D, O'Connor PG, et al. Buprenorphine/naloxone treatment in primary care is associated with decreased human immunodeficiency virus risk behaviors. J Subst Abus Treat. 2008;35:87–92.
21. Schwarz R, Zelenev A, Bruce RD, Altice FL. Retention on buprenorphine treatment reduces emergency department utilization, but not hospitalization, among treatment-seeking patients with opioid dependence. J Subst Abus Treat. 2012;43:451–7.
22. Yokell MA, Zaller ND, Green TC, Rich JD. Buprenorphine and buprenorphine/naloxone diversion, misuse, and illicit use: an international review. Curr Drug Abuse Rev. 2011;4:28–41.
23. Lofwall MR, Walsh SL. A review of buprenorphine diversion and misuse: the current evidence base and experiences from around the world. J Addict Med. 2014;8:315–26.
24. Lavonas EJ, Severtson SG, Martinez EM, Bucher-Bartelson B, Le Lait MC, Green JL, et al. Abuse and diversion of buprenorphine sublingual tablets and film. J Subst Abus Treat. 2014;47:27–34.
25. U.S. Drug Enforcement Administration, Office of Diversion Control. National forensic laboratory information system special report: opiates and related drugs reported in NFLIS, 2009–2014. Springfield, VA: U.S. Drug Enforcement Administration; 2015.
26. Office of Diversion Control. National Forensic Laboratory Information System (NFLIS) special report: methadone and buprenorphine, 2003–2008. Washington, DC: U.S. Drug Enforcement Administration; 2009.
27. Srinivasan V, Wielbo D, Tebbett IR. Analgesic effects of codeine-6-glucuronide after intravenous administration. Eur J Pain. 1997;1:185–90.
28. Vree TB, van Dongen RT, Koopman-Kimenai PM. Codeine analgesia is due to codeine-6-glucuronide, not morphine. Int J Clin Pract. 2000;54:395–8.
29. Guay DR, Awni WM, Findlay JW, Halstenson CE, Abraham PA, Opsahl JA, et al. Pharmacokinetics and pharmacodynamics of codeine in end-stage renal disease. Clin Pharmacol Ther. 1988;43:63–71.
30. Takahama K, Shirasaki T. Central and peripheral mechanisms of narcotic antitussives: codeine-sensitive and -resistant coughs. Cough. 2007;3:8.
31. Nelson L, Schwaner R. Transdermal fentanyl: pharmacology and toxicology. J Med Toxicol. 2009;5:230–41.
32. Streisand JB, Varvel JR, Stanski DR, Le Maire L, Ashburn MA, Hague BI, et al. Absorption and bioavailability of oral transmucosal fentanyl citrate. Anesthesiology. 1991;75:223–39.
33. Navani DM, Yoburn BC. In vivo activity of norhydrocodone: an active metabolite of hydrocodone. J Pharmacol Exp Ther. 2013;347:497–505.
34. Vuilleumier PH, Stamer UM, Landau R. Pharmacogenomic considerations in opioid analgesia. Pharmacogenom Personal Med. 2012;5:73–87.
35. Inciardi JA, Surratt HL, Lugo Y, Cicero TJ. The diversion of prescription opioid analgesics. Law Enforc Exec Forum. 2007;7:127–41.
36. Vallner JJ, Stewart JT, Kotzan JA, Kirsten EB, Honigberg IL. Pharmacokinetics and bioavailability of hydromorphone following intravenous and oral administration to human subjects. J Clin Pharmacol. 1981;21:152–6.
37. Mather LE, Smith MT. Clinical pharmacology and adverse effects. In: Stein C, editor. Opioids in pain control: basic and clinical aspects. Cambridge: Cambridge University Press; 1999. p. 188–211.

38. Prommer E. Levorphanol: revisiting an underutilized analgesic. Palliat Care. 2011;8:7–10.
39. Pham TC, Fudin J, Raffa RB. Is levorphanol a better option than methadone? Pain Med. 2015;16:1673–9.
40. Kominek C, Brooks A, Fudin J. The forgotten opioid–could levorphanol levitate above methadone misadventure? Pain Week J. 2016;4:28–34.
41. Yaksh TL, Wallace MS. Opioids, analgesia, and pain management. In: Brunton L, editor. Goodman and Gilman's pharmacologic basis of therapeutics. New York: McGraw-Hill; 2011. p. 481–525.
42. Jackson KC, Smith HS. Optimizing pharmacologic outcomes: drug selection. In: Smith HS, editor. Opioid therapy in the twenty-first century. Oxford: Oxford University Press; 2013. p. 43–68.
43. Centers for Disease Control. Vital signs: risk for overdose from methadone used for pain relief — United States, 1999–2010. MMWR. 2012;61:493–7.
44. Trescot AM, Datta S, Lee M, Hansen H. Opioid pharmacology. Pain Physician. 2008;11(2 Suppl):S133–53.
45. Brown R, Kraus C, Fleming M, Reddy S. Methadone: applied pharmacology and use as adjunctive treatment in chronic pain. Postgrad Med J. 2004;80:654–9.
46. Chang Y, Fang WB, Lin SN, Moody DE. Stereo-selective metabolism of methadone by human liver microsomes and cDNA-expressed cytochrome P450s: a reconciliation. Basic Clin Pharmacol Toxicol. 2011;108:55–62.
47. Ansermot N, Albayrak O, Schläpfer J. Substitution of (R,S)-methadone by (R)-methadone: impact on QTc interval. Arch Intern Med. 2010;170(6):529–36.
48. Wang D, Teichtahl H, Drummer O, Goodman C, Cherry G, Cunnington D, et al. Central sleep apnea in stable methadone maintenance treatment patients. Chest. 2005;128:1348–56.
49. Haroutiunian S, McNicol ED, Lipman AG. Methadone for chronic non-cancer pain in adults. Cochrane Database Syst Rev. 2012;11:CD008025. doi:10.1002/14651858.CD008025.pub2.
50. Marsch LA. The efficacy of methadone maintenance interventions in reducing illicit opiate use, HIV risk behavior and criminality: a meta-analysis. Addiction. 1998;93:515–32.
51. Mattick RP, Breen C, Kimber J, Davoli M. Methadone maintenance therapy versus no opioid replacement therapy for opioid dependence. Cochrane Database Syst Rev. 2003;2:CD002209.
52. Metzger DS, Woody GE, McLellan AT, O'Brien CP, Druley P, Navaline H, et al. Human immunodeficiency virus seroconversion among intravenous drug users in- and out-of-treatment: an 18- month prospective follow-up. J Acquir Immune Defic Syndr. 1993;6:1049–56.
53. Gowing L, Farrell M, Bornemann R, Ali R. Substitution treatment of injecting opioid users for prevention of HIV infection. Cochrane Database Syst Rev. 2004;4:CD004145.
54. Strain EC, Stitzer ML, Liebson IA, Bigelow GE. Dose-response effects of methadone in the treatment of opioid dependence. Ann Intern Med. 1993;119:23–37.
55. Strain EC, Bigelow GE, Liebson IA, Stitzer ML. Moderate- vs high-dose methadone in the treatment of opioid dependence. A randomized trial. JAMA. 1999;281:1000–5.
56. Faggiano F, Vigna-Taglianti F, Versino E, Lemma P. Methadone maintenance at different dosages for opioid dependence. Cochrane Database Syst Rev. 2003;3:CD002208.
57. Simpson DD, Sells SB. Effectiveness of treatment for drug abuse: an overview of the DARP research program. Adv Alcohol Subst Abuse. 1982;2:7–29.
58. Condelli WS, Dunteman GH. Exposure to methadone programs and heroin use. Am J Drug Alcohol Abuse. 1993;19:65–78.
59. International Narcotics Control Board. Narcotic drugs 2014, vol. 21. New York: United Nations; 2015. p. 30. isbn: 9789210481571
60. Woods BD, Sladen RN. Perioperative considerations for the patient with asthma and bronchospasm. Br J Anaesth. 2009;103(suppl 1):i57–65.
61. Ellingsrud C, Agewall S. Morphine in the treatment of acute pulmonary oedema — why? Int J Cardiol. 2016;202:870–3.
62. Hall M, Griffiths R, Appadu B. Is morphine indicated in acute pulmonary oedema? Emerg Med J. 2005;22:391.

63. Nielsen CK, Ross FB, Lotfipour S, Saini KS, Edwards SR, Smith MT. Oxycodone and morphine have distinctly different pharmacological profiles: radioligand binding and behavioural studies in two rat models of neuropathic pain. Pain. 2007;132:289–300s.
64. Samer CF, Daali Y, Wagner M, Hopfgartner G, Eap CB, Rebsamen MC, et al. Genetic polymorphisms and drug interactions modulating CYP2D6 and CYP3A activities have a major effect on oxycodone analgesic efficacy and safety. Br J Pharmacol. 2010;160:919–30.
65. Riley J, Eisenberg E, Müller-Schwefe G, Drewes AM, Arendt-Nielsen L. Oxycodone: a review of its use in the management of pain. Curr Med Res Opin. 2008;24:175–92.
66. King SJ, Reid C, Forbes K, Hanks G. A systematic review of oxycodone in the management of cancer pain. Palliat Med. 2011;25:454–70.
67. Schmidt-Hansen M, Bennett MI, Arnold S, Bromham N, Hilgart JS. Oxycodone for cancer-related pain. Cochrane Database Syst Rev. 2015;2:CD003870. doi:10.1002/14651858.CD003870.pub5.
68. Ma H, Liu Y, Huang L, Zeng XT, Jin SH, Yue GJ, et al. The adverse events of oxycodone in cancer-related pain a systematic review and meta-analysis of randomized controlled trials. Medicine. 2016;95:1–9.
69. Olesen AE, Staahl C, Arendt-Nielsen L, Drewes AM. Different effects of morphine and oxycodone in experimentally evoked hyperalgesia: a human translational study. Br J Clin Pharmacol. 2010;70:189–200.
70. Gaskell H, Moore RA, Derry S, Stannard C. Oxycodone for neuropathic pain and fibromyalgia in adults. Cochrane Database Syst Rev. 2014;6:CD010692. doi:10.1002/14651858.CD010692.pub2.
71. International Narcotics Control Board. Narcotic drugs: estimated world requirements for 2009; statistics for 2007. Report E/INCB/2008/2 (PDF). New York: United Nations; 2009. isbn:978-92-1-048124-3.
72. Kenan K, Mack K, Paulozzi L. Trends in prescriptions for oxycodone and other commonly used opioids in the United States, 2000-2010. Open Medicine. 2012;6:41–7.
73. Substance Abuse and Mental Health Services Administration. Results from the 2013 national survey on drug use and health: summary of national findings, NSDUH series H-48, HHS publication no. (SMA) 14-4863. Rockville, MD: Substance Abuse and Mental Health Services Administration; 2014.
74. Wightman R, Perrone J, Portelli I, Nelson L. Likeability and abuse liability of commonly prescribed opioids. J Med Toxicol. 2012;8:335–40.
75. Cicero TJ, Ellis MS, Paradis A, Ortbal Z. Determinants of fentanyl and other potent mu-agonist misuse in opioid-dependent individuals. Pharmacoepidemiol Drug Saf. 2010;19:1057–63.
76. Jones JD, VOsburg SK, Manubay JM, Comer SD. Oxycodone abuse in New York city: characteristics of intravenous and intranasal users. Am J Addict. 2011;20:190–5.
77. Substance Abuse and Mental Health Services Administration. The DAWN report: trends in emergency department visits involving non-medical use of narcotic pain relievers. Rockville, MD: Office of Applied Studies; 2010.
78. Butler S, Black R, Cassidy T, Dailey TM, Budman SH. Abuse risks and routes of administration of different prescription opioid compounds and formulations. Harm Reduct J. 2011;8:29–45.
79. Uddin F. Hope in fort hope: first nations community is winning the battle against prescription drug abuse. Can Fam Physician. 2013;59:391–3.
80. Young AM, Havens JR. Transition from first illicit drug use to first injection drug use among rural appalachian drug users: a cross-sectional comparison and retrospective survival analysis. Addiction. 2012;107:587–96.
81. Pollini RA, Banta-Green CJ, Cuevas-Mota J, Metzner M, Teshale E, Garfein RS. Problematic use of prescription-type opioids prior to heroin use among young heroin injectors. Subst Abuse Rehabil. 2011;2:173–80.
82. Lankenau SE, Teti M, Silva K. Initiation into prescription opioid misuse amongst young injection drug users. Int J Drug Policy. 2012;23:37–44.

83. Mars SG, Bourgois P, Karandino G, Montero F, Ciccarone D. "every 'never' I ever said came true": transitions from opioid pills to heroin injecting. Int J Drug Policy. 2014;25:257–66.
84. Anonymous. New guidelines create an 'oxy-free' ED. ED Manag. 2010;22:136–7.
85. Sloan P. Review of oral oxymorphone in the management of pain. Ther Clin Risk Manag. 2008;4:777–87.
86. Gimbel J, Ahdieh H. The efficacy and safety of oral immediate-release oxymorphone for postsurgical pain. Anesth Analg. 2004;99:1472–7.
87. Raffa RB, Buschmann H, Christoph T, Eichenbaum G, Englberger W, Flores CM, et al. Mechanistic and functional differentiation of tapentadol and tramadol. Expert Opin Pharmacother. 2012;13:1437–49.
88. Vadivelu N, Timchenko A, Huang Y, Sinatra R. Tapentadol extended-release for treatment of chronic pain: a review. J Pain Res. 2011;4:211–8.
89. Schröder W, Tzschentke TM, Terlinden R, De Vry J, Jahnel U, Christoph T, et al. Synergistic interaction between the two mechanisms of action of tapentadol in analgesia. J Pharmacol Exp Ther. 2011;337:312–20.
90. Riemsma R, Forbes C, Harker J, Worthy G, Misso K, Schäfer M, et al. Systematic review of tapentadol in chronic severe pain. Curr Med Res Opin. 2011;27:1907–30.
91. Dart RC, Cicero TJ, Surratt HL, Rosenblum A, Bartelson BB, Adams EH. Assessment of the abuse of tapentadol immediate release: the first 24 months. J Opioid Manag. 2012;8:395–402.
92. Butler SF, McNaughton EC, Black RA. Tapentadol abuse potential: a postmarketing evaluation using a sample of individuals evaluated for substance abuse treatment. Pain Med. 2015;16:119–30.
93. McNaughton EC, Black RA, Weber SE, Butler SF. Assessing abuse potential of new analgesic medications following market release: an evaluation of internet discussion of tapentadol abuse. Pain Med. 2015;16:131–40.
94. Grond S, Sablotzki A. Clinical pharmacology of tramadol. Clin Pharmacokinet. 2004;43:879–923.
95. Hara K, Minami K, Sata T. The effects of tramadol and its metabolite on glycine, gamma-aminobutyric acid A, and N-methyl-D-aspartate receptors expressed in Xenopus oocytes. Anesth Analg. 2005;100:1400–5.
96. Lassen D, Damkier P, Brøsen K. The pharmacogenetics of tramadol. Clin Pharmacokinet. 2015;54:825–36.
97. Christoph T, Kögel B, Strassburger W, Schug SA. Tramadol has a better potency ratio relative to morphine in neuropathic than in nociceptive pain models. Drugs R D. 2007;8:51–7.
98. Hollingshead J, Dühmke RM, Cornblath DR. Tramadol for neuropathic pain. Cochrane Database Syst Rev. 2008;(2):CD003726. doi:10.1002/14651858.CD003726.pub3.
99. Potschka H, Friderichs E, Löscher W. Anticonvulsant and proconvulsant effects of tramadol, its enantiomers and its M1 metabolite in the rat kindling model of epilepsy. Br J Pharmacol. 2000;131:203–12.
100. Senay EC, Adams EH, Geller A, Inciardi JA, Muñoz A, Schnoll SH, et al. Physical dependence on ultram (tramadol hydrochloride): both opioid-like and atypical withdrawal symptoms occur. Drug Alcohol Depend. 2003;69:233–41.
101. World Health Organization Expert Committee on Drug Dependence. Tramadol: Update Review Report. 2014. Available from: http://www.who.int/medicines/areas/quality_safety/6_1_Update.pdf.

Chapter 5
Attenuating the Agent: Reducing Opioid "Virulence"

Two young men in a remote village were abusing an extended-release oxycodone product via crushing the pills and "smoking" the powder, inhaling the fumes via a pipe. An argument ensued between the two of them, and one of the young men shot his associate several times in the abdomen with a 9 mm pistol. By report, the two men resolved their differences shortly thereafter and resumed smoking their oxycodone together. A few hours later, the assailant turned the gun upon himself and took his own life. The man shot in the abdomen then sought medical attention and was air evacuated and transferred to the regional trauma center where he underwent exploratory laparotomy, removal of projectiles, and excision/repair of injured bowel. He survived this incident.

Introduction

One theoretical approach to end an epidemic is to eliminate the agent.

This is neither realistic nor in all likelihood would it be in the best interest of the host population, in many cases. First of all, the agents are ubiquitous. Secondly, most microbes play some role in the larger balance of the ecosystem, and their elimination may have far-reaching negative consequences. Thirdly, mutation rates coupled with short propagation times invariably result in new pathogenic strains, or antimicrobial-resistant strains, as we have learned over the last few decades in the infectious disease realm.

Many of these considerations apply to the opioid as agent as well. Blanket elimination is impossible without destroying every poppy plant and chemical laboratory on the planet. Opioids do provide a necessary and useful role, and their elimination would have far-reaching negative consequences. Human nature is such that when one abusable substance is rendered inaccessible, another is often substituted.

H.B. McAnally, *Opioid Dependence*, DOI 10.1007/978-3-319-47497-7_5

An alternate approach addressing the agent is to somehow attenuate its virulence without eliminating it. Since the post-World War II period and Dr. Jonas Salk's inactivated and Dr. Albert Sabin's "live-attenuated" poliovirus vaccines, alteration of normal microbial pathogenic capacity has been the mainstay of infectious disease prevention, by means of stimulating host immune defenses via vaccination. More recently, "antivirulence therapies" aimed at altering agent virulence factor production, expression, regulation, etc. are under intensive research and development as classic twentieth century antimicrobial therapeutic approaches seem doomed to failure as resistance inevitably overcomes antibiotics. Some of these approaches include targeting adherence and protective (biofilm) mechanisms, enhancing competition for resources by increasing commensal organisms, interfering with "quorum sensing" and signaling among pathogens, "quorum quenching" agents, and other novel approaches [1–3].

This sort of multifaceted "outside-the-box thinking" must be applied to the development of novel analgesics as well if we hope to reduce human dependence upon exogenous opioids. Classic approaches (such as extended-release/long-acting formulations and abuse-deterrent/tamper-resistant technologies, discussed in greater detail below) have not proven successful on a wide scale in containing the opioid epidemic.

Nora Volkow's 2014 Congressional Address highlighted the need for the development of novel analgesic therapies that "circumvent the brain reward pathways, thereby greatly reducing abuse potential" [4]. In considering antivirulence strategies, one must first define and understand virulence. A succinct, recent definition highlighting both the concept of virulence along a spectrum and also its essentially broad context is "the relative capacity of a microbe to cause damage in a host [5]." These authors also make the point that the virulence of an agent may be dependent upon individual host vulnerability which varies as well. Host damage caused by opioids has been reviewed in Chap. 3 and ranges from mildly annoying side effects to death from respiratory depression and in some cases cardiac arrest. Significant morbidity affecting nearly every physiologic system is common but varies from individual to individual. Obese individuals with compromised airways and those with ultra-rapid CYP2D6 metabolizer status are more prone to respiratory arrest, and individuals with certain psychosocial risk factors (as discussed in greater detail in Chap. 9) are more prone to dependence and addiction. However, while the vulnerability to and outcome of opioid morbidity (including dependence and addiction) and mortality are variable, their correlation with increased exposure is not only intuitive but borne out in the literature. In addition, the correlation between abuse potential and increased exposure is well-established. Thus, while death (or addiction) may result from one single exposure and many chronic users survive and escape addiction, in general reducing abuse potential is a key strategy in attenuating virulence, as Dr. Volkow points out.

Brief Overview of Opioid Addiction Biology

Before examining past, present, and future mechanisms of reducing opioid virulence, a cursory review of current neurobiological theory of (psychological) substance dependence and addiction, along with proposed mechanisms whereby opioids "hijack" the proposed circuitry, is in order. A more comprehensive overview is presented in Chap. 9, with behavioral and societal theories broadening the discussion. It should be noted at the outset of any exploration of proposed addiction biology that:

- Interspecies differences limit extrapolation of animal neuroanatomic and neurophysiologic research to humans.
- There are profound and even diametrically opposed differences in response to the same stimulus within the same animal model depending on whether the subjects are awake or anesthetized [6].
- Human and nonhuman primate higher function confers complexity to the process of dependence and addiction not represented in lower species. Animals are incapable of understanding negative consequences of addictive behavior, and the added layers of cognitive, emotional, relational, and spiritual stresses that addiction confers to humans are simply not represented.

Current understanding of the neurobiology of reward motivation assigns a central role to dopaminergic neurons within the *ventral tegmental area (VTA)* of the midbrain. VTA dopaminergic neurons project superiorly along the *medial forebrain bundle* (nicknamed the "hedonic highway" [7]) to various limbic and executive areas including the:

- *Amygdala* – within the temporal lobe, this limbic structure is involved in emotional processing and memory.
- *Ventral striatum* (*nucleus accumbens*, NAc) – this basal ganglia structure is held to be the central region mediating motivation for pursuing rewarding substances or activities. The pathway between VTA and NAc is known as the *mesolimbic pathway* (shown in green in Fig. 5.1) and has long been held to be the key link in natural and exogenous reward/reinforcement and addiction.
- *Anterior cingulate cortex* – this paralimbic region is involved in the anticipation of reward and plays a key role in integrating emotions with painful stimuli as well.
- *Prefrontal cortex (PFC)* – this "executive center" of the brain is involved in decision-making based on integration of sensory and limbic inputs as well as memory and is thought to be a critical area for reinforcing drug effects.

Intracerebral dopamine agonists induce both self-administration and conditioned place preference (CPP) in rodents [9–12], and dopamine antagonism causes aversive behaviors in both animal and human subjects [13–15]. Virtually all drugs of abuse and other pleasurable stimuli are believed to exert hedonic effect via mesolimbic dopamine.

Opioid-induced reward (including euphoria) is thought to be mediated via cerebral mu-opioid receptors (MOR) [16–18]. MOR are ubiquitous throughout the brain, but extensive research in animal subjects has shown that there are specific regions, in particular the VTA, whose MOR appear particularly important to the reward/reinforcement phenomenon that is universally accepted as fundamental to the development of addiction [19–22]. Evidence for the centrality of the VTA in

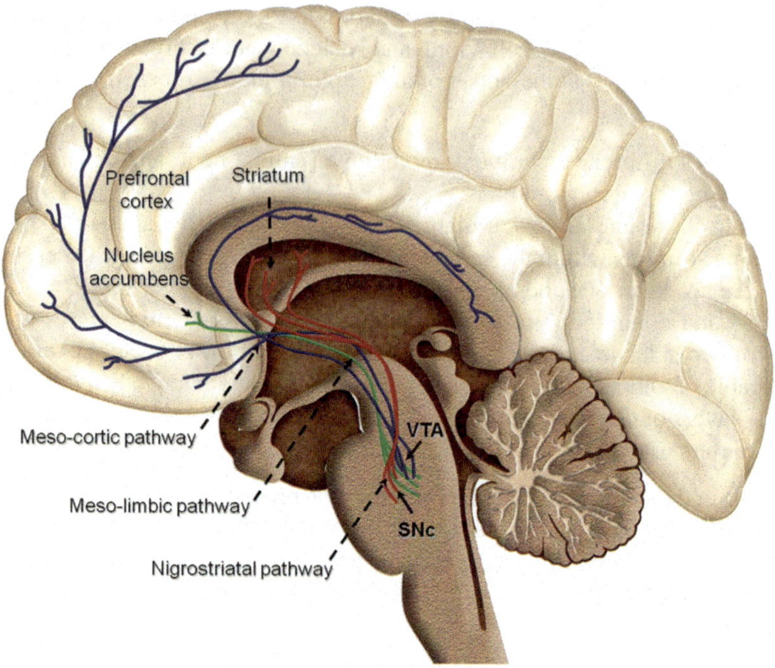

Fig. 5.1 Reward and addiction pathways in the brain. SNc, substantia nigra; VTA, ventral tegmental area. Reprinted from Ref. [8]. ©Arias-Carrión et al. (2010). http://www.biomedcentral.com/1755-7682/3/24/, CC BY 3.0, https://commons.wikimedia.org/w/index.php?curid=44695433

opioid dependence is both positive (intra-VTA opioid administration induces both self-administration and CPP in rodents [20, 22–24]) and negative (intra-VTA opioid antagonists or genetic MOR knockout results in loss of these behaviors [21, 25]).

Dopaminergic transmission to mesolimbic targets including the NAc is effected by VTA MOR agonism [26, 27], and thus a synthesis of these data has resulted in opioid-VTA MOR-mesolimbic dopaminergism being widely accepted as the foundational biologic paradigm for opioid addiction [28–30].

However, several recent lines of evidence indicate that the picture is much more complicated than this. First of all, ample evidence indicates that not all NAc dopaminergism is rewarding; several agents (delta-opioid receptor agonists, cholecystokinin, glial-derived neurotrophic factor) increase dopamine in the NAc but do not produce CPP [6], and furthermore even the administration of MOR antagonists sufficient to cause place aversion also results in NAc dopamine increases [31, 32]. Second, evidence is accumulating that opioid reinforcement can occur in the absence of mesolimbic dopaminergism [33–36]. Interestingly, dopaminergic neuronal activity in response to MOR agonism has been shown to increase in anesthetized animals but decrease in awake animals [6]. Similarly, MOR-mediated CPP inhibition by dopamine antagonism has been shown in opioid-dependent rodents whereas opioid-naïve animals do not lose CPP [37]. Finally, stimulation of VTA dopaminergic neurons has been shown to also result in release of other neurotransmitters including glutamate and GABA [38–40].

While our understanding of the complexities of addiction neurobiology (let alone behavior) is in its infancy, it is at least a useful construct to imagine a correlation between a substance's capacity to agonize midbrain MOR and effect pleasurable dopaminergic (or other) transmission to limbic and higher cortical structures and its virulence.

Overview of Virulence Attenuation Strategies

Historic and current approaches to attenuating opioid virulence are organized in this chapter into two categories:

1. Modifying existing mu-opioid receptor (MOR) agonists
2. Other approaches

The second category is necessarily and by design broad, indicating the diversity of approaches available. It is also intended to highlight the distinction between "out-of-the-box" thinking and more restricted efforts typified by the first category. This is not to disparage efforts to reduce virulence by altering delivery of currently extant agents; there is great practicality in utilizing agents already known to be (relatively) safe and efficacious. Such approaches however have little promise for improvement over the current situation besides limiting the potential for non-sanctioned routes of abuse. Development of novel opioid-mediated strategies will be necessary to effectively harness the full, balanced potential of the intricate and wonderful endogenous analgesic system we possess. Development of non-opioid-mediated strategies (e.g., *N*-methyl D-aspartate blockers, cannabidiol analogs) of course will provide complementary or alternative means of potent analgesia but are outside the scope of this work.

Modifying Existing Central MOR Agonists

Extended-Release/Long-Acting Opioids

The development of *extended-release* or *long-acting* (*ER/LA*) opioids, in addition to providing more stable pharmacokinetics and theoretically improved baseline analgesia, has also been thought to reduce the virulence of opioids. Synonyms include *controlled-release*, *sustained-release*, and time-release technology. These formulations are engineered pharmaceutically to provide more stable plasma and target site concentrations of the drug over a prolonged period. Inherent in this strategy is a greater amount of active drug presented per single vehicle, which is typically intended to effect analgesia over a 12–24 h period. Common mechanisms include embedding the agent within a poorly soluble or insoluble matrix from which it must diffuse or microencapsulation of the agent with a slowly dissolving "coat."

From a practical standpoint, individuals with malabsorptive syndromes (which are increasing in this country due to bariatric surgical operations) likely enjoy significantly less bioavailability of ER/LA formulations although there are not yet robust studies supporting this assumption.

Current ER/LA opioids in oral form include hydrocodone, hydromorphone, morphine, oxycodone, oxymorphone, tapentadol, and tramadol. Another means of achieving this sort of stable pharmacokinetics is via a transdermal delivery system, such as is used with certain lipophilic agents such as fentanyl and buprenorphine; this route circumvents the issues of oral absorption and may also confer reduced psychological dependence by eliminating pill-taking behavior.

Different arguments have been made in support of ER/LA opioid therapy, including the theory that chronic pain conditions should be treated with "round-the-clock" steady-state analgesia. From a virulence reduction standpoint, ER/LA agents result in lower peak plasma levels which have been thought to confer increased safety [41] although this may not be the case in situations of compromised metabolism, i.e., hepatic or renal insufficiency. Two large recent reviews have provided evidence that ER/LA agents may in fact be associated with a higher incidence of morbidity and mortality [42, 43].

As far as abuse liability, rapid onset or immediate-release drugs have been shown repeatedly to be preferred by abusers [44–48]—presumably as they result in more dramatic/dynamic presentation of dopamine from the VTA to the NAc and other limbic reward centers—drugs with a rapid elimination rate have also been associated with greater self-administration [44, 45]. Conversely, ER/LA formulations are believed to confer a lower risk of psychological (not physical) dependence and addiction and have been touted as conferring lower abuse liability [41, 49] although other data have called this conclusion into question as well [50, 51].

Ironically, the current opioid crisis in this country is often attributed to ER/LA oxycodone (Purdue's OxyContin) which entered the American market in 1996. The mining injury-rich and depressed socioeconomic climate of rural Appalachia is credited with facilitating a demographic ripe for substance abuse and addiction, and here the drug enjoyed particularly rapid adoption among prescribers thanks to aggressive marketing and subsidization. Individuals quickly discovered how to defeat the time-release mechanism by crushing and insufflating or injecting the powder, delivering a large dose of oxycodone (up to 160 mg from one tablet, equivalent to over 300 mg of morphine with a typical hospital inpatient dose being 2–4 mg of intravenous morphine) instantly. Rates of abuse, overdose and death, and crime soared over the next decade in what the Office of National Drug Control Policy has termed the Appalachia High Intensity Drug Trafficking Area, which includes 67 counties in Kentucky, Tennessee, and West Virginia. OxyContin became the top-selling pharmaceutical opioid in history, earning Purdue $35 billion between 1996 and 2015 [52]. After numerous investigations and lawsuits, three top officials ultimately pleaded guilty in 2007 to misleading the public about the drug's risk of addiction and paid $634.5 million in fines; in the late 2015 Purdue settled with the

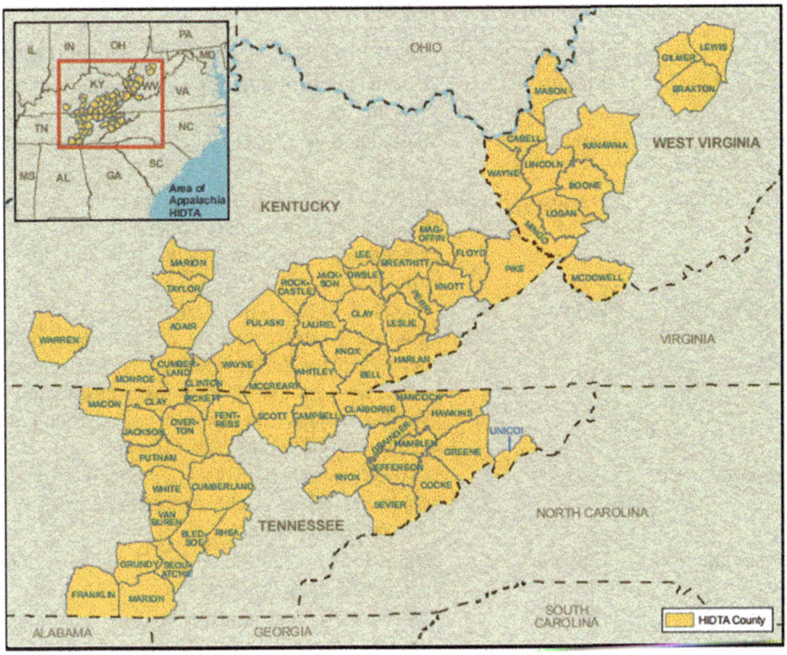

Fig. 5.2 Appalachia High Intensity Drug Trafficking Area. National Drug Intelligence Center, US Department of Justice

State of Kentucky for another $24 million in damages, and several other lawsuits remain in court (Fig. 5.2).

In 2012, the US Food and Drug Administration (FDA) initiated a *Risk Evaluation and Mitigation Strategy (REMS)* requiring ER/LA opioid manufacturers to make available prescribing training for healthcare professionals who prescribe ER/LA opioids and also to distribute educational materials to prescribers and patients on the safe use of these powerful pain medications.

Abuse-Deterrent/Tamper-Resistant Formulations

The OxyContin experience resulted in increased interest in/pressure to formulate higher-dose opioids in a vehicle that would prevent abusers from circumventing the time-release mechanisms, rendering them essentially immediate-release preparations of supratherapeutic doses. Common mechanisms for defeating ER/LA technology by abusers have included crushing and snorting or dissolving in water or solvents and injecting.

Abuse-deterrent or *tamper-resistant* strategies have multiplied over the past decade and include diverse tactics such as altering the physical formulation, adding aversive agents activated upon alteration or administration by non-indicated routes, and

Table 5.1 Abuse-deterrent/tamper-resistant opioids

Drug	Brand name	Mechanism of abuse deterrence/tamper resistance
Buprenorphine	Probuphine®	Partial agonist, MOR "blocker," subdermal implant system
Buprenorphine-naloxone	Suboxone®	Partial agonist, MOR "blocker," integrated naloxone
Hydrocodone ER	Hysingla®	RESISTEC® polymer matrix controls release and renders tablet difficult to crush and forms viscous gel when dissolved in aqueous solutions, hampering injection
Hydrocodone ER	Zohydro®	BeadTek® mixture of inactive beads, active immediate release, and active ER hydrocodone beads. Inactive beads maintain the 12 hr release properties of the drug when taken as directed but will immediately form a viscous gel when crushed and dissolved in liquids or solvents
Hydromorphone ER	Exalgo®	OROS® osmotic delivery system facilitates controlled release and also crush and extraction resistance properties
Morphine-naltrexone	Embeda®	Naltrexone is sequestered in micropellets' cores and is released upon crushing
Oxycodone	Oxaydo®	AVERSION® matrix forms viscous gelatinous mixture hampering injection; if crushed and snorted, sodium lauryl sulfate will cause nasal discomfort
Oxycodone ER	OxyContin®	INTAC® hydrophilic matrix controls release and forms a gel that cannot be easily injected or snorted if crushed or dissolved in solutions and resists extraction of active drug via solvents
Oxymorphone ER	Opana ER®	INTAC® hydrophilic matrix controls release and forms a gel that cannot be easily injected or snorted if crushed or dissolved in solutions and resists extraction of active drug via solvents
Tapentadol ER	Nucynta ER®	INTAC® hydrophilic matrix controls release and forms a gel that cannot be easily injected or snorted if crushed or dissolved in solutions and resists extraction of active drug via solvents

implant formulation in the case of buprenorphine. Currently available formulations are listed in Table 5.1.

Tamper Resistance

Several physical component mechanisms exist to discourage tampering, including formulation as extremely hard tablets that are resistant to crushing, and embedding active drug within a matrix such as polyethylene oxide that forms a viscous gel when exposed to water or solvent, hampering injection.

According to the National Poison Data System, "abuse exposures" related to OxyContin decreased by 36% in the 1-year period following the reformulation with INTAC tamper-resistant technology [53], and according to the manufacturer's adverse events database, related deaths are decreased by 82% from the year prior to the third year after reformulation [54].

Aversive Technology

Aversive technology has primarily taken the form of adding MOR antagonists (naloxone or naltrexone) into the formulation with the therapeutic opioid to deter administration by alternate/non-indicated routes. In the case of Suboxone® or generic buprenorphine/naloxone, sublingual (or accidental enteric) administration results in minimal antagonist activity due to the low bioavailability of naloxone by those routes; however, injection of dissolved agent results in significant antagonist effects and can precipitate profound opioid withdrawal. Similarly, in the case of Embeda® (ER/LA morphine with naltrexone), the naltrexone component is sequestered in the core of the micropellets and is released upon crushing.

The AVERSION® technology of Oxaydo® further discourages crushing and insufflation by the presence of inactive ingredients that cause nasal discomfort.

Implant Systems

While tamper-resistant technology undoubtedly discourages abuse by non-indicated routes, it does not have the capability of deterring abuse by indicated routes, i.e., individuals can ingest greater quantities orally without suffering the consequences of sequestered aversive agent release, etc. Depot/time-release intramuscular injections or implant systems are one response to this liability, although (except in the case of buprenorphine, discussed below) they still do not discourage/prevent individuals from obtaining and using other opioids.

The only currently approved opioid implant system (aside from intrathecal pump systems which are not discussed in this book) is a buprenorphine implant (Probuphine®) manufactured by Braeburn, which releases 80 mg of buprenorphine over the course of 6 months. It is a solid, matchstick-sized implant made from a mixture of ethylene-vinyl acetate (EVA) and buprenorphine. While undoubtedly advantageous in improving compliance with buprenorphine treatment for opioid dependence/reducing illicit use, this system may be problematic in terms of conferring unwanted MOR blockade in cases of trauma or emergency surgery.

Federal Oversight

The original OxyContin formulation was touted/labeled as being abuse-deterrent; after it became evident that individuals were abusing the product, Purdue removed the claim of abuse deterrence from the label, which was regranted after reformulation.

Since then, the FDA has exerted significantly greater oversight into the approval and marketing of abuse-deterrent formulations and recently released guidelines on the matter to the pharmaceutical industry [55].

Required processes include:

1. Laboratory-based in vitro manipulation and extraction studies (Category 1)
2. Pharmacokinetic studies (Category 2)
3. Clinical abuse potential studies (Category 3)
4. Postmarket impact studies (Category 4)

The FDA has also stated that it will require advisory committee meetings for all new non-abuse-deterrent opioids and has made clear that their intent is to facilitate eventual transition away from non-abuse-deterrent opioids.

Prodrugs

Another approach to reducing abuse proposed by the FDA [55] is the development of *prodrugs*. Prodrugs are less active or inactive precursor molecules that require biophysical alteration (generally by enzymatic cleavage) for transformation into active agents [56]. Prodrugs requiring gastrointestinal enzymatic activation may reduce parenteral abuse by eliminating therapeutic or recreational efficacy by non-indicated routes. However, prodrugs yielding MOR agonists as we know them today are unlikely to reduce abuse by excessive oral administration nor inherently circumvent the adverse effect profile of excessive or unbalanced MOR activation including euphoria, respiratory depression, etc.

"Outside-the-Box" Approaches

Partial Agonists

Partial mu-opioid receptor (MOR) agonists have been explored and trialed for almost half a century as a means of reducing adverse physical or psychiatric effects. Relative agonism is defined by in vitro studies comparing agents to a "full agonist" or one with maximally known efficacy. Reduced efficacy at the MOR confers a so-called ceiling effect beyond which further administration yields insignificant or at least significantly diminishing additive benefit; adverse effects mediated by the partially activated MOR are proportionately reduced but not eliminated [57]. Enthusiasm for this class of medication in terms of reduced respiratory depression and abuse liability and dependence has waxed and waned over the years [58–62]. Butorphanol, nalbuphine, and pentazocine are three older partial MOR agonists used in various "niche" arenas (e.g., butorphanol is still commonly used as a parenteral analgesic in many labor and delivery suites; nalbuphine is still used as a parenteral antipruritic to combat neuraxial opioid-mediated pruritus by many anesthesiologists), but by and large these agents have not enjoyed widespread adoption. This is in part due to the psychomimetic effects of kappa-opioid receptor (KOR) agonism that all three agents possess.

Buprenorphine (the pharmacology of which is discussed in greater detail in Chap. 4) is a partial agonist at the MOR and an antagonist at the KOR, which latter property eliminates the psychomimetic effects associated with the agents listed above. In fact, the KOR antagonism of buprenorphine has been shown confer significant antidepressant effects, and a therapeutic indication for treatment of refractory depression has been called for by the psychiatric community [63, 64]. Buprenorphine also possesses the lowest receptor dissociation constant [65, 66] (i.e., highest tenacity for the MOR) among currently available opioids, which is also relevant in terms of reducing adverse effects in that the agent effectively "blocks" other MOR agonists from exerting effects. This has led to its widespread use in treating opioid dependence/addiction; once an individual's MOR are occupied by buprenorphine, therapeutic or hedonic/euphoric effects of other MOR agonists including heroin are subverted.

The addition of naloxone to buprenorphine (introduced in the previous section on abuse deterrence/tamper resistance) does not alter the inherent effects conferred by its partial agonist or receptor dissociation qualities.

Peripheral Agonists

Restricting opioid agonism to the periphery is one means of limiting centrally mediated adverse effects, including euphoria and the development of dependence. Whether or not such an approach can provide meaningful analgesia remains to be seen but has been intensively investigated and remains an elegant and intriguing direction.

Peripheral opioid effects are thought to be most pronounced in states of tissue inflammation [67–69], and this phenomenon correlates with observation of increased peripheral opioid receptor synthesis/expression in states of inflammation [70–72].

Besides obviation of central activity, this "limited efficacy" may be beneficial in the sense of restricting self-administration to states of nociceptive pain where pathologic peripheral inflammation is present (e.g., rheumatoid arthritis) and reducing the desirability of the agent in states of "exclusively" centrally mediated states.

Selective peripheral MOR agonism has been utilized for decades for non-analgesic purposes, i.e., antidiarrheal activity. Loperamide is a well-known MOR agonist with virtually no central effect due to rapid CNS efflux transportation. This agent has been investigated in rodent models of peripheral analgesia and has shown some analgesic efficacy in this environment [73, 74]; however, these results cannot be reliably translated into primate or human experience, and furthermore effective analgesia from loperamide even in rodents is limited by short duration of action and very high toxicity with effective doses [75]. Other experimental peripheral MOR-selective agonists remain under investigation.

Peripheral kappa-opioid receptor (KOR) agonism has been investigated for several years as a means to selectively effect visceral analgesia, given the preponderance of KOR in the gut and associated organs [76]. KOR agonists have also been shown for years to exert extraordinary powerful anti-inflammatory effect [67], but their efficacy has heretofore been limited by centrally mediated adverse effects, predominantly psychogenic, as discussed in previous chapters. Selective peripheral KOR agonists may provide a means of harnessing this anti-inflammatory/analgesic benefit without dysphoria or euphoria, dependence, etc. [77]. At least one peripheral KOR agonist (CR845) at the time of this writing is in clinical trial investigating safety and efficacy of the intravenous form in postoperative pain (https://clinicaltrials.gov/ct2/show/NCT02542384); a recent trial investigating safety and efficacy of the oral form in hip and knee osteoarthritis has been completed but not yet reported on (https://clinicaltrials.gov/ct2/show/NCT02524197).

Peripheral delta-opioid receptor (DOR) agonists have not shown much analgesic efficacy in isolation; however, joint DOR-MOR agonism in the periphery has been shown to exert analgesic effects in non-inflamed states in rats [78].

Atypical Strategies

Several approaches to developing novel agents with reduced or even absent abuse and adverse effect liability are being pursued. This quest is not new, and historic efforts have been nicely documented in Corbett et al.'s 2006 review [79]. Recent advances in the understanding of the complex activities and interactions of the endogenous opioid system with other physiologic systems will undoubtedly facilitate new and safer means of harnessing and isolating the analgesic properties of this ubiquitous and dynamic ligand-receptor family. It should be kept in mind that one of many limitations of most "bench-level" research in this area is the consistent difference in interspecies response to many ligands or modifiers [80]. Clinical experience also demonstrates even within the smallest sample size that among humans, profoundly different responses are common. These issues of course necessitate and underlie the clinical trial system. Some current areas of exploration include:

- Enkephalinase inhibitors
- Endomorphin analogs
- Nociceptin/orphanin FQ receptor (NOR) ligands
- Other G-protein-coupled receptor (GPCR) manipulations
- Heteromeric ligands
- Glial modifiers

Enkephalinase Inhibitors

Enkephalin analogs have not found clinical application to date for various reasons as discussed in Chap. 2. Part of the reason the enkephalin/DOR system has received little clinical attention is the fact that the natural ligand possesses an extremely short half-life/duration of action and thus has little utility in its natural state. For many years, efforts to harness this system have focused on inhibiting their degradation by enkephalinases [81] but have been hampered for the most part by limited to no oral activity. Within the past decade however, *dual enkephalinase inhibitors (DENKIs)* which are a heterogeneous group of compounds designed to block the activity of membrane-bound peptidases (neprilysin/neutral endopeptidase and aminopeptidase N) have been engineered to increase oral bioavailability and show significant analgesic effect in various pain models in various species [82]. DENKI prodrugs have also recently been described that have even greater oral bioavailability and duration of action and show promising effect in animal models with essentially no adverse effects [83] as respiratory depression, euphoria, etc. are not mediated by DOR either centrally nor in the periphery. Seizures, one of the more concerning adverse effects of earlier synthetic DOR agonists, have not been reported with DENKIs either.

Endomorphin Analogs

Endomorphins (described in greater detail in Chap. 2) are tremendously MOR-specific and display significant analgesic effect. Interestingly, despite their high affinity and efficacy at the MOR, they confer markedly less respiratory depression at equianalgesic doses to other MOR agonists [84]. They are not, however, devoid of reward/reinforcing properties and thus may still possess abuse liability [24].

Zadina's (the scientist who discovered endomorphins) group at Tulane is developing endomorphin analogs demonstrating greater analgesia and reduced sedation/psychomotor effect, respiratory depression, tolerance, and reward/reinforcing behavior compared to morphine. Differential effects on glial activation are one mechanism postulated to account for this improvement in efficacy: adverse effect ratio [85].

Targeting the N/OFQ Receptor

Despite initial characterization of the N/OFQ receptor (NOR) as facilitating pronociceptive activity, it has become clear that the activity of this receptor and its ligands is exceedingly complex, as described in greater detail in Chap. 2, and includes antinociceptive activity as well. NOR ligands have been developed and demonstrated to exert analgesic effects in primates in various pain models, without respiratory depression or reward/reinforcement behavior [80, 86].

Other GPCR Manipulations

Yet another novel approach to virulence attenuation is that of "manipulating" the receptor, selecting desired effects (i.e., analgesia), and eliminating undesired/adverse effects. One proposed solution utilizing this sort of functional selectivity is the development of agents that interact with the GPCR (practically speaking the

MOR) in "biased agonism" whereby the ligand will activate and stabilize the receptor in a conformational state favoring certain downstream/intracellular signaling activity (e.g., G-protein-mediated adenylate cyclase activity) at the expense of other signaling (e.g., β-arrestin 2 activity). Evidence from animal models (i.e., β-arrestin 2 knockout mice) suggests that such biased agonism may confer improved analgesic efficacy with reduced adverse effects [87–89].

Another, more directly "manipulative" approach that has actually made significantly more headway developmentally is that of employing "allosteric modifiers" at the MOR to select for desired effects. An allosteric modifier is one that binds to a site on the receptor distinct from the (orthosteric) site where the "main" ligand is, e.g., opioid binds. Such modifiers may exert positive or negative modulation on the ability of the orthosteric agonist to bind to/exert effect on the receptor; the term "positive allosteric modulator" (PAM) is currently being used in the literature to describe the former. PAMs may confer synergistic effect if administered with opioid agents or may be used solely and independently to facilitate and amplify the effect of endogenous ligands [89] and have been isolated and are under investigation. It may be that these PAMs are binding to the intracellular G-protein site and effecting G-protein activity at the expense of β-arrestin 2 activity, in essence effecting biased agonism by the orthosteric ligand as described above.

Heteromeric Ligands

As discussed in Chap. 2, there is increasing evidence that opioid receptors are capable of joining into multimers with homologous receptors, other opioid receptors, or other GPCR, with subsequent variance in ligand binding, receptor signaling, and trafficking properties [90–94]. Differential effects including improved analgesia and reduced adverse effects have been described by some investigators, while increased adverse effects have been described by others. MOR-DOR heteromerization has been the most extensively investigated pairing, and a heterogeneous group of ligands have been developed to interact with this heteromer in hopes of producing novel opioid agonists with reduced adverse effects. Different ligands appear capable of eliciting various functional selectivity (e.g., G-protein signaling at the expense of β-arrestin signaling) and also of serving as allosteric modulators [94].

Blocking Opioid-Induced Glial Activation

Opioid exposure (and chronic, especially neuropathic pain states) cumulatively increases glial activation resulting in a number of undesirable effects including pronociception and pain sensitization and tolerance to/reduced analgesic efficacy of the drug [95]. There is some evidence that even opioid reward/reinforcement is mediated in part by glia [95–97]. These effects are mediated primarily by the Toll-like receptor (TLR) family; TLR4 has been extensively studied as the key player in opioid glial activation. TLR4 blockade and other suppressions of glial activation by a variety of structurally and mechanistically different means have been shown in animal studies to enhance opioid analgesia: adverse effect ratios and also palliate opioid withdrawal symptoms; there is also evidence that opioid reward/reinforcement properties are attenuated as well [97–100]. These interesting directions await human investigation.

Summary

One strategy in addressing the opioid epidemic is to decrease or attenuate the "virulence" of the agent, i.e., render opioids less "pathogenic." Historic approaches to such attenuation have largely focused on altering existing and commercially available drugs by converting them to an extended-release form and equipping them with tamper-resistant and abuse-deterrent properties. While certainly not without merit, these approaches cannot prevent misuse or abuse by excessive consumption and do not alter the fundamental characteristics of the agent (e.g., propensity to cause euphoria, dependence and addiction, respiratory suppression). They can only affect the delivery of the agent. Novel modifications or alternative strategies using the endogenous opioid system, such as peripheral-only agonists, endogenous ligand protease inhibitors (e.g., dual enkephalinase inhibitors), heteromeric ligands with biased agonism, allosteric modifiers, and agents targeting glia may provide safer analgesics and in effect reduce the population of virulent agents.

References

1. Brannon JR, Hadjifrangiskou M. The arsenal of pathogens and antivirulence therapeutic strategies for disarming them. Drug Des Devel Ther. 2016;10:1795–806.
2. Heras B, Scanlon MJ, Martin JL. Targeting virulence not viability in the search for future antibacterials. Br J Clin Pharmacol. 2015;79:208–15.
3. Blaser MJ. The microbiome revolution. J Clin Invest. 2014;124:4162–5.
4. Volkow ND. Prescription opioid and heroin abuse. Presentation to the house committee on energy and commerce subcommittee on oversight and investigations. 2014. Available from: https://www.drugabuse.gov/about-nida/legislative-activities/testimony-to-congress/2015/prescription-opioid-heroin-abuse.e.
5. Pirofski A, Casadevall A. Q and a what is a pathogen? A question that begs the point. BMC Biol. 2012;10:6.
6. Fields HL, Margolis EB. Understanding opioid reward. Trends Neurosci. 2015;38:217–25.
7. Clark DL, Boutros NN, Mendez MF. The brain and behavior: an introduction to behavioral neuroanatomy. 3rd ed. New York: Cambridge University Press; 2010.
8. Arias-Carrión O, Stamelou M, Murillo-Rodríguez E, Menéndez-González M, Pöppel E. Dopaminergic reward system: a short integrative review. Int Arch Med. 2010;3:24.
9. Wise RA, Gardner EL. Functional anatomy of substance-related disorders. In: D'haenen H, den Boer JA, Willner P, editors. Biological psychiatry. New York: Wiley; 2002. p. 509–22.

10. Corbett D, Wise RA. Intracranial self-stimulation in relation to the ascending dopaminergic systems of the midbrain: a moveable electrode mapping study. Brain Res. 1980;185:1–15.
11. Wise RA, Bozarth MA. Action of drugs of abuse on brain reward systems: an update with specific attention to opiates. Pharmacol Biochem Behav. 1982;17:239–43.
12. Bozarth MA, Wise RA. Neural substrates of opiate reinforcement. Prog Neuro-Psychopharmacol Biol Psychiatry. 1983;7(4–6):569–75.
13. Gardner EL. Introduction: addiction and brain reward and anti-reward pathways. Adv Psychosom Med. 2011;30:22–60.
14. Schechter MD, Meechan SM. Conditioned place aversion produced by dopamine release inhibition. Eur J Pharmacol. 1994;260:133–7.
15. Shippenberg TS, Bals-Kubik R, Huber A, Herz A. Neuroanatomical substrates mediating the aversive effects of D-1dopamine receptor antagonists. Psychopharmacology. 1991;103:209–14.
16. Gruber SA, Silveri MM, Yurgelun-Todd DA. Neuropsychological consequences of opiate use. Neuropsychol Rev. 2007;17:299–315.
17. Le Merrer J, Becker JA, Befort K, Kieffer BL. Reward processing by the opioid system in the brain. Physiol Rev. 2009;89:1379–412.
18. Ting-A-Kee R, van der Kooy D. The neurobiology of opiate motivation. Cold Spring Harb Perspect Med. 2012;2:a012096.
19. Britt MD, Wise RA. Ventral tegmental site of opiate reward: antagonism by a hydrophilic opiate receptor blocker. Brain Res. 1983;258:105–8.
20. Wise RA. Opiate reward: sites and substrates. Neurosci Biobehav Rev. 1989;13:129–33.
21. Olmstead MC, Franklin KB. The development of a conditioned place preference to morphine: effects of microinjections into various CNS sites. Behav Neurosci. 1997;111:1324–34.
22. McBride WJ, Murphy JM, Ikemoto S. Localization of brain reinforcement mechanisms: intracranial self-administration and intracranial place-conditioning studies. Behav Brain Res. 1999;101:129–52.
23. Bozarth MA, Wise RA. Intracranial self-administration of morphine into the ventral tegmental area in rats. Life Sci. 1981;28:551–5.
24. Zangen A, Ikemoto S, Zadina JE, Wise RA. Rewarding and psychomotor stimulant effects of endomorphin-1: anteroposterior differences within the ventral tegmental area and lack of effect in nucleus accumbens. J Neurosci. 2002;22:7225–33.
25. Zhang Y, Landthaler M, Schlussman SD, Yuferov V, Ho A, Tuschl T, et al. Mu opioid receptor knockdown in the substantia nigra/ventral tegmental area by synthetic small interfering RNA blocks the rewarding and locomotor effects of heroin. Neuroscience. 2009;158:474–83.
26. Gysling K, Wang RY. Morphine-induced activation of A10 dopamine neurons in the rat. Brain Res. 1983;277:119–27.
27. Johnson SW, North RA. Opioids excite dopamine neurons by hyperpolarization of local interneurons. J Neurosci. 1992;12:483–8.
28. Bozarth MA, Wise RA. Heroin reward is dependent on a dopaminergic substrate. Life Sci. 1981;29:1881–6.
29. Wise RA. Neurobiology of addiction. Curr Opin Neurobiol. 1996;6:243–51.
30. Ford CP, Mark GP, Williams JT. Properties and opioid inhibition of mesolimbic dopamine neurons vary according to target location. J Neurosci. 2006;26:2788–97.
31. Devine DP, Leone P, Wise RA. Mesolimbic dopamine neurotransmission is increased by administration of mu-opioid receptor antagonists. Eur J Pharmacol. 1993;243:55–64.
32. Shippenberg TS, Bals-Kubik R. Involvement of the mesolimbic dopamine system in mediating the aversive effects of opioid antagonists in the rat. Behav Pharmacol. 1995;6:99–106.
33. Bechara A, van der Kooy D. A single brain stem substrate mediates the motivational effects of both opiates and food in nondeprived rats but not in deprived rats. Behav Neurosci. 1992;106:351–63.

34. Olmstead MC, Munn EM, Franklin KB, Wise RA. Effects of pedunculopontine tegmental nucleus lesions on responding for intravenous heroin under different schedules of reinforcement. J Neurosci. 1998;18:5035–44.
35. Laviolette SR, Gallegos RA, Henriksen SJ, van der Kooy D. Opiate state controls bi-directional reward signaling via $GABA_A$ receptors in the ventral tegmental area. Nat Neurosci. 2004;7:160–9.
36. Hnasko TS, Sotak BN, Palmiter RD. Morphine reward in dopamine-deficient mice. Nature. 2005;438:854–7.
37. Nader K, van der Kooy D. Deprivation state switches the neurobiological substrates mediating opiate reward in the ventral tegmental area. J Neurosci. 1997;17:383–90.
38. Tecuapetla F, Patel JC, Xenias H, English D, Tadros I, Shah F, et al. Glutamatergic signaling by mesolimbic dopamine neurons in the nucleus accumbens. J Neurosci. 2010;30:7105–10.
39. Gorelova N, Mulholland PJ, Chandler LJ, Seamans JK. The glutamatergic component of the mesocortical pathway emanating from different subregions of the ventral midbrain. Cereb Cortex. 2012;22:327–36.
40. Root DH, Mejias-Aponte CA, Zhang S, Wang HL, Hoffman AF, Lupica CR, et al. Single rodent mesohabenular axons release glutamate and GABA. Nat Neurosci. 2014;17:1543–51.
41. Brennan MJ. Update on prescription extended-release opioids and appropriate patient selection. J Multidiscip Healthc. 2013;6:265–80.
42. Miller M, Barber CW, Leatherman S, Fonda J, Hermos JA, Cho K, et al. Prescription opioid duration of action and the risk of unintentional overdose among patients receiving opioid therapy. JAMA Intern Med. 2015;175:608–15.
43. Ray WA, Chung CP, Murray KT, Hall K, Stein CM. Prescription of long-acting opioids and mortality in patients with chronic noncancer pain. JAMA. 2016;315:2415–23.
44. Busto U, Sellers EM. Pharmacokinetic determinants of drug abuse and dependence. A conceptual perspective. Clin Pharmacokinet. 1986;11:144–53.
45. Farré M, Camí J. Pharmacokinetic considerations in abuse liability evaluation. Br J Addict. 1991;86:1601–6.
46. Comer SD, Ashworth JB, Sullivan MA, Vosburg SK, Saccone PA, Foltin RW. Relationship between rate of infusion and reinforcing strength of oxycodone in humans. J Opioid Manag. 2009;5:203–12.
47. Butler SF, Fernandez KC, Chang A, Benoit C, Morey LC, Black R, et al. Measuring attractiveness for abuse of prescription opioids. Pain Med. 2010;11:67–80.
48. Allain F, Minogianis EA, Roberts DC, Samaha AN. How fast and how often: the pharmacokinetics of drug use are decisive in addiction. Neurosci Biobehav Rev. 2015;56:166–79.
49. McCarberg BH, Barkin RL. Long-acting opioids for chronic pain: pharmacotherapeutic opportunities to enhance compliance, quality of life, and analgesia. Am J Ther. 2001;8:181–6.
50. Manchikanti L, Manchukonda R, Pampati V, Damron KS. Evaluation of abuse of prescription and illicit drugs in chronic pain patients receiving short-acting (hydrocodone) or long-acting (methadone) opioids. Pain Physician. 2005;8(3):257–61.
51. Wilsey BL, Fishman S, Li CS, Storment J, Albanese A. Markers of abuse liability of short-vs long acting opioids in chronic pain patients: a randomized cross-over trial. Pharmacol Biochem Behav. 2009;94:98–107.
52. Morrell A. The oxycontin clan: The $14 billion newcomer to Forbes 2015 list of richest U.S. families. Forbes Magazine, 1 Jul 2015. Available from http://www.forbes.com/sites/alexmorrell/2015/07/01/the-oxycontin-clan-the-14-billion-newcomer-to-forbes-2015-list-of-richest-u-s-families/#3b403fecc0e2.
53. Coplan PM, Kale H, Sandstrom L, Landau C, Chilcoat HD. Changes in oxycodone and heroin exposures in the National Poison Data System after introduction of extended-release oxycodone with abuse-deterrent characteristics. Pharmacoepidemiol Drug Saf. 2013;22:1274–82.

54. Sessler NE, Downing JM, Kale H, Chilcoat HD, Baumgartner TF, Coplan PM. Reductions in reported deaths following the introduction of extended-release oxycodone (OxyContin) with an abuse-deterrent formulation. Pharmacoepidemiol Drug Saf. 2014;23:1238–46.
55. U.S. Department of Health and Human Services Food and Drug Administration Center for Drug Evaluation and Research (CDER), Clinical Medical. Abuse-deterrent opioids—evaluation and labeling guidance for industry. Silver Spring, MD: Office of Communications Division of Drug Information; 2015.
56. Gudin JA, Nalamachu SR. An overview of prodrug technology and its application for developing abuse-deterrent opioids. Postgrad Med. 2016;128:97–105.
57. Yaksh TL, Wallace MS. Opioids, analgesia, and pain management. In: Brunton L, editor. Goodman and Gilman's pharmacologic basis of therapeutics. New York: McGraw–Hill; 2011. p. 481–525.
58. Lasagna L. Benefit-risk ratio of agonist-antagonist analgesics. Drug Alcohol Depend. 1987;20:385–93.
59. Hanks GW. The clinical usefulness of agonist-antagonistic opioid analgesics in chronic pain. Drug Alcohol Depend. 1987;20:339–46.
60. Hoskin PJ, Hanks GW. Opioid agonist-antagonist drugs in acute and chronic pain states. Drugs. 1991;41:326–44.
61. Ohlsen RI, Pilowsky LS. The place of partial agonism in psychiatry: recent developments. J Psychopharmacol. 2005;19:408–13.
62. Helm S, Trescot AM, Colson J, Sehgal N, Silverman S. Opioid antagonists, partial agonists, and agonists/antagonists: the role of office-based detoxification. Pain Physician. 2008;11:225–35.
63. Bodkin JA, Zornberg GL, Lukas SE, Cole JO. Buprenorphine treatment of refractory depression. J Clin Psychopharmacol. 1995;15(1):49–57.
64. Karp JF, Butters MA, Begley AE, Miller MD, Lenze EJ, Blumberger DM, et al. Safety, tolerability, and clinical effect of low-dose buprenorphine for treatment-resistant depression in midlife and older adults. J Clin Psychiatry. 2014;75(8):e785–93. doi:10.4088/JCP.13m08725.
65. Bai SA, Xiang Q, Finn A. Evaluation of the pharmacokinetics of single- and multiple-dose buprenorphine Buccal film in healthy volunteers. Clin Ther. 2016;38:358–69.
66. Yassen A, Olofsen E, van Dorp E, Sarton E, Teppema L, Danhof M, et al. Mechanism-based pharmacokinetic-pharmacodynamic modelling of the reversal of buprenorphine-induced respiratory depression by naloxone: a study in healthy volunteers. Clin Pharmacokinet. 2007;46:965–80.
67. Walker JS. Anti-inflammatory effects of opioids. Adv Exp Med Biol. 2003;521:148–60.
68. Sehgal N, Smith HS, Manchikanti L. Peripherally acting opioids and clinical implications for pain control. Pain Physician. 2011;14:249–58.
69. Vadivelu N, Mitra S, Hines RL. Peripheral opioid receptor agonists for analgesia: a comprehensive review. J Opioid Manag. 2011;7:55–68.
70. Zöllner C, Shaqura MA, Bopaiah CP, Mousa S, Stein C, Schafer M. Painful inflammation-induced increase in mu-opioid receptor binding and G-protein coupling in primary afferent neurons. Mol Pharmacol. 2003;64:202–10.
71. Philippe D, Chakass D, Thuru X, Zerbib P, Tsicopoulos A, Geboes K, et al. Mu opioid receptor expression is increased in inflammatory bowel diseases: implications for homeostatic intestinal inflammation. Gut. 2006;55:815–23.
72. Nunéz S, Lee JS, Zhang Y, Bai G, Ro JY. Role of peripheral mu-opioid receptors in inflammatory orofacial muscle pain. Neuroscience. 2007;146:1346–54.
73. Menéndez L, Lastra A, Meana A, Hidalgo A, Baamonde A. Analgesic effects of loperamide in bone cancer pain in mice. Pharmacol Biochem Behav. 2005;81:114–21.
74. Chung C, Carteret AF, McKelvy AD, Ringkamp M, Yang F, Hartke T, et al. Analgesic properties of loperamide differ following systemic and local administration to rats after spinal nerve injury. Eur J Pain. 2012;16:1021–32.

75. Khalefa BI, Shaqura M, Al-Khrasani M, Fürst S, Mousa SA, Schäfer M. Relative contributions of peripheral versus supraspinal or spinal opioid receptors to the antinociception of systemic opioids. Eur J Pain. 2012;16:690–705.
76. Rivière PJ-M. Peripheral kappa-opioid agonists for visceral pain. Brit J Pharmacol. 2004;141:1331–4.
77. Albert-Vartanian A, Boyd MR, Hall AL, Morgado SJ, Nguyen E, Nguyen VP, et al. Will peripherally restricted kappa-opioid receptor agonists (pKORAs) relieve pain with less opioid adverse effects and abuse potential? J Clin Pharm Ther. 2016;41:371–82.
78. Schramm CL, Honda CN. Co-administration of delta- and mu-opioid receptor agonists promotes peripheral opioid receptor function. Pain. 2010;151:763–70.
79. Corbett AD, Henderson G, McKnight AT, Paterson SJ. 75 years of opioid research: the exciting but vain quest for the holy grail. Brit J Pharmacol. 2006;147(Suppl 1):S153–62.
80. Lin AP, Ko M-C. The therapeutic potential of nociceptin/orphanin FQ receptor agonists as analgesics without abuse liability. ACS Chem Neurosci. 2013;4:214–24.
81. Thanawala V, Kadam VJ, Ghosh R. Enkephalinase inhibitors: potential agents for the management of pain. Curr Drug Targets. 2008;9:887–94.
82. Poras H, Bonnard E, Dangé E, Fournié-Zaluski MC, Roques BP. New orally active dual enkephalinase inhibitors (DENKIs) for central and peripheral pain treatment. J Med Chem. 2014;57:5748–63.
83. Bonnard E, Poras H, Nadal X, Maldonado R, Fournié-Zaluski M-C, Roques BP. Long-lasting oral analgesic effects of *N*-protected aminophosphinic dual enkephalinase inhibitors (DENKIs) in peripherally controlled pain. Pharmacol Res Perspect. 2015;3(2):e00116. doi:10.1002/prp2.116.
84. Zadina JE. Isolation and distribution of endomorphins in the central nervous system. Japan J Pharmacol. 2002;89:203–8.
85. Zadina JE, Nilges MR, Morgenweck J, Zhang X, Hackler L, Fasold MB. Endomorphin analog analgesics with reduced abuse liability, respiratory depression, motor impairment, tolerance, and glial activation relative to morphine. Neuropharmacology. 2016;105:215–27.
86. Zaveri NT. Nociceptin opioid receptor (NOP) as a therapeutic target: progress in translation from preclinical research to clinical utility. J Med Chem. 2016;59(15):7011–28. doi:10.1021/acs.jmedchem.5b01499.
87. Walwyn WM, Miottob KA, Evans CJ. Opioid pharmaceuticals and addiction: the issues, and research directions seeking solutions. Drug Alcohol Depend. 2010;108:156–65.
88. Thompson GL, Kelly E, Christopoulos A, Canals M. Novel GPCR paradigms at the mu-opioid receptor. Brit J Pharmacol. 2015;172:287–96.
89. Burford NT, Traynor JR, Alt A. Positive allosteric modifiers of the mu-opioid receptor: a novel approach for future pain medications. Brit J Pharmacol. 2015;172:277–86.
90. Van Rijn RM, Whistler JL, Waldhoer M. Novel pharmaco-types and trafficking-types induced by opioid receptor heteromerization. Curr Opin Pharmacol. 2010;10(1):73–9.
91. Al-Hasani R, Bruchas MR. Molecular mechanisms of opioid receptor-dependent signaling and behavior. Anesthesiology. 2011;115(6):1363–81.
92. Costantino CM, Gomes I, Stockton SD, Lim MP, Devi LA. Opioid receptor heteromers in analgesia. Expert Rev. Mol Med. 2012;14:e9. doi:10.1017/erm.2012.5.
93. Fujita W, Gomes I, Devi LA. Revolution in GPCR signalling: opioid receptor heteromers as novel therapeutic targets: IUPHAR review 10. Brit J Pharmacol. 2014;171(18):4155–76.
94. Fujita W, Gomes I, Devi LA. Heteromers of μ-δ opioid receptors: new pharmacology and novel therapeutic possibilities. Brit J Pharmacol. 2015;172(2):375–87.
95. Hutchinson MR, Bland ST, Johnson KW, Rice KC, Maier SF, Watkins LR. Opioid-induced glial activation: mechanisms of activation and implications for opioid analgesia, dependence, and reward. ScientificWorldJournal. 2007;7:98–111.
96. Watkins LR, Hutchinson MR, Rice KC, Maier SF. The "toll" of opioid-induced glial activation: improving the clinical efficacy of opioids by targeting glia. Trends Pharmacol Sci. 2009;30:581–91.

97. Bland ST, Hutchinson MR, Maier SF, Watkins LR, Johnson KW. The glial activation inhibitor AV411 reduces morphine-induced nucleus accumbens dopamine release. Brain Behav Immun. 2009;23:492–7.
98. Hutchinson MR, Lewis SS, Coats BD, Skyba DA, Crysdale NY, Berkelhammer DL, et al. Reduction of opioid withdrawal and potentiation of acute opioid analgesia by systemic AV411 (ibudilast). Brain Behav Immun. 2009;23:240–50.
99. Eidson LN, Murphy AZ. Blockade of toll-like receptor 4 attenuates morphine tolerance and facilitates the pain relieving properties of morphine. J Neurosci. 2013;33(40):15952–63.
100. Han Y, Jiang C, Tang J, Wang C, Wu P, Zhang G, et al. Resveratrol reduces morphine tolerance by inhibiting microglial activation via AMPK signalling. Eur J Pain. 2014;18:1458–70.

Part III
Focusing on the Vector

"Skepticism is as much the result of knowledge, as knowledge is of skepticism. To be content with what we at present know, is, for the most part, to shut our ears against conviction; since, from the very gradual character of our education, we must continually forget, and emancipate ourselves from, knowledge previously acquired; we must set aside old notions and embrace fresh ones; and, as we learn, we must be daily unlearning something which it has cost us no small labour and anxiety to acquire."

-- Homer, *The Iliad*

Chapter 6
Best Practices Education, Part I: Pain Physiology, Psychology, and Alternatives to Opioids

A gynecologist colleague requests that a thoracic epidural catheter be placed for perioperative pain management for a planned laparoscopic supracervical hysterectomy for a 32-year-old female suffering from intractable chronic pelvic pain thought to be caused by endometriosis which was diagnosed via prior laparoscopy. Thinking this an unusual request (epidurals are typically reserved for more painful operations with large incisions and especially supraumbilical incisions which may compromise diaphragmatic excursion by respiratory splinting), you probe for a little more detail. Your colleague simply says, "just go see her in Bay 4."

When you arrive to assess the patient, there are concerned family members surrounding the bed of a somnolent and dysphoric young woman with pinpoint pupils. Upon further questioning, you ascertain that she has seen multiple physicians for complaints of chronic pelvic pain and was initially started on opioid therapy by her primary care physician who subsequently referred her to a local pain management clinic who has escalated her regimen to extended-release morphine sulfate 120 mg twice a day and hydrocodone-acetaminophen 10 mg/325 mg six per day. She is also using alprazolam as an anxiolytic and carisoprodol as a "muscle relaxant."

After further evaluation and discussion, you agree to place a thoracic epidural catheter which is used to provide preemptive analgesia prior to incision and continued via infusion for the next 3 days while she is in the hospital. During this time, you also provide a morphine PCA with no basal rate and a

H.B. McAnally, *Opioid Dependence*, DOI 10.1007/978-3-319-47497-7_6

total hourly lockout rate at 16 mg/h for the first day, transitioning to Percocet p.o. the second day when she is taking solids. Scheduled lorazepam and clonidine are also provided. She denies any abdominopelvic pain and consistently evidences bilateral sensory block from roughly T6 to L2 levels with an epidural infusion of ropivacaine. She suffers mild opioid withdrawal symptoms primarily consisting of tachycardia and some agitation during the first 2 days, but by the third day, she displays a dramatically improved mental status and bright affect and expresses gratitude for your care.

Two weeks later when you follow up with her by telephone, she is excited to report that she destroyed her remaining opioids at home and vows "never to take that stuff again!" She is also excited to report that she has a job interview.

Introduction

Transmission of an infectious agent frequently requires a vector, which entity serves as a reservoir for the agent, either symptomatically or asymptomatically. Common examples include anopheles mosquitoes carrying *Plasmodium falciparum* or deer ticks harboring *Borrelia burgdorferi*. Unique among epidemics to date, this agent (opioids) is "transmitted" primarily by those to whom the well-being of the individual and also the community is entrusted. As such, a thorough understanding of opioids is essential for every prescriber, and so we began with basic opioid biology and pharmacology in Chaps. 2, 3, and 4. Knowing *about* the drugs is not enough however; the prescriber must know *why*, *when*, and *how* to use them and, perhaps of greater importance, *when not to*. These specific questions are addressed in the two chapters that follow.

Altering "transmission" of opioids via professional vectors is a laborious but not insurmountable task. Recent intensive provider educational and regulatory approaches (discussed in Chaps. 7 and 8) have begun to show a temporal association at least with reduction in opioid prescribing and possibly in some morbidity and mortality outcome measures as well. There has in fact been a shift noticed by emergency department physicians and law enforcement within the past couple years toward "street" opioids such as heroin, as the procurement of prescription drugs obtained illicitly is becoming more difficult. (While it is within the realm of responsibility of the physician to educate and treat patients who abuse street drugs, controlling the transmission of such remains the responsibility of law enforcement and as such is not discussed in this book.) At any rate, the often-quoted analogy of a pendulum swinging back and forth between poles of liberal vs. conservative prescription of opioids for pain seems to be traversing back toward the guarded at present. While this undoubtedly represents a public health triumph in many regards, with reductions in morbidity and mortality, it must not be forgotten that in the majority of cases, opioid-dependent individuals suffer from various predisposing chronic pain states.

In the United States, the prevalence of chronic pain has been estimated at 100 million individuals [1]. This of course ranges from aggravating single-limb osteoarthritic pain and dysfunction to global, entire-body states of agony. Associated disability which also varies tremendously among persons with the same apparent pathology further adds to the misery of the individual and often the family and in some cases society as well. As the preface to the Institute of Medicine's (IOM) landmark 2011 monograph, "Relieving Pain in America" states:

> The magnitude of the pain suffered by individuals and the associated costs constitute a crisis for America, both human and economic…. [1]

To underscore the seriousness of the issue, if empathy for suffering is not enough, it should be noted by all practitioners of every healthcare discipline that suicide is two to three times more prevalent in the chronic pain population than the general population [2, 3].

As physicians, we are ethically and professionally responsible to alleviate pain and suffering whenever possible. Understanding the multifaceted nature of both pain and suffering (biopsychosocial-spiritual) is essential to accurate assessment and thus effective treatment. Unfortunately, the training of most physicians and mid-level providers is sadly lacking in at least one of these dimensions, and these deficits have been highlighted recently as a major issue requiring educational and even certification-oriented overhaul [4]. To quote the IOM report again:

> Many health care providers lack a comprehensive perspective on pain… We believe pain arises in the nervous system but represents a complex and evolving interplay of biological, behavioral, environmental, and societal factors that go beyond simple explanation. Knowledge of pain needs to be enriched from the molecular and genetic to the cellular, neural network, and systems levels. It is necessary to understand how the settings and surroundings in which pain occurs and is experienced have an impact on its biology. [1]

The recently unveiled National Pain Strategy [4] emphasizes as one of its core foci the remediation of what comprises a substantial deficit in provider knowledge and competency of how pain works and how to treat it.

This chapter is divided into two main components: first is a basic primer on pain physiology and pathophysiology and psychology. It is certainly not intended to serve as an exhaustive treatise on the subject; for more complete sources, the reader is referred to the excellent textbooks by Wall and Melzack [5], Bonica [6], and Deer [7], among others. Physical pain has classically been held to be a cardinal symptom of inflammation and many other disease processes; while many champion the notion that chronic pain is a disease in its own right [1], it remains evident that pain is always a symptom. As such, any complaint of pain requires thoughtful history taking and physical examination (both of which in themselves are often therapeutic for patients whose complaints have not been addressed to their satisfaction), frequently the formulation of a differential diagnosis, and then frank discussion about natural history and therapeutic options.

The second half of the chapter focuses on multimodal pain therapy—alternatives to opioids. Prevention (discussed in greater detail in Chap. 11) must undergird every effort of the physician to help the patient complaining of pain. Poor dietary choices, tobacco and alcohol use, sleep deprivation, sedentary lifestyle, and many other physical insults are in many cases contributory if not causative of a great many pain states. Psychological dysfunctions (including anxiety and stress, cognitive distortions, and deeper underlying emotional wounds) often amplify—if not initiate—chronic pain. A proper viewpoint on the spirituality of the individual and how that spirituality relates to their pain experience is essential to treating the whole person. Concurrent with efforts aimed addressing these issues, rational treatment must apply (or at least offer) interventions that maximize the benefit-risk ratio not only for the individual intervention in question but for the entire treatment plan, whether or not opioids are part of that plan.

Pain Basic Science Primer

Before briefly discussing common therapeutic modalities for treating pain, it is important to take a step back and examine what we think we know about pain. Everyone knows what pain is, but no one can fully explain it. Definitions are generally circular ("It hurts!"). The following International Association for the Study of Pain (IASP) definition of pain seems excessively vague at first glance but, as we will see shortly, is of necessity very nonspecific:

> An unpleasant sensory and emotional experience associated with actual or potential tissue damage, or described in terms of such damage. [8]

Nociception and the Cartesian Model

As with most scientific ideas, the conceptualization of what pain is has undergone numerous paradigm revolutions since the Renaissance. In 1664 Rene Descartes proposed that pain may have more to do with physical stimulus and cerebral perception than prior constructs based on metaphysical, spiritual/moral, or other ethereal factors (Fig. 6.1). The basic assumption that insult to the physical integrity of the organism is transmitted and translated into the subjective experience of pain is so entrenched in our thinking 450 years later that it is difficult for most to conceive of a model of pain that differs much from this. Furthermore, laboratory and clinical investigation have verified and elaborated on the basic injury stimulus-pain response pattern to the point that it is very nearly dogma that if pain is present, i.e., "organic" pathophysiology, tissue damage is responsible for it.

This simplest of frameworks, cause and effect, of course has quite a bit of truth to it. In the conscious patient, *nociception* (the activation of and communication

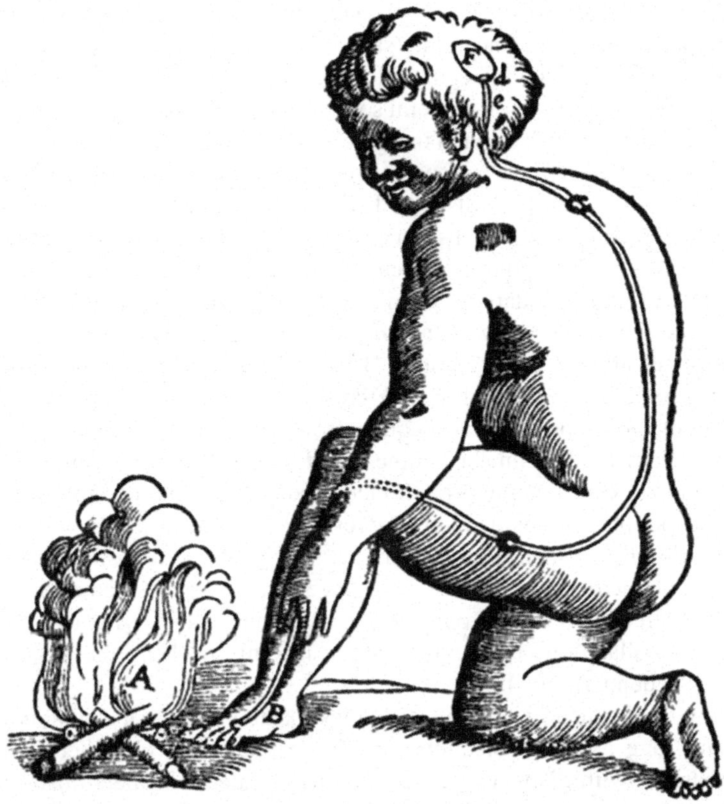

Fig. 6.1 "For example, if the fire A is close to the foot B, the small particles of fire, which as you know move very swiftly, are able to move as well the part of the skin which they touch on the foot. In this way, by pulling at the little thread cc, which you see attached there, they at the same instant open e, which is the entry for the pore d, which is where this small thread terminates; just as, by pulling one end of a cord, you ring a bell which hangs at the other end… Now when the entry of the pore, or the little tube, de, has thus been opened, the animal spirits flow into it from the cavity F, and through it they are carried partly into the muscles which serve to pull the foot back from the fire, partly into those which serve to turn the eyes and the head to look at it, and partly into those which serve to move the hands forward and to turn the whole body for its defense." Descartes' Traité de l'homme, 1664. US Public Domain

from peripheral pain receptors on specialized nerves described in more detail below) is a real and in many cases sufficient cause for the experience of pain, especially acute pain. (The criteria of consciousness applied in the previous sentence are based upon the currently accepted definition of pain as a conscious subjective experience.) Evidence supporting the importance of nociception is consistently found in the operating room when the administration of intravenous opioids or ketamine or institution of conductive nerve block to a sedated/anesthetized patient results in normalization of vital signs and suppression of EEG activity and unconscious aversive behavior. Not to mention, almost everyone has slammed their finger in a car door or stubbed their toe and experienced the (subjective) effect.

Understanding pain should begin with understanding nociception. Somatic nociception, which arises from non-visceral sources, is discussed first; visceral nociception is functionally very similar but more complicated due to richer autonomic communication. *Nociceptors* are specialized receptors on sensory neurons among the Aδ- and C-fiber families (discussed in greater detail below) that generate an afferent action potential in response to a specific noxious stimulus. This process of *transduction* occurs in response to mechanical, thermal, or chemical stimuli generally associated with tissue damage and is initiated by transmembrane cationic channels such as *transient receptor potential* (*TRP*) and tetrodotoxin-resistant or tetrodotoxin-sensitive sodium channels. Besides activation by initial stimulus, nociceptors may be sensitized (with lowered thresholds or in some cases even "awakening" of "silent" nociceptors) by subsequent local inflammatory mediators including arachidonic acid, bradykinin, histamine, serotonin, substance P, calcitonin gene-related peptide (CGRP), nerve growth factor, potassium, hydrogen ions, and other factors. This peripheral sensitization may result in the phenomenon of *hyperalgesia* (pain sensed with less-than-normal stimulus intensity) and *allodynia* (painful perception of a typically non-painful stimulus such as light touch). Besides pain (*dolor*), these mediators elicit other cardinal inflammatory symptoms and signs including vasodilatation and extravasation leading to heat (*calor*), erythema (*rubror*), and edema (*tumor*).

These first-order neurons, with cell bodies located in the paraspinal dorsal root ganglia and long axonal projections to the periphery, are classified as *Aδ-* and *C-fiber* neurons, with distinct roles. Larger, myelinated Aδ fibers (also known as "fast pain fibers") conduct relatively rapidly and provide fairly precise pain localization due to a small receptive field. Sharp, stabbing, acute sensations comprise the message carried by the fast pain fibers. In contrast, unmyelinated C fibers ("slow pain fibers") which outnumber their Aδ counterparts 2:1 conduct much more slowly and confer less precise localization of pain. Slow pain fibers conduct aching, sore, and burning pain. Both sets of afferents enter the dorsal horn of the spinal cord (along with other sensory traffic) either directly or after a one-to-two segment rostrocaudal deviation through *Lissauer's tract* and synapse with their second-order neuron (also known as projection neurons) in specific gray matter regions delineated as the *Rexed laminae*.

Aδ fibers synapse primarily in lamina I (also laminae II, V, and X) and communicate with their projection neurons primarily by means of glutamate. Aspartate is another excitatory neurotransmitter involved in communication between first-order and projection neurons, and multiple other facilitatory (e.g., substance P, CGRP) or inhibitory (e.g., gamma-aminobutyric acid) neurotransmitters are involved in enhancing or suppressing transmission, as discussed in greater detail below. Projection neurons synapsing with the Aδ fibers generally decussate at the level of cord entry and ascend via the *spinothalamic/anterolateral tract* to the thalamus (ventroposterolateral nucleus or VPL). Similarly, primary Aδ afferents from the head and face relay their messages via the trigeminal system, descending in the brainstem to the medullary spinal trigeminal nucleus (nucleus caudalis), synapsing with a second-order neuron that also decussates and joins the spinothalamic tract to ascend to the thalamus (ventroposterior medial nucleus or VPM). From the thalamus, these fast pain pathways project via third-order neurons to the somatosensory cortex and are represented along with other sensory traffic somatotopically on the postcentral gyrus (Fig. 6.2).

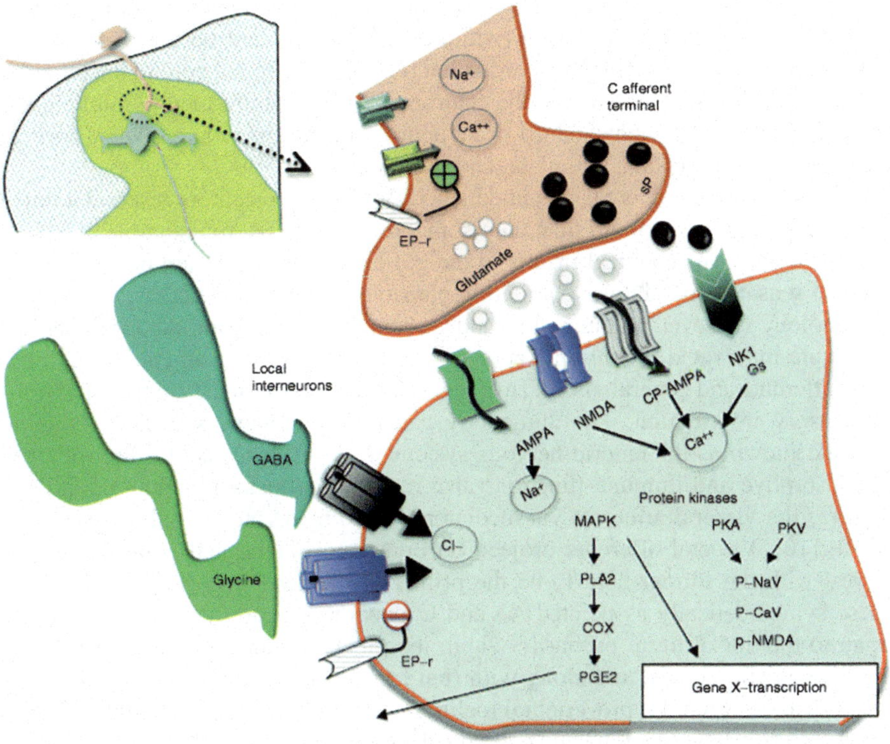

Fig. 6.2 This schematic provides an overview of the organization of the events transpiring at the level of the first-order synapse. (1) As indicated, the presynaptic effects of depolarization lead to opening of voltage-sensitive calcium and sodium channels with increases in intracellular sodium and calcium and mobilization and release of transmitters (*sP* and glutamate). (2) These act upon eponymous receptors (see text), leading to depolarization and increase in intracellular calcium. (3) Activation of kinases which phosphorylate a variety of channels and receptors activates intracellular enzyme cascades such as for PLA2 and increasing gene transcription. (4) Release of products such as prostanoids (*PGE2*) which can act upon the local membrane through their eponymous receptors (*EP-r*) where presynaptically they enhance the opening of voltage-sensitive calcium channels and postsynaptically reduce the activity of glycine receptors. (5). As indicated in addition, the first-order synapse is regulated by inhibitor interneurons such as those release GABA and glycine. These interneurons can be activated by afferent collaterals and by descending pathways to downregulate the excitability of this synapse. Reprinted from Comprehensive Treatment of Chronic Pain by Medical, Interventional, and Integrative Approaches, A Survey of Systems Involved in Nociceptive Processing, 2013, Yaksh TL, Wiese AJ. With permission of Springer

C fibers are a more functionally heterogeneous group than their Aδ counterparts, with a greater diversity of both activating stimuli and output message (see Todd and Koerber's excellent summary of C-fiber biology [9]). They generally synapse in lamina II, also known as the *substantia gelatinosa* (and to a lesser extent in laminae I and V) and communicate primarily with the interneurons that make up the primary population of that lamina, via both substance P and glutamate. Many of their ultimate second-order afferents (especially those in lamina V) are often described as "polymodal" or "wide dynamic range" neurons, indicating their ability to receive sensory messages from multiple input sources besides nociceptors. Some of these projection neurons then decussate (while others do not) and both ascend via the *paleospinothalamic tract* in the anterolateral region of the spinal cord to the reticular formation of the brainstem and to the centromedian and parafascicular intralaminar thalamic nuclei, from whence third-order neurons project to a more diverse cortical audience including insula, cingulate, and frontal cortices.

Visceral nociception is far less understood. Visceral nociceptors respond a much more limited array of stimuli than their somatic counterparts; for example, it is well known that most mechanical insults to the gut including cutting are not perceived. Visceral sensation is relatively limited in physiologic states to detecting distension; in pathology however inflammation and ischemia produce pain. Abdominopelvic organs are innervated by multiple networks including parasympathetic and sympathetic efferents and general visceral afferent (C, Aδ, and Aβ) fibers carrying polymodal sensory information. The alimentary canal also contains a dedicated neural network known as the enteric nervous system, which besides controlling motility and absorptive and immune functions also modulates local inflammation and can sensitize the visceral afferents via mediators including serotonin, substance P, and CGRP [10]. Visceral afferents project via both sympathetic and parasympathetic nerves, with the former held to be the primary pathway for visceral nociception. These sympathetically associated Aδ and C fibers run a tortuous course from the organ to the dorsal horn, primarily within the greater splanchnic, lumbar colonic, and hypogastric nerves, and along with (but in reverse order to) their sympathetic counterparts traverse the prevertebral (celiac, superior, and inferior mesenteric) ganglia and paravertebral ganglia and enter the dorsal ramus via rami communicantes to their cell bodies located in the dorsal root ganglia. From there, the pathway is analogous to that of somatic afferents, entering the dorsal horn and synapsing with a second-order neuron generally in Rexed laminae I, V, or X [11, 12]. The second-order neuron then ascends to the thalamus, in particular the posterolateral nucleus [10]. Visceral afferents also accompany parasympathetic (vagal and pelvic) nerves; these appear to be relatively more important than their sympathetic-associated counterparts in mediating sensory (including nociceptive) information from lower structures including the colorectum, urinary bladder, and genitalia [10]. Finally, recent human and animal evidence also point to a significant dorsal column visceral nociceptive pathway [10] that may be even more important in mediating visceral pain than are spinothalamic or spinoreticular tracts. This pathway has no known somatic correlate, as the dorsal columns mediate only somatic tactile and proprioceptive sense, to our current knowledge.

The distinction between "somatic" vs. "visceral" pain based is especially clinically relevant when evaluating pain in the thorax and abdomen. Abdominal pain, for example, can arise from either internal organs (generally poorly localized and more frequently associated with autonomic phenomena) or from somatic sources such as the abdominal wall or an intercostal nerve (more clearly delineated). The concept of *referred pain* should be addressed briefly as well, which is a phenomenon whereby pain arising from pathology in one region is perceived in a somatically distinct (and sometimes distant) region. Referred pain is most commonly considered as a visceral phenomenon (e.g., right scapular pain with cholecystitis, jaw claudication, and left arm pain with myocardial ischemia); however, a wealth of data and experience indicate that somatic pain generators such as zygapophyseal joints [13] and myofascial trigger points [14] also refer pain elsewhere. Visceral pain referral is thought to occur as the result of convergent or shared pathways between visceral and somatic afferents at the dorsal horn, with some evidence for brain-level convergence as well [15].

While in no way intended to disparage the genius of Descartes and his groundbreaking theories at the time, the caption in Fig. 6.1 is also reproduced from his classic treatise to illustrate the possibility that 400 some years from now, people may look back on our current theories and models as equally quaint.

Neuropathic Pain and Central Sensitization

Neuropathic pain is currently defined by the IASP as "Pain caused by a lesion or disease of the somatosensory nervous system…Neuropathic pain is a clinical description (and not a diagnosis) which requires a demonstrable lesion or a disease that satisfies established neurological diagnostic criteria" [8]. The term "non-nociceptive pain" is often errantly used as a synonym for neuropathic pain; this imprecise nomenclative admixture is discouraged, as much non-nociceptive pain falls outside the realm of objective neurologic pathology.

Neuropathic pain is often characterized by spontaneous and often lancinating pain and multiple other fairly consistent symptoms (e.g., burning sensation, dysesthesias) and signs (e.g., hyperalgesia and allodynia, temporal summation). Neuropathic pain encompasses both well-localized/anatomically defined syndromes such as carpal tunnel syndrome, sciatica, and tic douloureux and more widespread (typically distal extremity) burning pain seen in advanced diabetes, hypothyroidism, vitamin B12 deficiency and with neurotoxicity from alcohol, heavy metals, or chemotherapeutic agents. CNS lesions such as spinal cord or thalamic/cortical lesions may confer even more generalized and devastating pain states. Proposed mechanisms underlying the genesis and perpetuation of neuropathic pain include [16–19]:

- Persistent inflammatory state at the site of the lesion or upstream sites (e.g., dorsal root ganglion) may sensitize/lower the nociceptive threshold of the primary afferent.

- Increased TRP and sodium channel expression on primary afferents, with decreased action potential threshold/increased excitability, and frequently ectopic potential generation.
- Increased adrenoreceptors (α_1 and α_2) with increased sympathetic sensitivity.
- Activation of *N*-methyl-D-aspartate (NMDA) receptors in the dorsal horn leading to "windup" (increasing sensitivity to nonincreasing stimulus intensity) and lowered threshold/tonic activation of secondary afferents.
- Loss of descending inhibition (discussed in greater detail below).
- "Invasion" of Aβ afferents into the Rexed lamina II with normally non-nociceptive primary afferent stimuli now evoking pain (allodynia).
- Recruitment of typically non-nociceptive secondary afferents into a nociceptive state.
- Microglial activation/sensitization with resultant CNS pro-inflammatory effects.

Inherent in this construct is the apparent active and dynamic role that both peripheral and central nervous systems play not only in communicating and interpreting pain but also in amplifying and even generating it. No longer viewed as merely a passive relay from the periphery to the brain, nocineurons (and microglia) are now being seen as effectors and modulators of many if not most chronic pain states. While not included in this primer for the sake of brevity, our growing understanding of the critical role microglia play in the chronification or control of pain is deserving of much greater attention, and the reader is referred to the excellent review by Beggs and Salter [20] and others for an introduction to the topic.

Taking the concept of CNS participation in the pain experience a step further, the phenomenon of *central sensitization* first described by Woolf in 1983 [21] has greatly expanded our understanding of chronic pain. Nociception (and neuropathic pain) is not the full story by any means; non-psychogenic pain can occur in the absence of nociception (or neuropathic pain per IASP definition). Central sensitization provides a plausible explanation for the subjective phenomena of many pain states disproportionate to (even occurring in the absence of) any discernible pathology, along with related features of allodynia. Objective evidence for central sensitization states include changes in functional MRI signal and electrophysiologic parameters (potential amplitudes) [22]. Essentially the theory (with ample animal and human evidence) posits that a reduction in pain threshold has occurred within the CNS such that previously insufficiently noxious or non-noxious stimuli are now painful (hyperalgesia and allodynia, respectively). In Dr. Woolf's words, "The net effect of central sensitization is to recruit previously subthreshold synaptic inputs to nociceptive neurons, generating an increased or augmented action potential output: a state of facilitation, potentiation, augmentation, or amplification" [23]. Proposed mechanisms underlying this state are similar to those presented above for neuropathic pain and include [22, 23]:

- Reduced secondary afferent thresholds
- Reduced inhibition

- Expansion of secondary nocineuron receptive field
- Transformation of secondary nocineurons to wide dynamic range neurons capable of activation by formerly innocuous stimuli
- Glial contributions

Glutamate (via NMDA and other receptors) is currently thought to be the most important protagonist in the development of central sensitization, effecting these pathologic changes via the establishment of supranormal intracellular calcium levels [23]. However, many other familiar factors such as substance P, CGRP, brain-derived neurotrophic factor, bradykinin, and nitric oxide are invoked in facilitating these changes, which may occur in numerous brain structures as well and are not limited to the dorsal horn [23].

Many chronic pain conditions, including migraines, TMJ disorders, fibromyalgia, osteoarthritic and chronic low back pain, interstitial cystitis, and many neuropathic pain states including complex regional pain syndrome (formerly known as reflex sympathetic dystrophy or causalgia) are now thought to represent manifestations of a central sensitized state. Functional abdominal pain, chronic pelvic pain, and other visceral pain states are also now considered to reflect a centrally sensitized state [24].

Cancer Pain

Cancer is frequently associated with severe chronic pain; it is estimated that over 2/3 of patients with advanced cancer suffer from significant pain related to the disease [25]. Multiple pathogenic (and iatrogenic) processes are responsible for the pain associated with cancer, including [26]:

- Local pressure and destruction from the primary tumor
- Release of several inflammatory mediators (including bradykinin, nerve growth factor, proteases, tumor necrosis factor α, various interleukins, and cytokines)
- Peripheral neuronal injury and alterations of the dorsal root ganglion and neo-neurogenesis and neuroma formation with upregulated sodium channels and ectopic activity
- Epidural compression of spinal nerve roots from tumor mass effect (this occurs in up to 10% of cancer patients, and persistent or dramatic back pain complaints require thorough investigation and workup)
- Central sensitization with upregulated NMDA and AMPA activity
- Osteoclastic activity at bone sites, facilitated by the acidic environment generated by cancer cells
- Neuropathy from chemotherapeutic agents (especially vinca alkaloids, the taxanes, and platinum-based compounds)

Neural Plasticity and Chronic Pain

Much recent research has focused on the contribution of neural plasticity to chronic pain, with the former defined by the National Institutes of Health's 2009 Blueprint for Neuroscience Research Workshop as:

> The ability of the nervous system to respond to intrinsic or extrinsic stimuli by reorganizing its structure, function and connections. [27]

While these changes can occur at any level of the CNS including the dorsal horn as introduced above, that which occurs in the brain is the focus of this section. Distortion of size and other geographic perceptions of injured body parts have been documented for centuries, with phantom limb pain perhaps being the most salient example. Reorganization of the primary somatosensory cortex in response to both acute and chronic pain has been shown over the past two decades to underlie these phenomena [28–31], with the recent application of noninvasive imaging modalities demonstrating functional [32–34] and even anatomic changes [35–38] within the brain in various chronic pain states. Fortunately, it has been demonstrated consistently that these distortions and cortical reorganizations can be undone with adequate therapy [39]. A recurring observation with chronification of pain is that of enhanced and in many cases spontaneous activity in the cortical-limbic circuitry [40–42] and in particular the anterior cingulate cortex, which is associated with a significant emotional component [43]; this has led many to conclude that much if not most chronic pain represents a learned state or:

> Persistence of the memory of pain and/or the inability to extinguish the memory of pain evoked by an initial inciting injury. [41]

Perception and Modulation

Arithmetic is necessary in constructing a ledger or a house; however, arithmetic, calculus, astrodynamics, and even general relativity are also required to build a vessel and send it to the Moon or Mars and back. The simple Cartesian model may be sufficient to explain acute nociceptive or even neuropathic pain, but falls quite short of explaining the complexities of most chronic pain and suffering, or why such immense variability in subjective experience exists between people afflicted by identical pathology. Not only can pain occur without nociception (or neuropathic pain); nociception can also occur without pain. In the conscious individual, it is quite clear that intangible and immeasurable factors can override or sufficiently modify the simple physical stimulus-response model of pain, as evidenced by Asian fire walkers, Native American Sun dancers, and elite athletes of all disciplines and regions (Fig. 6.3).

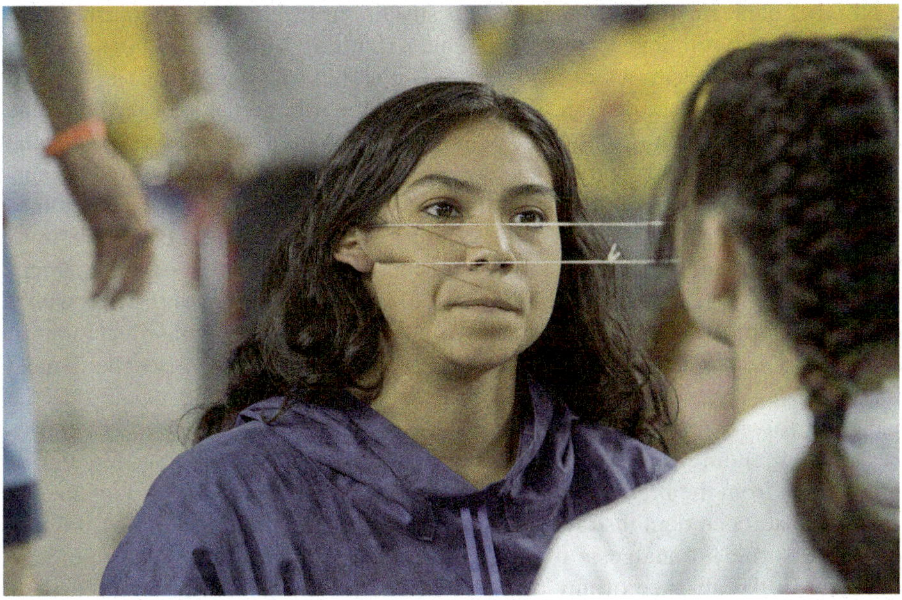

Fig. 6.3 Ear pull at the 2007 World Eskimo Indian Olympics, held in Anchorage, Alaska Reprinted with permission from Patrick Endres, AlaskaPhotoGraphics

Gate Control Theory

Widely regarded as the most seminal work of the twentieth century in understanding pain, Melzack and Wall's landmark 1965 publication [44] described a "gate control system" exerting dynamic and variable influence on synaptic transmission between first- and second-order pain afferents. What have come to be known as interneurons were postulated as assessing and responding to competing inputs from both peripheral non-nociceptive afferents as well as from brain regions to allow or prohibit nociceptive stimuli from proceeding rostrally. The gate control theory expanded our understanding of the role of the central nervous system in processing and even influencing pain. In Dr. Melzack's words, it:

> Forced the medical and biological sciences to accept the brain as an active system that filters, selects and modulates inputs. The dorsal horns, too, were not merely passive transmission stations but sites at which dynamic activities (inhibition, excitation and modulation) occurred. [45]

Prior to our (yet superficial) understanding of the neurobiology of pain, practitioners across the world for millennia have used various means of modifying pain perception with sometimes astounding success (witness the reports of efficacy of mesmerism or acupuncture in facilitating operations without allopathic anesthesia). Dr. Henry Beecher (introduced in Chap. 2) was the first in the modern era of medicine to document and report on the potency of psychological factors in modifying pain. He observed that soldiers sustaining severe wartime injuries were often apparently unmoved by their trauma, exhibiting little pain behavior in the acute and subacute phases of their injury [46]. This was noted to be in marked contradistinction to similar injuries sustained by civilians outside of the war zone and also in sharp contrast to pain behaviors later demonstrated by these same soldiers in response to minor nociceptive stimuli such as venipuncture. He surmised that the profound emotional influences of surviving potentially lethal combat, the knowledge that they would be returning home, and the camaraderie of their fellows, among other factors all contributed to suppression of pain perception [47]. We now understand that these soldiers' stoic responses to what would otherwise typically elicit significant pain response were a manifestation of *descending modulation*. (As a side note, it is fascinating that Dr. Beecher's most important legacy is the placebo-controlled trial, as we now understand that the factors involved in mediating the placebo response are those involved in the process of descending modulation.) By the 1950s, it was evident that descending projections from the brain could modulate afferent traffic [48, 49], and by the late 1960s, it had been demonstrated that focal electrical stimulation of the midbrain produced sufficient analgesia to allow for highly noxious surgical procedures to transpire in the absence of any other anesthetic [50]. This (invasive and experimental) phenomenon has been replicated in humans, allowing preservation of general cognitive as well as motor function while eliminating the perception of pain [51, 52]. Intensive investigation over the subsequent half century has revealed a complex bidirectional (descending and ascending) modulating network that functions to suppress or enhance pain transmission according to a host of competing inputs and the needs of the organism [53, 54]. Teleologically, it makes sense that pain, despite being a vital "sense," must be triaged along with other inputs such as hunger or thirst or the need for sleep. Accordingly, the system may function to augment the pain message when amplification is required for benefit or to dampen the pain message when competing needs (e.g., running from a predator) supersede. Pathologically, the amplification of the system may be seen in many chronic pain states as introduced in the previous section on neuroplastic pain and sensitization. Conversely, enhancement (or simple utilization) of the system's ability to suppress pain may be harnessed therapeutically, as practitioners of spirituality, meditation, exercise, and various healing arts have done throughout recorded history.

From a neurobiologic standpoint, we now have evidence that a vast convergence of input from higher centers including the prefrontal cortex, anterior cingulate cortex, insula, amygdala, and hypothalamus can act to up- or downregulate pain [55]. Our current understanding of the system assigns a primary effector role to the periaqueductal gray (PAG) region of the midbrain and rostroventral medulla (RVM). The PAG-RVM appears to exert its influence primarily via serotonergic and noradrenergic direction of interneurons in the superficial dorsal horn that serve as intermediaries between C-fiber afferents and projection neurons [53, 54]. This, in essence, fulfills the "gate control system" predicted by Melzack and Wall in 1965.

The Biopsychosocial Model and Pain Psychology

The biopsychosocial model, a term coined by George Engel in 1977 [56], was not developed to explain chronic pain, but it has become so axiomatic that no serious (or effective) assessment of chronic pain, let alone treatment attempt, can be made without consideration of the psychological and social (and many believe spiritual) factors involved in the individual's suffering. Pain involves multiple psychological appraisals on the part of the individual, including degree of threat, relative salience, relative value/reward, and the degree of ability to control or cope with the sensation. While in-depth psychological evaluation and treatment are outside the scope of this work and the practice of most physicians, there is a growing realization among the medical community (echoed in the assessments and recommendation of policymakers at every level) that without attention to the cognitive and emotional aspects of and contributors to chronic pain, treatment will fail.

The rates of comorbid anxiety, depression, posttraumatic stress disorder, and substance abuse (as well as numerous personality disorders) have long been known to be disproportionately high in the chronic pain population, and while many patients are still reluctant to admit to any psychological dysfunction at all, let alone its centrality in perpetuating (if not generating) pain, the data are incontrovertible. Certain common threads are observed so frequently that they bear mention here:

- While descriptive statistics are fraught with difficulty in the psychosocial sciences, depression, anxiety, and posttraumatic stress disorder are highly overrepresented in the chronic pain population [57] and regardless of which is "chicken vs. egg," the successful treatment of chronic pain generally must co-occur with its partner illness(es).
- A history of abuse, especially childhood sexual abuse, is also disproportionate among the chronic pain population [58–60] and is likely related to hypervigilance and alterations in perception/interpretation of physical stimuli as threatening.
- Suicide is two to three times more prevalent in the chronic pain population than the general population [2, 3].
- Cognitive distortions (e.g., catastrophic thinking), lack of self-efficacy, and avoidant/disengaging coping strategies are highly associated with chronic pain [61–64].

Beyond the overwhelming anecdotal evidence, numerous individual studies and reviews [65–68] support equivalent if not greater benefit in many cases from psychological interventions (including stress reduction efforts, cognitive-behavioral treatment, acceptance and commitment or "mindfulness" approaches) compared to or in addition to physical modalities. As with virtually all therapies, equivocal evidence also exists [69, 70], yet the overall current consensus opinion as reflected in guidelines at every level, including the Institute of Medicine's highly cited 2011 report [1], the Veterans Health Administration Pain Management Directive [71] and the recently released National Pain Strategy [4] highlights the need for greater application of psychological assessment and treatment, and specifically fostering greater self-efficacy in addressing chronic pain.

Sociological assessment is likewise outside the scope of this work, not to mention the author's expertise; however, it bears mention again that in many cases the contributions from relationships, employment status, cultural factors, etc. may well overpower any biologic pathology or lack thereof. Secondary gain issues, whether motivated by desire for attention, comfort and ease, money, etc., are inherently social issues and are likely frequently underappreciated in the evaluation of chronic pain. This statement is not intended to foster cynicism in the practitioner by any means, but rather to remind us that if we are to best serve our patients, accuracy in diagnosis must extend beyond the medical.

Non-opioid Pain Management

We who treat pain—whether at a primary care or specialty level—are responsible to our patients to assess and address not only their chief complaint but the multiple underlying comorbidities that may be present with a rational and effective plan, which generally requires far more than a simple prescription. A well-established and honored guideline as discussed in more detail below and in the next chapter is to reserve the use of opioids for:

> Intractable ... pain that is not adequately managed with more conservative or interventional methods. [72]

It behooves us therefore to be as knowledgeable and proficient as possible in offering (directly or by referral) other modes of treatment.

Prevention and Multimodal Care

Tailoring pain management to address all salient pathologic contributors, including overall health deficiencies; organic "pain generator(s)," if applicable; and psychosocial dysfunction, is logical and essential if the practitioner is to be of any use to the suffering patient.

There are three principles of pain management (and medicine in general) that we share with all of the medical students, residents, and fellows that we interact with:

1. First, do no harm.
2. Second, don't enable the patient to do themselves harm (bearing in mind that successful behavior modification requires evoking the initiative and motivation of the individual) [73, 74]. To quote the National Pain Strategy [4]:

> Prevention of acute and chronic pain, especially primary prevention strategies, needs greater emphasis throughout the health care system, the NPS recognizes that opportunities

to prevent the conditions and events that lead to chronic pain, such as those associated with the work place and lifestyles must not be missed. Furthermore, evidence-based strategies to intervene early to prevent acute pain from becoming a chronic condition and the research to develop them are needed.

3. Third, diagnose and treat accurately. Remember that pain is a symptom/experience, not a diagnosis, and teasing out the underlying issues (of body, mind, heart, soul, and spirit) is essential to effective treatment.

   At the simplest, Cartesian level, applying both:

a. Preventive efforts toward reducing self-destructive issues such as poor diet and obesity, sedentary lifestyle, poor posture and mechanics, smoking, poor sleep hygiene, etc.
b. Therapeutic efforts aimed at applicable organic pathology

form the basic and generally most readily acceptable/palatable interventions that most patients will at least concede intellectual assent to.

It is the rare chronic pain patient who does not report some degree of sleep disturbance, and in our experience, the majority also perceive an association between poor sleep and increased pain. Counseling regarding sleep hygiene and the necessity of adequate slow-wave sleep for psychological and physical healing are discussed, especially with those who suffer along the fibromyalgia spectrum. I can recall only one patient with fibromyalgia out of hundreds that reported more than a few hours of broken sleep per night, and sleep deprivation is currently held to be integral to the pathophysiology of that condition among many experts. Screening for and treating obstructive sleep apnea is vital and may not only save a life from acute respiratory failure or cor pulmonale but almost universally helps facilitate weight loss and improves pain.

Smoking cessation is discussed at every visit with patients who smoke. Besides the obligatory references to cardiovascular, pulmonary, and oncologic risk reduction, we appeal to data showing that cigarettes increase pain; patients seem to care more about that issue oftentimes.

Dietary modification to eliminate excesses of pro-inflammatory components (e.g., refined sugars including high-fructose corn syrup, trans fats and hydrogenated oils, unbalanced polyunsaturated fatty acid, i.e., excessive omega-6, alcohol, various preservatives) may be the most profound intervention the provider can offer an American patient. A 2-month gluten-free challenge in the right individual may completely change the course of their disease management and pain. Most physicians need to learn a lot more about nutrition.

Physical exercise is essential not only for weight reduction, insulin sensitization, maintenance of bone mineral density, etc. but also restoration of normal somatosensory mapping/overcoming somatic distortion. We spend at least 10 min with almost every low back pain patient going over the pathophysiology of lumbar intervertebral discs, how the posterior annulus is the weakest area and vulnerable to tearing and protrusion with twisting and bending, and deconditioning, poor posture and flexion mechanics, etc. Instruction on proper pelvic anteversion and lumbar lordosis, and "hip-hinging," and an isometric and dynamic core strengthening program are offered. We frequently refer to a physical therapist for more expert evaluation and treatment of kinesiologic disturbances. We frequently quote Pete Egoscue ("we hurt because of motion starvation" [75]), and the more experience we gather working with patients in chronic pain, the more convinced we are of the accuracy of this statement. Not only does exercise confer significant benefits in terms of cardiopulmonary and vascular conditioning, endocrine homeostasis, etc., we tell our patients it may also offer the best means of "conditioning" the endogenous opioid system as well as the best means of maintenance of "normal" somatosensory processing. If the CNS is regularly occupied with processing the usual spectrum of sensory input including proprioception and also with governing the usual spectrum of locomotion, it is logical to deduce (and empirically evident) that it has less room and time to be "hijacked" by a chronic pain state.

Simple analgesics such as acetaminophen and NSAIDs are often overlooked by physicians who assume patients are using them. Patients may not be using them or may be using too much of them. Similarly, the use of cold and heat modalities, topical formulations of menthol or capsaicin, or compounded admixtures of local anesthetics, NSAIDs, membrane stabilizers, etc. or the use of TENS units may provide symptomatic relief greater than that of opioids. I will never forget one patient who was referred to me by their distraught primary care provider; the patient was (ostensibly) using over 1000 mg morphine equivalents per day. In the process of weaning the patient off of opioids, we instituted an NSAID and the patient remarked at next visit with great surprise, "that [stuff] actually *works* [for pain]!"

Membrane stabilizers (anticonvulsants) have proven benefit in neuropathic pain and have a relatively good therapeutic window. Gabapentin, pregabalin (which we generally prefer for its improved bioavailability and cleaner side effect profile as well as apparent improvement in slow-wave sleep facilitation and mood stabilization/anxiolysis), and older agents such as topiramate and oxcarbazepine may be very useful primary or adjunctive agents. Magnesium is a membrane stabilizer as well as NMDA blocker and has multifaceted benefit in many patients, conferring migraine prophylaxis and improved bowel hygiene in addition to pain relief. Various complementary/alternative agents such as omega-3 fatty acids and alpha-lipoic acid may have significant benefit in neuropathic pain states as well.

Antidepressants, especially the serotonin and norepinephrine reuptake inhibitor (SNRI) class, also have proven benefit in neuropathic and also in non-neuropathic pain states. Vigilance for concurrent tramadol or tapentadol, or amphetamine, or multiple antidepressant prescriptions is essential to avoid seizures or serotonin syndrome.

Interventional procedures ranging from steroid injections into joints including the zygapophyseal (facet) joints or the epidural space, nerve blockade or modulation by pulsed radiofrequency application, neurolysis by chemical or thermal (or cryoablation) means, spinal cord stimulation, and others may provide significant or even complete relief of pain in appropriate situations.

Referral to other specialties (e.g., orthopedics, neurosurgery, rheumatology, general surgery, gastroenterology, gynecology, psychiatry, etc.) is of course often indicated.

Opioid Alternatives/Multimodal Analgesia in the Perioperative Setting

Perioperative pain (POP) represents a unique situation (it is iatrogenic and generally elective) of potentially severe acute pain with a strong potential likelihood of chronification. While opioids have historically been the primary (if not sole) means of controlling POP, as discussed in greater detail in the next chapter, they are increasingly viewed as "rescue agents" with numerous non-opioid "first line" or at least adjunctive alternatives [76, 77] receiving greater attention and utility.

The use of regional anesthesia (e.g., continuous epidural analgesia, brachial plexus, or lumbosacral plexus blocks) is safer now than ever with ultrasound technology to guide needle placement and may render entire limbs or even the trunk insensate for days if managed properly.

N-methyl-D-aspartate (NMDA) receptor blockade, with corresponding reduction in windup and central sensitization, has long been a focus of anesthesiologists in the operative setting, with ketamine historically being the agent of choice (if not the sole agent available). Low-dose ketamine continues to display the best efficacy among the NMDA blockers in terms of improved perioperative analgesia and reduced opioid consumption; however, multiple alternatives (e.g., dextromethorphan, magnesium, memantine) may also be useful [78, 79].

Alpha-2 agonists such as dexmedetomidine are being increasingly used as sedatives in the operating room and intensive care environment and also display analgesic efficacy with opioid sparing [80, 81].

The perioperative use of both gabapentinoids (gabapentin, pregabalin) and cyclooxygenase-2 inhibitors (celecoxib) have become well-established over the past decade also, with ample evidence of decreased perioperative and CPSP, as well as perioperative opioid consumption and its adverse effects [82–84].

The perioperative use of nonsteroidal anti-inflammatory agents (NSAIDs) including cyclooxygenase-2 inhibitors (COX2I) has been a contentious issue for decades, given these agents' inevitable disruption of normal coagulation and also uncertainty as to whether they retard bone and general wound-healing. However, the past decade has seen increasing use of perioperative NSAIDs and even preoperative use of COX2I for preemptive analgesic and postoperative opioid-sparing benefits [85, 86]. The opioid-sparing effect of ketorolac is well-documented [87]; recent reviews of NSAID [88] or NSAID in combination with acetaminophen [89] have shown analgesic efficacy equivalent to or greater than that of oxycodone 15 mg [90].

Psychosocial Assessment and Therapy

Just as a simplistic Cartesian model is insufficient to explain chronic pain, so too any attempt to diagnose and treat the patient suffering with it from an exclusively biological viewpoint is inadequate and arguably unethical. Effective pain management requires significant and intensive investigation and relationship-building with the patient to better ascertain psychosocial factors that underlie virtually all chronic pain to some extent. While this task is usually best carried out by behavioral health professionals if possible, we as physicians are not excused from exercising the time, effort, and genuine care necessary to understand to the best of our ability all of the factors afflicting the human being in the exam room or procedure suite who has put their trust in us to help alleviate their suffering. Sir William Osler's famous statement, "It is much more important to know what sort of a patient has a disease than what sort of a disease a patient has," may be more applicable in the setting of chronic pain than in any other.

One thing we tell most of our complex chronic pain patients (those who suffer with comorbid psychiatric pathology including but not limited to depression, anxiety, and suboptimal coping strategies if not outright substance dependence) is that "while my scope of practice [comprises the physical], I've done this long enough to know that if we don't address [cognitive, emotional and spiritual issues concurrently] you will never get better." It is the very rare patient that refutes this.

Patient Education and Fostering Self-Efficacy

We have observed in our practice that which has been known for centuries if not millennia: education and empowerment may confer a significant advantage in coping with pain. This statement of course has its caveats; a little knowledge can be a dangerous thing, and greater knowledge can sometimes foster undue attention or preoccupation. However, we believe as a general rule that the more truth an individual possesses, the greater their defenses are against anxiety and other cognitive distortions (including catastrophic thinking, kinesiophobia, disability mindset, etc.) which may represent the greatest scourges of pain in their life. Even interventions that may superficially seem oriented in a disparate direction (e.g., acceptance and commitment therapy, mindfulness, prayer, and spiritual disciplines) are not intended to foster naïveté but rather the separation and suppression of worry and fear that exploit ignorance at least as much as understanding.

Again, while every physician has a responsibility to recognize psychosocial pathology and suggest treatment/initiate appropriate referral, the complexities of human nature generally render these issues best treated by professionals in the behavioral health and counseling fields. Basic mastery of pain physiology (the subject of this chapter) however is the responsibility of all physicians, and education of the patient about the physical factors associated with why they hurt should always be as thorough as possible in our opinion. The data would seem to support this conviction [91, 92] with evidence of markedly better outcomes in terms of pain coping and functional improvements with a little education. Again, the National Pain Strategy recognizes the importance of these efforts at a public health level as well:

> People with pain would have access to educational materials and learn effective approaches for pain self-management programs to prevent, cope with, and reduce pain and its disability… Patients, including those with low literacy or communication disabilities, would have access to information they can understand about the benefits and risks of treatment options. [4]

Closely associated with education [93] is self-efficacy, defined by Dr. Albert Bandura as "one's belief in one's ability to succeed in specific situations or accomplish a task" [94] and an increasingly recognized predictor of effective management if not even triumph over chronic pain [95, 96]. Cultivation of self-efficacy may be as complicated a task as raising a child and may well require a "village" of behavioral health professionals, physiotherapists, and spiritual directors not to mention family and other close relationships. However, the indispensable role of the physician in both education and encouragement cannot be overstated. "Doctor" after all means teacher in Latin, and the purpose of teaching is not only to transmit knowledge but to facilitate positive change and growth.

Finally, even a brief introductory discussion on the teleologic purpose of pain (education beyond the "what" and "how" of pain to include the "why") may pay long-term dividends in the management of pain or at least suffering. Even restricting the discussion to the physical realm, taking the time to enlighten a patient to the vital allostatic role pain plays, and helping them reframe the experience of nociception as a beneficial and protective sense may facilitate acceptance and commitment, mindfulness, or spiritual growth that helps to disarm pain of its suffering aspects by undermining learned helplessness/victimization, catastrophization, etc.

Spirituality of Pain and Suffering

Western academia is "late to the party" when it comes to acknowledging, let alone understanding the role that pain plays in an individual's or society's spiritual framework and conversely the role that spirituality and religion play in providing meaning and coping for human beings of every race and culture. This is inevitable, for science can only deal with that which is observable and reproducible, and the spirituality and religions of the world appeal to faith, which by definition relies on trust in the unseen (perhaps not so different really than one's conviction that the Mariana trench or black holes exist without personal verification). The five largest and most established religions of the world (Christianity, Islam, Hinduism, Buddhism, and Judaism) all assign a tremendous importance to the human experiences of pain and suffering, ranging from punitive to constructive, and also prescribe interpretations and responses to these experiences.

It is at one level ironic that pain is complained about the most in the developed world and in particular in the West, when we have achieved the highest general level of ease and comfort in known history. To quote Dr. Paul Brand, a pioneering missionary surgeon in India in the past century (whose work with lepers led to groundbreaking understanding of diabetic neuropathy):

> …as a society gains the ability to limit suffering, it loses the ability to cope with what suffering remains…the "less advanced" societies do not fear physical pain as much… These traditional cultures may lack modern analgesics, but the beliefs and family support systems built into everyday life help equip individuals to cope with pain. The average Indian villager knows suffering well, expects it, and accepts it as an unavoidable challenge of life. In a remarkable way the people of India have learned to control pain at the level of the mind and spirit, and have developed endurance that we in the West find hard to understand. Westerners, in contrast, tend to view suffering as an injustice or failure, an infringement on their guaranteed right to happiness. [97]

Many other Western-trained healthcare providers (including this author) have observed far fewer pain behaviors and apparent suffering in third-world patients with significant pathology or injuries. While the sociocultural explanations for this are varied and complex, it does beg the question whether a correlation between reduction in pain resilience/coping (or even increase in perception) and decreasing individual and societal spiritual foundation exists.

Regardless, given that over 75% of the world's population reportedly identify with one of these five faiths, to ignore the role that spirituality and religion play in an individual's pain experience is ignorant at best and arrogant at worst. To quote one of the leading researchers in the field, "Regardless of their own belief system, physicians should not allow their own bias to blind them to the possibility that spiritual/religious beliefs play an important role for their patients [98]." In a larger context, it seems the acme of hubris (and unfortunately historically the hallmark of academia) to exclude the transcendent from attempts to interpret and respond to so universal yet inexplicably variable an experience as pain.

Fortunately for Western healthcare, recent pain management literature reflects a growing awareness and acceptance of the value of spirituality and religion [98–100]. Spiritual and religious practices have been shown to correlate with improved mental and physical health, including both coping with illness as well as improved medical outcomes [101–103]. Far from reflecting a strictly passive and avoidant state, spiritual and religious beliefs and practices correlate strongly with an active/adaptive coping strategy [99] and those who adopt positive spiritual coping practices such as looking to God for strength and support display higher pain tolerance [91, 92, 102, 104, 105] as well as better mood and satisfaction with life in the presence of pain [100, 106, 107]. Further stratifying by view of God, it has been demonstrated that those who are experiencing pain and see God as forgiving and kind have lower pain intensity and are higher-functioning as compared with those who see God as harsh or abandoning [102, 104, 108].

While it is no more incumbent upon the physician to be expert in matters of faith and spirituality than psychology, sensitivity to and nonjudgmentalism of patients' religious and spiritual beliefs and practices are imperative for optimal medical care, especially in a matter as personal and individual as pain management. Regulatory bodies are beginning to adopt a more proactive stance in this arena; for example, the Joint Commission lists spiritual assessment as one of its standards for hospital accreditation [109], and both the American Psychiatric Association and the American Psychological Association have rendered instruction/guidelines for its members to the same end [110, 111].

Summary

Knowing why and when to prescribe opioids is facilitated by a basic understanding of pain physiology and psychology and the treatment modalities that are best oriented toward those processes. Acute pain usually begins with nociception or sensation and is transmitted by both the peripheral and central nervous system to higher centers for processing and perception and also for modulation of the incoming message. Growing evidence suggests that chronic pain may not always follow these pathways but may in fact find its genesis within these higher centers including the limbic system and the cortex. Besides tolerance, adverse effects, and hyperalgesia, opioids simply are not right for many chronic pain conditions based upon their pathophysiology.

Pain management should always require much thought and should consider the individual's problem(s) in light of what is known about pain physiology/pathophysiology and psychology and tailor therapy accordingly. Educating the patient on basic physiologic and psychologic aspects of their pain is often therapeutic in its own right and correlates with increased self-efficacy, which is increasingly seen as contributory to optimal outcomes. Multimodal therapies (including attenuation of detrimental lifestyle, behavioral health interventions, spiritual support, physiotherapy interventions, and non-opioid pharmacotherapeutics) should be presented as primary rather than adjunctive.

References

1. Institute of Medicine. Relieving pain in america: a blueprint for transforming prevention, care, education and research. Washington, D.C.: National Academies Press; 2011.
2. Fishbain DA, Goldberg M, Rosomoff RS, Rosomoff H. Completed suicide in chronic pain. Clin J Pain. 1991;7:29–36.
3. Tang NK, Crane C. Suicidality in chronic pain: a review of the prevalence, risk factors and psychological links. Psychol Med. 2006;36:575–86.
4. United States Department of Health and Human Services. National pain strategy: a comprehensive population health-level strategy for pain. Downloaded from: https://iprcc.nih.gov/docs/HHSNational_Pain_Strategy.pdf.
5. McMahon SB, Koltzenburg M, Tracey I, Turk D, editors. Wall & Melzack's textbook of pain. 6th ed. Philadelphia: Elsevier; 2013.

6. Fishman SM, Ballantyne JC, Rathmell JP, editors. Bonica's management of pain. 4th ed. Baltimore: Lippincott, Williams & Wilkins; 2010.
7. Deer TR, Leong MS, Buvanendran A, Gordin V, Kim PS, Panchal SJ, Ray AL, editors. Comprehensive treatment of chronic pain by medical, interventional and integrative approaches: the american academy of pain medicine textbook on patient management. New York: Springer; 2013.
8. Merskey H, Bogduk N. Part III: pain terms, a current list with definitions and notes on usage. In: Classification of chronic pain, IASP task force on taxonomy. 2nd ed. Seattle: IASP Press; 1994. p. 209–14.
9. Todd AJ, Koerber HR. Neuroanatomical substrates of spinal nociception. In: McMahon SB, Koltzenburg M, Tracey I, Turk D, editors. Wall & Melzack's textbook of pain. 6th ed. Philadelphia: Elsevier; 2013. p. 77–93.
10. Vermeulen W, De Man JG, Pelckmans PA, De Winter BY. Neuroanatomy of lower gastrointestinal pain disorders. World J Gastroenterol. 2014;20:1005–20.
11. Gebhart GF. Visceral pain−−peripheral sensitization. Gut. 2000;47(Suppl IV):iv54–iv2.
12. Robinson DR, Gebhart GF. Inside information–the unique features of visceral sensation. Mol Interv. 2008;8(5):242–53.
13. Bogduk N. Low back pain. In: Bogduk N, editor. Clinical and radiological anatomy of the lumbar spine. 5th ed. London: Elsevier; 2012. p. 173–205.
14. Simons DG. General overview. In: Simons DG, Travell JG, Simons LS, editors. Travell & Simons' myofascial pain and dysfunction: the trigger point manual, Upper half of body, vol. 1. 2nd ed. Philadelphia: Lippincott Williams & Wilkins; 1999. p. 11–93.
15. Griffin R, Fink E, Brenner GJ. Functional neuroanatomy of the nociceptive system. In: Fishman SM, Ballantyne JC, Rathmell JP, editors. Bonica's management of pain. 4th ed. Baltimore: Lippincott, Williams & Wilkins; 2010. p. 98–119.
16. Baron R. Mechanisms of disease: neuropathic pain – a clinical perspective. Nat Clin Pract Neurol. 2006;2:95–106.
17. Yaksh TL, Wiese AJ. A survey of systems involved in nociceptive processing. In: Deer TR, editor. Comprehensive treatment of chronic pain by medical, interventional, and integrative approaches. New York: Springer; 2013.
18. Ness T, Randich A. Substrates of spinal cord nociceptive processing. In: Fishman SM, Ballantyne JC, Rathmell JP, editors. Bonica's management of pain. 4th ed. Baltimore: Lippincott, Williams & Wilkins; 2010. p. 35–48.
19. Gangadharan V, Kuner R. Pain hypersensitivity mechanisms at a glance. Dis Model Mech. 2013;6:889–95.
20. Beggs S, Salter MW. Microglia: critical mediators of pain hypersensitivity after peripheral nerve injury. In: McMahon SB, Koltzenburg M, Tracey I, Turk D, editors. Wall & Melzack's textbook of pain. 6th ed. Philadelphia: Elsevier; 2013. p. 68–76.
21. Woolf CJ. Evidence for a central component of post-injury pain hypersensitivity. Nature. 1983;306:686–8.
22. Woolf CJ. Central sensitization: implications for the diagnosis and treatment of pain. Pain. 2011;152(Suppl 3):S2–15.
23. Latremoliere A, Woolf CJ. Central sensitization: a generator of pain hypersensitivity by central neural plasticity. J Pain. 2009;10:895–926.
24. Sengupta JN. Visceral pain: the neurophysiological mechanism. Handb Exp Pharmacol. 2009;194:31–74.
25. van den Beuken-van Everdingen MH, Hochstenbach LM, Joosten EA, Tjan-Heijnen VC, Janssen DJ. Update on prevalence of pain in patients with cancer: systematic review and meta-analysis. J Pain Symptom Manag. 2016;51:1070–90.
26. Mantyh PW. Cancer pain: causes, consequences, and therapeutic opportunities. In: McMahon SB, Koltzenburg M, Tracey I, Turk D, editors. Wall & Melzack's textbook of pain. 6th ed. Philadelphia: Elsevier; 2013. p. 1029–38.
27. Cramer SC, Sur M, Dobkin BH, O'Brien C, Sanger TD, Trojanowski JQ, et al. Harnessing neuroplasticity for clinical applications. Brain. 2011;134:1591–609.

28. Flor H, Braun C, Elbert T, Birbaumer N. Extensive reorganization of primary somatosensory cortex in chronic back pain patients. Neurosci Lett. 1997;224:5–8.
29. Tinazzi M, Zanette G, Volpato D, Testoni R, Bonato C, Manganotti P, Miniuissi C, Fiachi A. Neurophysiological evidence of neuroplasticity at multiple levels of the somatosensory system in patients with carpal tunnel syndrome. Brain. 1998;121(Pt 9):1785–94.
30. Soros P, Knecht S, Bantel C, Imai T, Wusten R, Pantev C, et al. Functional reorganization of the human primary somatosensory cortex after acute pain demonstrated by magnetoencephalography. Neurosci Lett. 2001;298:195–8.
31. Vartiainen N, Kirveskari E, Kallio-Laine K, Kalso E, Forss N. Cortical reorganization in primary somatosensory cortex in patients with unilateral chronic pain. J Pain. 2009;10:854–9.
32. Grachev ID, Fredrickson BE, Apkarian AV. Abnormal brain chemistry in chronic back pain: an in vivo proton magnetic resonance spectroscopy study. Pain. 2000;89:7–18.
33. Gussew A, Rzanny R, Gullmar D, Scholle HC, Reichenbach JR. 1H-MR spectroscopic detection of metabolic changes in pain processing brain regions in the presence of non-specific chronic low back pain. NeuroImage. 2011;54:1315–23.
34. Valdes M, Collado A, Bargallo N, Vazquez M, Rami L, Gomez E, et al. Increased glutamate/glutamine compounds in the brains of patients with fibromyalgia: a magnetic resonance spectroscopy study. Arthritis Rheum. 2010;62:1829–36.
35. Apkarian AV, Sosa Y, Sonty S, Levy RE, Harden RN, Parrish TB, et al. Chronic back pain is associated with decreased prefrontal and thalamic gray matter density. J Neurosci. 2004;24:10410–5.
36. Schmidt-Wilcke T, Leinisch E, Straube A, Kampfe N, Draganski B, Diener HC, et al. Gray matter decrease in patients with chronic tension type headache. Neurology. 2005;65:1483–6.
37. Kuchinad A, Schweinhardt P, Seminowicz DA, Wood PB, Chizh BA, Bushnell MC. Accelerated brain gray matter loss in fibromyalgia patients: premature aging of the brain? J Neurosci. 2007;27:4004–7.
38. Rodriguez-Raecke R, Niemeier A, Ihle K, Ruether W, May A. Brain gray matter decrease in chronic pain is the consequence and not the cause of pain. J Neurosci. 2009;29:13746–50.
39. Pelletier R, Higgins J, Bourbonnais D. Is neuroplasticity in the central nervous system the missing link to our understanding of chronic musculoskeletal disorders? BMC Musculoskelet Disord. 2015;16:25. doi:10.1186/s12891-015-0480-y.
40. Apkarian AV, Hashmi JA, Baliki MN. Pain and the brain: specificity and plasticity of the brain in clinical chronic pain. Pain. 2011;152(3 Suppl):S49–64.
41. Mansour AR, Farmer MA, Baliki MN, Apkarian AV. Chronic pain: the role of learning and brain plasticity. Restor Neurol Neurosci. 2014;32:129–39.
42. Parks EL, Gehal PY, Balikil MN, Katzl J, Schnitzerl TJ, Apkarian AV. Brain activity for chronic knee osteoarthritis: dissociating evoked pain from spontaneous pain. Eur J Pain. 2011;15:843.
43. Apkarian AV, Bushnell MC, Schweinhardt P. Representation of pain in the brain. In: McMahon SB, Koltzenburg M, Tracey I, Turk D, editors. Wall & Melzack's textbook of pain. 6th ed. Philadelphia: Elsevier; 2013. p. 111–28.
44. Melzack R, Wall PD. Pain mechanisms: a new theory. Science. 1965;150:971–9.
45. Melzack R. From the gate to the neuromatrix. Pain. 1999;(Suppl 6):S121–6.
46. Beecher HK. Relationship of significance of wound to pain experienced. JAMA. 1956;161:1609–13.
47. Beecher HK. Measurement of subjective responses. New York: Oxford University Press; 1959.
48. Hagbarth KE, Kerr DI. Central influences on spinal afferent conduction. J Neurophysiol. 1954;17:295–307.
49. Kuypers HG, Fleming WR, Farinholt JW. Descending projections to spinal motor and sensory cell groups in the monkey: cortex versus subcortex. Science. 1960;132:38–40.
50. Reynolds DV. Surgery in the rat during electrical analgesia induced by focal brain stimulation. Science. 1969;164:444–5.

51. Levy R, Deer TR, Henderson J. Intracranial neurostimulation for pain control: a review. Pain Physician. 2010;13:157–65.
52. Bittar RG, Kar-Purkayastha I, Owen SL, Bear RE, Green A, Wang S, et al. Deep brain stimulation for pain relief: a meta-analysis. J Clin Neurosci. 2005;12:515–9.
53. Heinricher MM, Fields HL. Central nervous system mechanisms of pain modulation, chapter 8. In: McMahon SB, Koltzenburg M, Tracey I, Turk D, editors. Wall & Melzack's textbook of pain. 6th ed. Philadelphia: Elsevier; 2013. p. 129–42.
54. Heinricher MM, Tavares I, Leith JL, Lumb BM. Descending control of nociception: specificity, recruitment and plasticity. Brain Res Rev. 2009;60:214–25.
55. Tracey I, Mantyh PW. The cerebral signature for pain perception and its modulation. Neuron. 2007;2:377–91.
56. Engel GL. The need for a new medical model: a challenge for biomedicine. Science. 1977;196:129–36.
57. Fishbain DA. Psychiatric pain-associated comorbidities. In: McMahon SB, Koltzenburg M, Tracey I, Turk DC, editors. Wall and Melzack's textbook of pain. Philadelphia: Elsevier; 2013. p. 273–82.
58. Springer KW, Sheridan J, Kuo D, Carnes M. The long-term health outcomes of childhood abuse: an overview and a call to action. J Gen Intern Med. 2003;18:864–70.
59. Irish L, Kobayashi I, Delahanty DL. Long-term physical health consequences of childhood sexual abuse: a meta-analytic review. J Pediatr Psychol. 2010;35:450–61.
60. Hart-Johnson T, Green CR. The impact of sexual or physical abuse history on pain-related outcomes among blacks and whites with chronic pain: gender influence. Pain Med. 2012;13:229–42.
61. Denison E, Åsenlöf P, Lindberg P. Self-efficacy, fear avoidance, and pain intensity as predictors of disability in subacute and chronic musculoskeletal pain patients in primary health care. Pain. 2004;111:245–52.
62. Weissman-Fogel I, Sprecher E, Pud D. Effects of catastrophizing on pain perception and pain modulation. Exp Brain Res. 2008;186:79–85.
63. Turk DC, Wilson HD. Fear of pain as a prognostic factor in chronic pain: conceptual models, assessment, and treatment implications. Curr Pain Headache Rep. 2010;14:88–95.
64. Linton SJ, Shaw WS. Impact of psychological factors in the experience of pain. Phys Ther. 2011;91:700–11.
65. Flor H, Fydrich T, Turk DC. Efficacy of multidisciplinary pain treatment centers: a meta-analytic review. Pain. 1992;49:221–30.
66. Hoffman BM, Papas RK, Chatkoff DK, Kerns RD. Meta-analysis of psychological interventions for chronic low back pain. Health Psychol. 2007;26:1–9.
67. Dixon KE, Keefe FJ, Scipio CD, Perri LM, Abernethy AP. Psychological interventions for arthritis pain management in adults: a meta-analysis. Health Psychol. 2007;26:241–50.
68. Kerns RD, Sellinger J, Goodin BR. Psychological treatment of chronic pain. Annu Rev Clin Psychol. 2011;7:411–34.
69. Williams ACDC, Eccleston C, Morley S. Psychological therapies for the management of chronic pain (excluding headache) in adults. Cochrane Database Syst Rev. 2012;11:CD007407. doi:10.1002/14651858.CD007407.pub3.
70. Ehde DM, Dillworth TM, Turner JA. Cognitive-behavioral therapy for individuals with chronic pain: efficacy, innovations, and directions for research. Am Psychol. 2014;4:153–66.
71. Department of Veterans Affairs. VHA Directive 2009–053: Pain management. Downloaded from: http://www.va.gov/painmanagement/docs/vha09paindirective.pdf.
72. American Academy of Pain Medicine. Use of opioids for the treatment of chronic pain: a statement from the American academy of pain medicine. 2013. http://www.painmed.org/files/use-of-opioids-for-the-treatment-of-chronic-pain.pdf.
73. Prochaska JO, Butterworth S, Redding CA, Burden V, Perrin N, Leo M, et al. Initial efficacy of MI, TTM tailoring, and HRI's in multiple behaviors for employee health promotion. Prev Med. 2008;46:226–31.

74. Miller WR, Rolnick S. Research evidence and the evolution of motivational interviewing. In: Miller WR, Rolnick S, editors. Motivational interviewing: helping people change. 3rd ed. New York: Guilford Press; 2013. p. 34–386.
75. Egoscue P, Gittines R. Pain free: a revolutionary method for stopping chronic pain. New York: Bantam Books; 1998.
76. Devin CJ, McGirt MJ. Best evidence in multimodal pain management in spine surgery and means of assessing postoperative pain and functional outcomes. J Clin Neurosci. 2015;22:930–8.
77. Gritsenko K, Khelemsky Y, Kaye AD, Vadivelu N, Urman RD. Multimodal therapy in perioperative analgesia. Best Pract Res Clin Anaesthesiol. 2014;28:59–79.
78. McCartney CJ, Sinha A, Katz J. A qualitative systematic review of the role of *N*-methyl-D-aspartate receptor antagonists in preventive analgesia. Anesth Analg. 2004;98:1385–400.
79. Suzuki M. Role of *N*-methyl-D-aspartate receptor antagonists in postoperative pain management. Curr Opin Anaesthesiol. 2009;22:618–22.
80. Carollo DS, Nossaman BD, Ramadhyani U. Dexmedetomidine: a review of clinical applications. Curr Opin Anaesthesiol. 2008;21:457–61.
81. Blaudszun G, Lysakowski C, Elia N, Tramèr MR. Effect of perioperative systemic α2 agonists on postoperative morphine consumption and pain intensity: systematic review and meta-analysis of randomized controlled trials. Anesthesiology. 2012;116:1312–22.
82. Ho KY, Gan TJ, Habib AS. Gabapentin and postoperative pain--a systematic review of randomized controlled trials. Pain. 2006;126:91–101.
83. Tiippana EM, Hamunen K, Kontinen VK, Kalso E. Do surgical patients benefit from perioperative gabapentin/pregabalin? A systematic review of efficacy and safety. Anesth Analg. 2007;104:1545–56.
84. Clarke H, Bonin RP, Orser BA, Englesakis M, Wijeysundera DN, Katz J. The prevention of chronic postsurgical pain using gabapentin and pregabalin: a combined systematic review and meta-analysis. Anesth Analg. 2012;115:428–42.
85. Straube S, Derry S, McQuay HJ, Moore RA. Effect of preoperative cox-II-selective NSAIDs (coxibs) on postoperative outcomes: a systematic review of randomized studies. Acta Anaesthesiol Scand. 2005;49:601–13.
86. Reuben SS. Update on the role of nonsteroidal anti-inflammatory drugs and coxibs in the management of acute pain. Curr Opin Anaesthesiol. 2007;20:440–50.
87. De Oliveira GS Jr, Agarwal D, Benzon HT. Perioperative single dose ketorolac to prevent postoperative pain: a meta-analysis of randomized trials. Anesth Analg. 2012;114:424–33.
88. Derry C, Derry S. Single dose oral naproxen and naproxen sodium for acute postoperative pain in adults. Cochrane Database Syst Rev. 2009;1:CD004234. Retrieved from: http://onlinelibrary.wiley.com/doi/10.1002/14651858.CD004234.pub3/pdf/standard
89. Derry C, Derry S, Moore R. Single dose oral ibuprofen plus paracetamol (acetaminophen) for acute postoperative pain (review). Cochrane Database Syst Rev. 2013;6:CD010210. doi:10.1002/14651858.CD010210.pub2.
90. Teater D. Evidence for the efficacy of pain medications. http://www.nsc.org/RxDrugOverdoseDocuments/Evidence-Efficacy-Pain-Medications.pdf.
91. Wachholtz AB, Pargament KI. Is spirituality a critical ingredient of meditation? Comparing the effects of spiritual meditation, secular meditation, and relaxation on spiritual, psychological, cardiac, and pain outcomes. J Behav Med. 2005;28:369–84.
92. Wachholtz A, Pearce M. Does spirituality as a coping mechanism help or hinder coping with chronic pain? Curr Pain Headache Rep. 2009;13:127–32.
93. Mackey LM, Doody C, Werner EL, Fullen B. Self-management skills in chronic disease management: what role does health literacy have? Med Decis Mak. 2016;36:741–59.
94. Bandura A. Self-efficacy: toward a unifying theory of behavioral change. Psychol Rev. 1977;84:191–215.
95. Jackson T, Wang Y, Wang Y, Fan H. Self-efficacy and chronic pain outcomes: a meta-analytic review. J Pain. 2014;15(8):800–14.

96. Delgado R, York A, Lee C, Crawford C, Buckenmaier C, Schoomaker E, et al. Assessing the quality, efficacy, and effectiveness of the current evidence base of active self-care complementary and integrative medicine therapies for the management of chronic pain: a rapid evidence assessment of the literature. Pain Med. 2014;15(Suppl 1):S9–S20.
97. Brand P, Yancey P. The gift of pains. Zondervan: Grand Rapids; 1997.
98. Büssing A, Michalsen A, Balzat HJ, Grünther RA, Ostermann T, Neugebauer EA, et al. Are spirituality and religiosity resources for patients with chronic pain conditions? Pain Med. 2009;10(2):327–39.
99. Dedeli O, Kaptan G. Spirituality and religion in pain and pain management. Health Psychol Res. 2013;1(3):e29. doi:10.4081/hpr.2013.e29.
100. Siddall P, Lovell M, MacLeod R. Spirituality: what is its role in pain medicine? Pain Med. 2015;16:51–60.
101. Yates JW, Chalmers BJ, St. James P, Follansbee M, McKegney FP. Religion in patients with advanced cancer. Med Pediatr Oncol. 1981;9:121–8.
102. Rippentrop EA, Altmaier EM, Chen JJ, Found EM, Keffala VJ. The relationship between religion/spirituality and physical health, mental health, and pain in a chronic pain population. Pain. 2005;116:311–21.
103. Koenig HG. Integrating spirituality into medical practice: a new era in medicine. In: Büssing A, Ostermann T, Glöckler M, Matthiessen PF, editors. Spiritualität, Krankheit und Heilung—Bedeutung und Ausdrucksformen der Spiritualität in der Medizin. Frankfurt: VAS-Verlag für Akademische Schriften; 2006. p. 232–41.
104. Bush EG, Rye MS, Brant CR, Emery E, Pargament KI, Riessinger CA. Religious coping with chronic pain. Appl Psychophysiol Biofeed. 1999;24:249–60.
105. Keefe FJ, Affleck G, Lefebvre J, Underwood L, Caldwell DS, Drew J, et al. Living with rheumatoid arthritis: the role of daily spirituality and daily religious and spiritual coping. J Pain. 2001;2:101–10.
106. Moreira-Almeida A, Koenig HG. Religiousness and spirituality in fibromyalgia and chronic pain patients. Curr Pain Headache Rep. 2008;12:327–32.
107. Dezutter J, Robertson LA, Luyckx K, Hutsebaut D. Life satisfaction in chronic pain patients: the stress-buffering role of the centrality of religion. J Sci Study Relig. 2010;49:507–16.
108. Dezutter J, Luyckx K, Schaap-Jonker H, Büssing A, Corveleyn J, Hutsebaut D. God image and happiness in chronic pain patients: the mediating role of disease interpretation. Pain Med. 2010;11:765–73.
109. The Joint Commission. Spiritual assessment. 2013. Available from: http://www.jointcommission.org/standards_information/jcfaqdetails.aspx?StandardsFAQId5290&StandardsFAQChapterId593.
110. American Psychiatric Association Board of Trustees. Guidelines regarding possible conflict between psychiatrists' religious commitment and pyschiatric practice. Am J Psychiatry. 1990;147:542.
111. American Psychological Association. Ethical principles of psychologists and code of conduct. 2010. http://www.apa.org/ethics/code/principles.pdf
112. Louw A, Diener I, Butler DS, Puentedura EJ. The effect of neuroscience education on pain, disability, anxiety, and stress in chronic musculoskeletal pain. Arch Phys Med Rehabil. 2011 Dec;92(12):2041–3.
113. Geneen LJ, Martin DJ, Adams N, Clarke C, Dunbar M, Jones D, et al. Effects of education to facilitate knowledge about chronic pain for adults: a systematic review with meta-analysis. Syst Rev. 2015;4:132. doi:10.1186/s13643-015-0120-5.

Chapter 7
Best Practices Education, Part II: Evidence for and Against Opioid Therapy

A 62-year-old female patient is referred to you by a colorectal surgeon in consultation regarding pain management for advanced (Stage IV) colorectal adenocarcinoma that has involved the majority of her lower pelvis, with metastases to the liver and brain. She complains of severe deep pelvic pain as well as perineal pain exacerbated by sitting, and dyschezia/tenesmus. Secondarily she also complains of lower segment posterior neck and shoulder girdle pain without radicular symptoms, and with a cramping/aching quality, for which she has found cyclobenzaprine to be moderately effective in relieving. Her past medical history is otherwise notable for hyperthyroidism and psoriatic arthritis. She has a remote history of opioid dependence as well and is very concerned about the referral to you, as she "doesn't want to be addicted again." She has however been using Percocet 10 mg/325 mg every 2–3 h. Scintigraphy shows no concerning osseous lesions; her liver function studies are within normal limits.

Together you and her decide on a pain management plan that includes:

1. Meloxicam 7.5 mg qd.
2. Gabapentin titrating up to effect from 300 mg qhs.
3. Fentanyl 37 mcg/h. Patch with hydromorphone 2 mg tablets q4 h PRN after explaining to her that in the context of terminal cancer with severe pain, opioid therapy is considered beneficial to not only improve quality of life but also potentially reduce pain-related immunosuppression.
4. Venlafaxine beginning in 2 weeks after assessing her response to the previous interventions. You explain to her that you don't want to start too many new agents simultaneously, so as to avoid confounding potential adverse effects.

H.B. McAnally, *Opioid Dependence*, DOI 10.1007/978-3-319-47497-7_7

5. Pudendal nerve and ganglion impar neurolysis, with possible superior and inferior hypogastric plexus neurolysis depending on her response to the former.
6. Referral for myofascial release/manual therapy for her cervicalgia/shoulder girdle pain.

Introduction

Opioids remain a prevalent therapeutic modality for a reason: They possess significant analgesic effects across a wide spectrum of painful conditions. Often referred to as "broad-spectrum analgesics," they reduce nociception and perception and enhance descending modulation with time-tested efficacy. Mounting evidence however suggests that as with most tools within medicine, there is a time and place for opioid therapy, and "blanket use" to treat pain of all shapes and sizes, for an indiscriminate duration, may be detrimental. Tolerance with resultant decrease in the benefit-risk ratio, adverse effects including hyperalgesia, and simple inefficacy in many situations mandate that the physician knows *why* and *when* to prescribe opioids (the subject of this chapter) and perhaps more importantly, *when not to* (Chap. 8 is devoted to *how*).

So why should the clinician prescribe opioids for pain? The first and most obvious reason is to relieve severe pain that cannot be relieved otherwise, assuming the risks do not outweigh the benefit. A well-established and honored guideline as discussed in more detail below and in the next chapter is to reserve the use of opioids for:

> Intractable … pain that is not adequately managed with more conservative or interventional methods. [1]

As introduced in the previous chapter, however, pain is a subjective and individual experience with heterogeneous (and generally multifactorial) etiology. Fatigue is similarly subjective and individualized and also shares a plethora of potential causes. Universally prescribing thyroid hormone replacement to all fatigued patients is inconceivable. Hypertension similarly has different etiologies (e.g., vascular, renal, cardiac, neuroendocrine factors) that contribute to varying degrees in any given individual, and while profound vasodilators such as sodium nitroprusside or phentolamine will effectively lower anyone's blood pressure, this may be not only overkill but literally lethal.

Granted, fatigue and hypertension do not share the same current public nor professional conviction regarding a "moral imperative" [2] for treatment that pain does, nor are they generally associated with the same degree of distress and emotional urgency experienced and communicated by most patients in pain. This is not intended in any way to make light of the pain and suffering of any individual. It is intended rather to highlight the fact that while it is second nature for physicians to approach fatigue or hypertension (or most clinical issues) with an analytical mindset, taking a good history and physical and ordering appropriate tests, and tailoring (hopefully evidence-based) therapy to that individual, the same is rarely true of dealing with patients in pain. Pain often brings with it a sense of urgency that can supersede the ration of both patient and physician, and these pressures are arguably greater upon the uninformed and untrained provider. A better understanding of the nature of pain was the intent of the previous chapter, and a better understanding of the efficacy (or lack) of opioids in treating pain is the thrust of this one.

The second reason—perhaps goal is a better word—for a physician to prescribe opioids, and one that has been highlighted recently in several consensus opinions and guidelines [1, 3–5], is to facilitate functional improvements in people who would otherwise be unable to achieve such improvement. This subject is addressed in greater detail in the next chapter.

Opioid prescribing patterns have historically swung in pendulum fashion between conservative and liberal practice, with competing societal concerns for personal and community damage versus inadequate treatment of pain and suffering. Lack of consensus opinion on any topic generally indicates incomplete collective knowledge and understanding of a subject, and this is arguably true of medicine in general. An often-quoted statistic is that roughly half of what we believe to be true isn't. Constant evaluation of past and present (as well as what the near future may hold) is necessary to offer sound advice and treatment to those who put their trust in us. As such, and in keeping with the current climate of evidence-based medicine, this chapter will attempt to present in greater detail the *why* and *when* (with some *when nots*, e.g., headache, fibromyalgia, etc.) of opioid prescribing for various scenarios, including:

- Acute pain, including perioperative pain
- Chronic "inflammatory" pain
- Chronic "neuropathic" pain
- Chronic visceral pain
- Cancer pain

within the context of recent literature review on therapeutic efficacy or lack thereof.

Opioid Therapy in Acute Pain

General Considerations

When should the physician (or if within legally defined scope of practice, the mid-level practitioner) prescribe opioids for acute pain? The relief of pain and suffering has always been recognized as a fundamental moral and ethical responsibility of the physician (within the confines of positive benefit-risk ratio, standards of care, legality, etc.) It has long been appreciated in acute care settings such as the emergency department and also in operative medicine/anesthesia that severe untreated pain may have highly negative physiologic consequences including hypertensive crises and their sequelae, myocardial ischemia due to demand/supply imbalance, etc. Quality of life, functionality, and overall well-being are also affected both in the short term and frequently long term, depending on how well the acute pain is treated [6, 7]. There is also evidence that how acute pain is managed frequently dictates

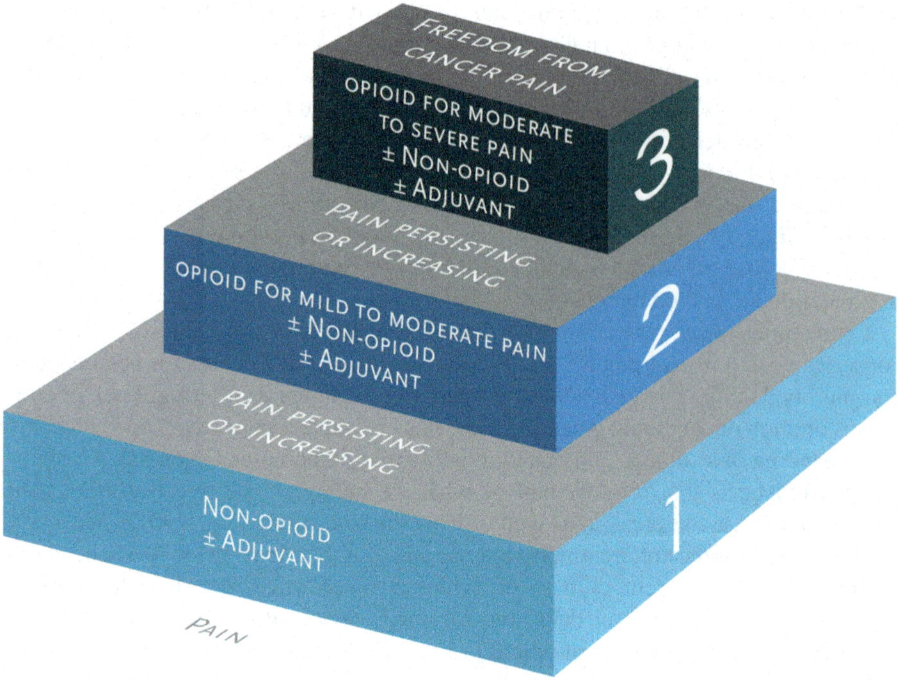

Fig. 7.1 World Health Organization analgesic ladder

whether or not the painful condition becomes chronic [7, 8], and our growing understanding of long-term neuronal potentiation and plasticity and sensitization provides a biologic rationale for effective acute pain relief whenever possible. Long-standing strategies such as preemptive analgesia (discussed in greater detail below) to prevent chronic postsurgical pain states [9] or immediate antiviral treatment of shingles to prevent post-herpetic neuralgia [10] illustrate the widespread utility of this principle (Fig. 7.1).

The use of opioids to treat severe acute pain with clearly demonstrable physical pathology is rarely contested (although application of a stepwise approach, e.g., the WHO ladder [see Figure 7.1], with opioid use reserved for severe and refractory pain, is certainly consistent with good practice of balancing risks, benefits, and alternatives). This stepwise approach, and the associated multimodal analgesic strategy, has been adopted by numerous organizations and federal agencies including the American Society of Anesthesiologists [11], the American Academy of Pain Management [12], the Washington State Agency Medical Directors' Group [3], the Institute for Clinical Systems Improvement [13], the US Military Joint Theater Trauma System [14], the Veterans Administration [15], and many others. Given what we know about the pathophysiology of pain (including the tremendous contributions of psychosocial-spiritual factors), there are ample opportunities for intervention upon acute pain including reductions in nociception and peripheral sensitization (e.g., cooling modalities, anti-inflammatories), transmission (e.g., local anesthetics, anticonvulsants), and perception and modulation (e.g., brief behavioral interventions and counseling/education, anxiolytics/sedatives, opioids). Such multimodal care not only improves analgesia but also reduces the risks of adverse effects of any one therapeutic class and in particular opioids.

The use of opioids to treat acute pain must also be carefully analyzed in light of comorbidities including respiratory, gastrointestinal (e.g., ileus, pancreatitis), renal and psychiatric pathology. Comorbidities aside, evidence also exists to support the limitation of opioids in certain situations that might otherwise seem innocuous, such as acute low back pain; the prescription of opioids for acute low back pain for greater than 1–2 weeks has been shown to predict greater loss of function and long-term disability [16, 17].

"Acute on chronic" pain occurring in the chronic pain patient, and especially the chronic pain patient on chronic opioid therapy (COT), is an exceptionally difficult situation to intervene upon to the satisfaction of both patient and provider [18, 19]. Such so-called breakthrough pain (borrowing from the oncologic lexicon) may in fact be better treated in many cases with a combination of basic injury treatment (e.g., rest, ice, elevation), non-opioid pharmacotherapeutics, brief counseling and anxiolytic techniques (e.g., diaphragmatic breathing, progressive muscle relaxation, and guided imagery), and other soothing activities (e.g., warm baths, massage, etc.)

In summary, opioid therapy has a time and place in the treatment of acute pain but only in the context of a multimodal approach, and with great care exercised toward the prevention of dependence, with a clearly delineated "exit strategy" (discussed in greater detail in Chap. 8).

Perioperative Opioid Therapy

A special subset of acute pain deserving unique consideration is perioperative pain, the majority of which is associated with elective procedures that can be anticipated and planned for. Perioperative pain (POP) is virtually universal, and the literature consistently reports a prevalence of chronic postsurgical pain (CPSP) in the neighborhood of 50%. Neuropathic pain and central sensitization are believed to represent a significant component of most CPSP states [20–24]. Increased POP intensity/poor (immediate) postsurgical pain control has been understood to be a risk factor for CPSP for decades and confirmed recently by robust investigations [25–27]. Increased POP also shares psychological confounders which are strong independent predictors of increased CPSP [26–31].

Opioids have enjoyed perioperative (including pre- and intraoperative) use for over 150 years in conjunction with sedative-hypnotic agents to facilitate surgery as well as relieve some of the severe associated pain. The concept of "balanced anesthesia" taught to every anesthesiologist in their training includes (generally intravenous, intraoperative) opioids within the admixture, as these agents have historically provided unparalleled efficacy in analgesia and sympatholysis, with widespread availability and low cost. The concept of preemptive analgesia (PEA) was first proposed by Dr. Patrick Wall (of gate theory fame, as discussed in the previous chapter)

[32] and later developed more fully by his protégé Dr. Clifford Woolf, who demonstrated that prevention of central sensitization underlies the mechanism of PEA [33]. In essence the theory states that adequate analgesia surrounding a traumatic insult (e.g., surgery) can prevent the chronification and amplification too often seen with a surgical operation. Initial interpretation and application of PEA were confined to the preoperative (including immediate pre-incision moment) period and focused on blunting or eliminating nociceptive input by means of systemic analgesics (e.g., intravenous opioids or ketamine) and/or local anesthetic. Despite widespread enthusiasm for the concept, the data did not support the efficacy of this (exclusively pre-incisional) strategy until expanded awareness of the ongoing contribution of low-level C-fiber transmission from the surgical wound is critical in maintaining the sensitized state, necessitating ongoing analgesia until adequate healing occurs [33]. Opioids have continued to represent the lion's share of PEA practice, as ongoing adequate local anesthetic blockade is technically challenging and logistically difficult and prolonged ketamine use (or rather cumulative excess) confers significant dissociation and psychosis. However, it has been recognized for quite some time, well prior to the onset of the current opioid epidemic, that:

> Until an opioid without side effects is available, opioid sparing strategies need to be adopted to ensure sufficient analgesia without sedation and nausea…. [33]

Increasing awareness of the importance of the perioperative arena as a significant contributor to the opioid epidemic has focused research on elucidating risk factors for prolonged postoperative opioid use (PPOU) [34]. Over 100 million surgical procedures are performed in the United States every year at present [35], and the prevalence of long-term opioid use in previously opioid-naïve patients following surgery appears to be on the order of 1:20–1:15 patients [36, 37]. This yields a rough incidence of 50,000 new individuals per year using chronic opioids. (The prevalence of chronic postoperative opioid use in opioid-experienced patients is substantially higher.)

The Toronto General Hospital Transitional Pain Service investigated risk factors for PPOU with a retrospective study of nearly 40,000 opioid-naïve Canadian patients undergoing major elective operations between 2003 and 2010 [38]. Patient-specific (not associated with type of operation or medical comorbidities including diabetes mellitus, congestive heart failure, or pulmonary disease) risk factors included younger age and lower household income. Preoperative use of benzodiazepines and antidepressants, as well as angiotensin-converting enzyme inhibitors, was also independently associated with PPOU.

Recent work done by the Stanford University Anesthesia and Pain Medicine Department has identified preoperative depression, self-perceived addiction vulnerability, and preoperative opioid use as risk factors for PPOU [39, 40]. An investigation of orthopedic trauma patients at the Massachusetts General Hospital also identified catastrophic thinking patterns, anxiety, depression, and post-traumatic stress disorder (PTSD) as predictors of prolonged (greater than 1–2 months) postoperative opioid use, with the former holding the strongest association [41].

A recent study done in a Veterans Administration patient population also reported PTSD as a risk factor for PPOU [42].

Multiple investigations have shown, not surprisingly, that preoperative use of opioids, whether licit or illicit, confers a high risk of PPOU [26, 39–41, 43–45]. Preoperative opioid use has also been universally documented (and dreaded by providers and nursing staff) as a poor predictor of adequate/satisfactory perioperative analgesia as well as patient safety; increasing awareness of the complexities of dealing with such "acute on chronic" pain may fortunately be driving practice toward improved preoperative assessment and a multimodal approach to perioperative analgesia [46–49], the latter of which was discussed in the previous chapter. (Also of interest to patients, surgeons, and hospitals alike should be the additional findings that preoperative opioid use is associated with worsened functional outcomes, decreased satisfaction with the operation, and increased length of stay/increased pain management referrals postoperatively [44, 50–52].)

Surgeons, anesthesiologists, and pain physicians all have an opportunity within this critical window to improve the health of their individual patients as well as institute more generalized strategies impacting the epidemic. Screening for patients at high risk of PPOU should be a standard part of the preoperative assessment [53] and discussed candidly with the patient. Given the strong correlation between psychodysfunctional diathesis and both increased CPSP and PPOU, it may be in the best interest of all parties involved, including the taxpayer, to explore on a large scale whether preoperative psychological clearance prior to elective operations yields improved outcomes. Such an approach has been routine for many years now for certain procedures such as spinal cord (dorsal column) stimulator implantation and bariatric operations. A more targeted approach, given the apparent associations between preoperative opioid use and depression, anxiety, PTSD, etc., using simple screening methods such as state-run prescription database monitoring systems (discussed in greater detail in the next chapter) to risk stratify patients into groups dictating the salience of preoperative psychological assessment and intervention may be "higher yield."

Second, increasing awareness of the paramount contributions of anxiety and catastrophization to CPSP mandates that education on expected perioperative pain/discomfort (which has been shown for over half a century to be beneficial [54, 55]) must continue to be emphasized and practiced by surgeons and their care teams. Consultation of behavioral health professionals for additional preoperative assistance with overcoming cognitive distortions may be uniquely effective [56].

Third, the use of non-opioid modalities to reduce POP has been advocated by anesthesiologists for over a quarter of a century. A significant practice shift among anesthesiologists and surgeons has occurred even within the past decade; whereas opioids have historically comprised the major, if not sole, pre-, intra-, and postoperative analgesics, they are increasingly viewed as "rescue agents" with numerous non-opioid "first-line" or at least adjunctive alternatives [57, 58] receiving greater attention and utility, as discussed in the previous chapter.

Opioid Therapy in Chronic Non-cancer Pain

The use of prescription opioids in chronic non-cancer pain (CNCP) was rare in the past century until the mid-1990s, when a constellation of factors including pressure from the parascientific community (ranging from the American Pain Society and Joint Commission to the Federation of State Medical Boards), aggressive marketing by pharmaceutical companies, lawsuits against physicians alleging inadequate analgesic prescribing, and increasingly emboldened requests from patients appear to have changed the "standard of care" in America. Dovetailing with this latter factor is the subtle leverage exerted upon many hospital-based physicians over the past decade by the Hospital Consumer Assessment of Healthcare Providers and Systems (HCAHPS) survey administered to patients upon discharge. Within the HCAHPS survey are questions on patient satisfaction related to pain management during their hospitalization, and as the Centers for Medicare and Medicaid Services (CMS) bases facility reimbursements in part on this survey, it has been argued recently that physician opioid-prescribing behavior has been influenced toward more liberal patterns by these incentives (or fear of sanction). CMS has recently announced its intent to remove the survey's pain management questions from its calculations of hospital reimbursement [59]. In the outpatient arena, physicians face similar pressures from burgeoning internet reviews, satisfaction ratings, etc. that can have tremendous impact on small practice viability [60].

Regardless of the causal factors involved, the past 20 years have seen an unprecedented degree of liberal prescribing of opioids for non-indicated complaints of all sorts; guilty parties include not only "pill-mills" but also well-meaning but poorly informed or equipped providers trying to please patients. In the author's opinion, a substantial contributor to the increase in patient requests for/provider compliance with opioid prescribing has been a widespread and complex breakdown of societal structure as a whole coupled with poorly reimbursed/funded/staffed behavioral health resources. Opioids are frequently requested (and prescribed) for psychological distress, and opioid dependence once established cements the pattern.

Reactionary attention toward an instruction on the topic of opioid use for CNCP has been commensurate with the magnitude of the societal issue. More detailed examination of these issues follows in the next chapter; for now, suffice it to say that it is once again becoming the general consensus within medicine at the midpoint of this decade that opioids for chronic non-cancer pain should be prescribed only:

- For moderate to severe pain with a plausible etiology that is recalcitrant to other forms of treatment
- When potential benefits outweigh the risks
- As part of a comprehensive treatment plan involving other primary modalities as applicable, with opioids as the adjunctive therapy
- With constant evaluation of benefit in terms of improved function vs. adverse effects
- With clear instructions as to patient responsibility for compliance, safe use, storage, non-diversion, etc.
- With exit strategy clearly delineated a priori

Objective measurement of pain is difficult at best, given that pain by definition is a subjective experience. In the operative and ICU environments, anesthesiologists and other intensivists use hemodynamic variables (or if neuromuscular function is not chemically paralyzed, respiratory effort and somatic movement) as surrogates for pain and discomfort. Postanesthesia care unit nurses learn very quickly to assess respiratory rate and pupil diameter when caring for recovering patients who are requesting more opioid analgesics (as well as assessing the patient for other potential causes of pain and discomfort such as a full bladder or rapidly expanding postoperative hematoma). Beyond these physiologic surrogates, more modern parameters such as biomarkers (e.g., cortisol levels) and biopotentials (e.g., electromyographic or electroencephalographic data) have been proposed [61] as means to help "measure" pain; at present such efforts are impractical and not cost-efficient. Near-infrared spectroscopy (a technology similar to pulse oximetry) can be used to analyze neuronal activity by means of cerebral blood flow and volume and may show promise as a noninvasive and efficient means of providing objective data.

Chronic non-cancer pain (CNCP) comprises a heterogeneous group of conditions, potentially sharing the common ground of central sensitization, but nonetheless with their own unique pathophysiology deserving consideration. In this chapter we will consider three separate entities of chronic "nociceptive" pain, neuropathic pain, and visceral pain.

Chronic "Nociceptive" Pain

Despite the suggestion that all chronic pain states are neuropathic by means of CNS alterations including central sensitization, in this section we will label traditionally understood "non-neuropathic" states as "nociceptive," in line with the traditional viewpoint that most such conditions (e.g., musculoskeletal pain) are a peripheral issue maintained by ongoing tissue insult with associated inflammation. This category, including chronic neck and low back pain, and appendicular orthopedic and rheumatologic disease states comprise the majority of chronic pain within the developed world. As mentioned above in the introduction to this section, the use of chronic opioid therapy for such chronic pain complaints was exceedingly rare prior to the last decade of the previous millennium, with a dramatic increase in liberal use over the past 20 years or so. The resulting crisis has encouraged considerable investigation into the efficacy (or lack thereof) of chronic opioid therapy in CNCP, and the results of most of these investigations are summarized below. Reviews focusing on neuropathic pain are presented in the section that follows.

In 2003, Chou et al. [62] published what is likely the first systematic review of opioid studies. This analysis specifically examined long-acting opioids in CNCP and evaluated 24 studies including 16 randomized clinical trials (RCTs). The review focused on whether long-acting opioids showed any benefit compared to short-acting opioids, in terms of pain relief, and also compared long-acting opioids against others in that class. Long-acting codeine, morphine, oxycodone, and fentanyl were represented in the studies; methadone and levorphanol were not. The study populations included musculoskeletal and neuropathic pain. No trial extended beyond 4 months. The authors concluded that there was insufficient evidence to prove that different long-acting opioids are associated with different efficacy or safety profiles. There was also insufficient evidence to determine whether long-acting opioids as a class are more effective or safer than short-acting opioids.

Kalso et al. in 2004 [63] provided a systematic review of 15 RCTs (*n* = 1025 patients) evaluating the use of various opioids (including morphine 30–120 mg, methadone 15 mg, and oxycodone 20–45 mg) vs. placebo in the treatment of both musculoskeletal and neuropathic CNCP states. Greater than 30% of reported improvement in pain was reported in the treatment groups regardless of etiology. The authors concluded that there was insufficient evidence to draw any conclusions regarding long-term efficacy due to the brevity of the trials involved (the majority involved no more than 8 weeks of study).

Devulder et al. in 2005 [64] reviewed 11 studies, comprising six RCTs and five observational studies, and reported moderate-quality evidence suggesting improvements in functional outcomes and quality of life in patients with CNCP treated with intermediate (12 weeks) to long-term (4 years) opioid therapy. Pain outcomes were not addressed, and the authors admit to the absence of solid, objective measured variables. Further, more rigorous investigations were recommended.

Furlan et al. in 2006 [65] published a meta-analysis of over 6000 patients in 41 RCTs with opioid treatment lasting up to 4 months. This interesting analysis showed an improvement in pain in patients treated with strong opioids (morphine and oxycodone) but no improvement in function. Conversely, patients treated with weak opioids (tramadol, codeine, and propoxyphene) or non-opioids (naproxen and nortriptyline) reported no improvement in pain but did show improvements in functional outcomes.

Martell et al. in 2007 [66] reviewed 15 studies (*n* = 1008 patients) including ten RCTs all examining the question of whether opioids (including tramadol, codeine, dextropropoxyphene, morphine, oxycodone, oxymorphone, or fentanyl) improved chronic low back pain. Data from four of the RCTs were pooled into a meta-analysis showing no statistically significant improvement in low back pain with opioid use; furthermore, a high prevalence of substance use disorder (up to 45%) was noted among the populations studied with up to 24% showing aberrant use of prescribed medications.

Trescot et al. provided guidelines from the American Society of Interventional Pain Physicians (ASIPP) in 2008 [67] including a broad analysis looking at the effectiveness of COT as a class but also evaluated evidence for specific agents. They concluded that weak evidence exists for some improvement in both pain and functional outcomes with the use of both morphine and fentanyl, but such evidence is lacking for other opioids, including the most commonly prescribed agents hydrocodone and oxycodone (and combination acetaminophen products).

Noble et al. in 2010 [68], in a Cochrane Review, examined 26 studies on COT in CNCP (only one which was an RCT) with nearly 5000 patients total. Meta-analysis technique was used when appropriate; they report that weak evidence suggested that patients who were able to tolerate long-term opioid therapy in the absence of limiting adverse effects (which group comprised the minority) experience clinically significant but unquantified pain relief, without any evidence of improvement in quality of life or functional outcomes.

Papaleontiou et al. (2010) performed a systematic review and meta-analysis of 31 RCTs and 12 observational studies comparing opioids to placebo or non-opioid analgesics in CNCP, with 10,545 patients in total [69]. Inclusion criteria included an age equal to or greater than 60 years old (mean age 64). The majority of studies were of 4 weeks' duration or less; roughly two-thirds of the studies evaluated low-potency opioids such as tramadol and codeine. While cautioning that the majority of studies were sponsored by the pharmaceutical industry, the authors report that in older adults with chronic pain and no significant comorbidity, short-term use of opioids is associated with reduction in pain intensity and better physical functioning but poorer mental health functioning. They also concluded that long-term safety, efficacy, and abuse potential of opioids in older adults require further study.

Whittle et al. in 2011 [70] in another Cochrane Review assessed 11 controlled trials ($n = 672$ patients) comparing opioid therapy to placebo or other non-opioid analgesics specifically for rheumatoid arthritis. They report a weak but statistically significant improvement in analgesia (with NNT of 6) from opioids compared to placebo, but none was seen comparing opioids to NSAIDs. They also concluded that there is lack of evidence of any benefit of opioid use beyond 6 weeks.

Furlan et al. in 2011 updated their earlier analysis with 21 additional studies for a total of 62 RCTs comparing opioids vs. placebo or other drugs for CNCP in 11,927 patients [71]. The purpose of this subsequent investigation was primarily to evaluate whether enriched enrollment randomized withdrawal trials (EERW, a type of RCT in which potential participants receive the study drug on a trial basis prior to randomization into the actual study) provided improved data quality by augmenting the pool with participants with improved tolerance; subanalyses focused on adverse effects and are discussed in Chap. 3. As far as efficacy, the authors report small effect size of positive benefit of opioids on function and medium effect size of positive benefit of opioids on pain; however, they note that the majority of studies lasted 6 weeks or less, were sponsored by the pharmaceutical industry, and contained a large number of dropout subjects. As such they advise that no conclusions can be drawn regarding long-term use.

In 2012 Manchikanti et al. updated the earlier ASIPP position paper from Trescot et al. referenced above and provided an extensive two-part reference, the first part of which [72] presented data on numerous topics including rates of nonmedical use/substance abuse, opioid prescribing patterns, adverse effect review, short- and long-term efficacy review, review of individual agents, and review of specific populations. There were no substantive changes between the conclusions drawn in 2008, with the society reporting fair evidence of pain relief and quality of life benefit for opioid therapy in the short term but limited evidence for benefit in long-term situations (>3 months) and fair evidence that chronic use or long-acting agents confer frequent complications.

Chaparro et al. in 2013 [73] in another Cochrane Review evaluated the role of opioids in chronic low back pain. Fifteen RCTs ($n = 5540$ patients) comparing opioids to placebo or non-opioid analgesics or antidepressants were included. Strong opioids (tapentadol, morphine, oxycodone, oxymorphone, hydromorphone) were shown to be more effective than placebo in lowering pain reports and improving function (with the caveat that the studies reviewed showed "limited interpretability of functional improvement). Compared to non-opioid analgesics and antidepressants, however, there were no statistically significant differences between the classes in terms of analgesia or functional improvement. The authors concluded that there are no good-quality data (placebo-controlled RCTs) supporting either safety or efficacy of COT in chronic low back pain.

Sehgal et al. in 2013 [74] synthesized data from 144 articles (including 14 RCTs exceeding 3 months' duration, 9 uncontrolled trials exceeding 3 months' duration, and 13 systematic reviews) and categorized their analysis by evidence for pain relief, functional improvement, and adverse effects. Their conclusions include:

- Among chronic pain patients who respond favorably to opioid therapy (which comprise fewer than half of the patients studied), an average of 30% decreased pain scores was reported.
- There is no evidence for long-term efficacy of COT, and conversely there is strong evidence of a high rate of adverse effects including death.
- Opioids show no superiority compared to non-opioid analgesics/adjuvant therapy (e.g., NSAIDs, antidepressants, and anticonvulsants) in terms of pain relief and functional improvement.
- Greater than 120 mg morphine equivalent dose per day and short-acting FDA Schedule II opioids increase misuse.

DaCosta et al. in 2014 [75] in another Cochrane review examined opioid use in osteoarthritic pain (hip and knee). A meta-analysis of 22 RCTs ($n = 8275$ patients) comparing opioid use (codeine, tapentadol, morphine, oxycodone, oxymorphone, hydromorphone, or fentanyl) vs. placebo or no treatment was performed, and a very weak benefit (improvement of 0.7 cm on a visual analog scale or 12% pain reduction; NNT = 10) in pain was seen, with an even smaller benefit seen in functional outcomes (improvement of 0.6 units on a 10-point scale; NNT = 11). All of these benefits diminished rapidly after 4 weeks.

Reinecke et al. (2015) performed a meta-analysis of 46 RCTs ($n = 10{,}742$ patients) evaluating treatment methodologies in CNCP [76]; 24 of these RCTs evaluated pharmacologic interventions involving both opioid and non-opioid drugs compared to placebo (the remainder evaluated physical and psychological therapy modalities). All studies lasted at least 3 weeks. The authors report that while a small statistically significant benefit of opioids on pain relief was shown, there was no significant difference between any of the modalities investigated.

Chou et al. (2015), in a study funded by the Agency for Healthcare Research and Quality, reviewed 39 studies including RCTs and observational studies that compared opioid therapy for at least 3 months vs. other modalities including placebo [77, 78]. While opioids were found to be moderately effective for pain relief in RCTs lasting generally 3 months or less, functional improvement evidence was less robust, and there were considerable dropout rates due to inefficacy or adverse effects. The authors note that no studies comparing opioids to no therapy, placebo, or other drug evaluated long-term (defined as >12 months) outcomes related to pain relief, functional improvement, or quality of life and caution that there is no evidence for long-term benefit.

This investigation was subsequently expanded with seven more studies and summary data presented in the 2016 Centers for Disease Control (CDC) Guideline for Prescribing Opioids [5]; the authors again report that insufficient data exist to answer the question of whether COT for CNCP is beneficial.

Summarizing all of the data currently available, no study to date has shown greater than 50% improvement in either analgesia or functional outcomes from chronic opioid therapy sustained over months to years, and as most of the studies show, there is a very high rate of adverse effects with COT. Those data were reviewed in Chap. 3. On the other hand, Ballantyne [79] and Trescot [67] have argued that restricting acceptable evidence to that presented by randomized controlled trials confers artificial constraints not generalizable to "real-world" clinical experience; RCTs are by necessity of short duration, generally limited to a specific disease state, and rely on poorly validatable categorical measurements of subjective outcomes. And finally, Smith and Pell, in their excellent 2003 editorial [80], remind us that RCTs and evidence-based medicine in toto should not provide the only guidance for clinical practice and that medicine is both science and art. Data by definition are plural, and good data reflects a very large sample size. Given the inherent heterogeneity of human beings, the complexity of pain itself, and the acknowledgment that "half of what we currently think to be true probably isn't," it appears safe to say that while for the vast majority of patients and conditions the evidence of harm from COT appears to outweigh the benefit, there are always exceptions to the mean ± two or three standard deviations.

Neuropathic Pain

As discussed above, there is a school of thought that holds that all chronic pain is essentially neuropathic, whether by means of peripheral sensitization of nociceptors, alterations within the dorsal horn of the spinal cord, or higher structures including the limbic and other cortical areas. The tremendous plasticity of neurons and glia is just beginning to be explored, and there is evidence that chronic pain may represent more "memory" than current event. Having said that, in this section we will restrict the discussion to conditions traditionally considered to be neuropathic in the sense of arising from injured nerves, such as peripheral neuropathies, post-herpetic neuralgia, and compressive neuropathies (e.g., certain radiculopathies).

There has been a general sense among physicians experienced in treating pain that the use of opioids in neuropathic pain states is generally not beneficial, or at least less beneficial than in "nociceptive" pain states [81, 82]. Multiple mechanisms have been postulated to account for this apparent inefficacy (many of which are putatively linked with opioid-induced hyperalgesia), and the excellent recent review by Smith summarizes most current hypotheses [82]. Regardless of the underlying mechanisms, our growing understanding of the incredibly complex interactions between psychological factors and the neuroendocrine and endogenous opioid systems supports the concept that perturbations in the allostasis of this otherwise finely balanced system by prolonged exposure to exogenous mu-agonists perpetuate or even exacerbate the pain experience.

Few studies and reviews have restricted their focus to chronic opioid therapy in neuropathic conditions; most major reviews are summarized below, with select individual trials discussed later in the section in the context of specific agents.

Ballantyne and Mao [83], in one of the earliest reviews of COT in CNCP, identified a handful of studies specifically investigating COT in neuropathic pain and concluded that opioid therapy in the short term provided improvement in pain scores including neuropathic pain conditions, although this spectrum required higher doses than non-neuropathic pain.

Eisenberg et al. in 2005 [84] conducted a review of 22 RCTs evaluating opioid use (codeine, meperidine, morphine, methadone, levorphanol, alfentanil, fentanyl) in neuropathic pain states. Fourteen of the trials lasted less than 24 h and yielded conflicting results; the remaining eight trials again reported roughly 30% improvement in pain compared to placebo but had a median duration of only 28 days.

Hollingshead et al. in a 2006 Cochrane review [85] reported on the results of examining the benefit of tramadol in treating neuropathic pain. Six randomized trials were included in their analysis, four of which compared tramadol to placebo and the other two to other drugs (clomipramine, morphine). The four placebo-controlled trials showed significant reduction in pain with tramadol, and three of these trials were further combined in a meta-analysis showing the number needed to treat with tramadol (compared to placebo) to reach at least 50% pain relief was 3.8 (95% confidence interval 2.8–6.3).

McNicol et al. in 2013 [86] reviewed 31 RCTs ($n = 1237$ patients) in which pure opioid agonists (excluding combination agents with acetaminophen or NSAIDs) were trialed against placebo in the treatment of neuropathic pain. Almost a third of these subjects were exposed to the opioid for 24 h or less, and these data were contradictory and inconclusive. The remaining two-thirds were studied for 3 months or less (the majority for fewer than 6 weeks), and meta-analysis showed small benefit (NNT = 4) from opioid vs. placebo if a cutoff of 33% improvement was used and, as would be expected, even less benefit (NNT = 5.9) if a 50% improvement criteria was used. The authors make the point that no improvement was seen in "many aspects of emotional or physical functioning" and also admit that significant pro-treatment bias likely skews the results of the study due to short duration of evaluation and other component study limitations.

Two recent Cochrane reviews [87, 88] examined whether oxycodone or hydromorphone was efficacious in neuropathic pain; the former showed "only very low quality evidence that oxycodone (as oxycodone MR) is of value in the treatment of painful diabetic neuropathy or postherpetic neuralgia [with] no evidence for other neuropathic pain conditions," and the latter showed no evidence of benefit from hydromorphone. Adverse events typical of opioids were common.

Exogenous opioids are of course heterogeneous as well, and both anecdotal and clinical trial evidences seem to suggest that some of these drugs work better than others in neuropathic pain. Those that seem to show the best efficacy include tramadol and tapentadol, methadone and levorphanol, and buprenorphine.

Tramadol has been shown in numerous studies (as summarized above) to be beneficial in neuropathic pain states. It is suggested that the serotonin and norepinephrine reuptake inhibition (SNRI) activity of this agent confers synergistic benefit with the weak mu-agonism of the molecule that results in a pharmacologic profile more effective than pure mu-agonists and without significant tolerance/hyperalgesia. It should be noted however that combining tramadol with other serotonergics (which are first line in neuropathic pain) confers a high risk of seizures or serotonin syndrome. Tapentadol, like tramadol, combines norepinephrine (without significant serotonin) reuptake inhibition with a mu-agonist, yielding particular benefit in neuropathic pain states [89, 90] with very good tolerability. The drug is new, and as of yet multiple post-marketing trials and systematic reviews have not corroborated early findings.

Methadone has shown benefit in neuropathic pain states as well, with numerous trials evidencing significant pain reduction with very little tolerance development [91–95]. This latter phenomenon is thought to be due to the NMDA-blocking function of the S-enantiomer. Low doses (10–20 mg/day) are often effective [91, 92] which is of particular interest in neuropathic pain given that first-line treatment agents (antidepressants) frequently either inhibit cytochrome P450 enzymes that metabolize methadone or prolong the QT interval in their own right. Buprenorphine has also been observed to exhibit significant benefit in neuropathic pain [96–99] including very difficult-to-treat conditions such as central pain syndrome [100] and phantom limb pain [101]. High-quality randomized control trial data are not extant at the time of this writing. Like methadone, buprenorphine appears to subvert typical opioid-induced hyperalgesia through mechanisms that are as of yet unclear but may have to do with its kappa-receptor antagonism.

As in any painful condition, opioid use for the treatment of neuropathic pain should be deferred until therapeutic failure of lower-risk agents has been established. First-line agents for the treatment of neuropathic pain include SNRIs (or tricyclic antidepressants, being mindful of increased adverse effects from these older drugs) and gabapentinoids [102–104] with strong consideration of topical agents (e.g., topical lidocaine patches, capsaicin cream) in select conditions, e.g., post-herpetic neuralgia. When opioids are introduced into the antineuropathic armamentarium, they should always be part of a multimodal regimen including first- and second-line agents as described above [105] and should always be considered a trial with ongoing assessment of benefit vs. harm.

Chronic Visceral Pain

Chronic abdominopelvic visceral pain encompasses several pathologic conditions (e.g., chronic pancreatitis, pain conditions related to the liver or gallbladder, inflammatory bowel disease, functional gastrointestinal disorders, endometriosis, interstitial cystitis, chronic pelvic pain without identifiable etiology, and others). Visceral nociception, as discussed in the previous chapter, remains fairly poorly understood at present, but given that most of the viscera lack perceptible sensitivity to stimuli other than distension, most chronic visceral pain is thought in general to represent a central sensitization state and in many cases likely has strong psychological overlay [106, 107, 108].

Acute abdominopelvic pain is generally deserving of urgent if not emergent evaluation, and as such most assessment takes place in the emergency department. Traditionally, opioids are used sparingly so as to not mask progression of symptoms that could signify imminent catastrophe. The use of chronic opioids to treat chronic visceral pain has increased significantly in the past two decades, along with other chronic pain conditions, but no rigorous investigations have singled out visceral pain for evaluation of either efficacy or harm from chronic opioid use.

Summary of Opioid Use in Chronic Non-cancer Pain

With the exception of certain agents showing benefit in certain neuropathic pain states, for the most part, the literature does not show benefit of chronic opioid therapy for chronic non-cancer pain. Given the high risk of harm with these agents, including perpetuation or worsening of pain, the decision to trial opioid therapy for CNPC should be a cautious one, with ongoing assessment for evidence of improved function and pain. As in any situation, reservation of opioids for cases where more conservative therapy has failed is wise, and if opioid therapy is agreed upon, it should also always be part of a multimodal regimen [109].

Knowing *when not to* prescribe opioids is perhaps even more imperative than knowing when and why to prescribe them. Certain conditions (e.g., headache, fibromyalgia) are almost invariably worsened by opioid therapy, and guidelines from national and international professional societies recommend against the use of opioids in these (and other) situations [110–113].

In terms of the individual patient, a careful risk-benefit ratio analysis taking into account comorbidities including at least psychiatric, respiratory, gastroenterologic, and renal conditions is mandatory each and every time; the oath to first do no harm is frequently transgressed by a thoughtless or hurried prescription. It is relatively easy to ascertain and explain to patients that severe respiratory or hepatic or renal disease contraindicates opioid therapy; making and communicating such decision in case of severe depression or other psychiatric malady, or in cases when self-medication of emotional suffering is suspected, are not generally as easy. The development of good rapport and patient engagement is essential to helping all patients, and those with psychiatric comorbidities are certainly no exception. Communicating a decision to not prescribe opioids can and should always be done in a manner that reflects both our professional standards of care and comfort and, at the same time, genuine compassion and concern for the well-being of the patient. In our experience, it is the rare patient that does not perceive and appreciate this, no matter how distasteful your decision is to them.

Withholding opioid prescription is frequently in the best interest of the community as well. While law enforcement is not within the purview of physicians, it is nonetheless incumbent upon us to be vigilant for any signs of certain illegal activities that endanger the health and well-being of the patient or others, for example, suspected child abuse situations. The diversion of prescribed opioids poses a grave danger to the community, and physicians bear some degree of responsibility for this and must at all times exercise due diligence and alter or curtail (or refuse to prescribe in the first place) opioid prescription when diversion is suspected. Readily available and appropriate means of surveillance for potential diversion include random pill counts, random urinalysis to confirm that the prescribed agent and/or metabolites are present in the urine, and the use of prescription database monitoring programs to screen for "doctor shopping." These and other considerations are discussed in greater detail in Chap. 8.

Opioid Therapy in Cancer Pain

Chronic opioid therapy in cancer (and other terminal states) remains prevalent and is much more widely accepted. Over two-thirds of patients with cancer suffer from pain associated with the disease, and significant psychological malaise is almost universal. Further complicating cancer pain are the facts that:

- Multiple distinct physical "pain generators" (median four, range one to seven [114]) are common.
- Multiple pathophysiologic processes are generally at work (as discussed in the previous chapter) often in varying stages, conferring mechanical, inflammatory, and neuropathic insults.

Awareness of a general progression, however, from early mechanical and inflammatory effect, to a later primarily neuropathic state (often compounded by chemotherapy) and in many cases ultimately osseous pain from bony metastases helps to tailor multimodal therapy, which is as important in cancer pain as in CNCP. Fortunately, the latter may respond well to bisphosphonates or inhibitors of osteoclastic receptor activator of nuclear factor κB ligand (RANKL) [115] as well as to radiotherapy.

The WHO analgesic ladder referenced at the beginning of the chapter and shown in Fig. 7.1 has been used for decades to guide opioid therapy in cancer, with good results (greater than 75% of patients reporting satisfactory analgesia) reported in a large observational study of over 2000 patients [116]. It should be noted that these data do not reflect opioid monotherapy results; rather the patients underwent multimodal pain therapy including antidepressant and anticonvulsant pharmacotherapy, corticosteroids, palliative antineoplastic treatment, nerve blocks or ablation, physiotherapy including transcutaneous electrical nerve stimulation, and psychotherapy.

National- and international-level guidelines [117–120] support both a staged and more accurately a tiered approach, with opioid potency tailored to match the severity of cancer pain; in other words, the patient with previously unassessed/untreated severe pain does not need to be subjected to initial trials of non-opioid analgesics or so-called Step II (weak) opioids prior to prescribing "Step III" (strong) opioids. As with non-cancer pain, however, the use of opioids should always occur within the context of a multimodal plan, and most recent guidelines reflect this wisdom.

One final area the clinician treating cancer patients is frequently called upon to prescribe opioids is in the management of dyspnea. Over half of all cancer patients suffer from dyspnea [121, 122]. As with pain, thorough workup and comprehensive treatment are required (e.g., oxygen, bronchodilators or diuretics, or thoracentesis may be warranted), but opioids have traditionally been used in this palliative setting and will likely continue to due to their unparalleled efficacy. Even this most universally accepted indication has been subjected to the rigors of modern clinical trials, and a recent systematic review [121] of eight RCTs (including four placebo-controlled RCTs) and six nonrandomized trials ($n = 424$ patients) showed "modest" evidence of benefit in relieving dyspnea. Additional analyses in some of the trials showed no significant hypercarbia or hypoxemia despite reductions in respiratory rate.

Guidelines from the major societies recommend the use of strong opioids (preferentially morphine as a first-line agent) in a multimodal approach to treat dyspnea associated with cancer [122–124].

Summary

Opioids are not a panacea for pain; tolerance renders them imperfect, and adverse effects (including hyperalgesia) often render them malicious. While they do possess tremendous potency for pain relief especially in naïve patients, in experienced/tolerant patients, the cold, hard facts are that they have yet to be shown to be efficacious for CNPC by rigorous examination. In the era of evidence-based medicine, several reviews of the efficacy of opioid therapy in various conditions and for various durations have been published, and the majority of the high-quality analyses extant at the time of this writing are summarized above. The objective consensus of these reviews is that for chronic non-cancer pain, there is currently no good evidence that chronic opioid use results in either improved pain control or functional outcomes beyond a 3- to 4-month period.

Providers should consider opioid prescription as a matter of last resort generally, after more conservative means have failed. When used, opioids must always be part of a multimodal approach tailored to the patient's pathology. The prescription of opioids for non-cancer pain, whether acute or chronic, should always be viewed as a trial, with continuous assessment of efficacy in facilitating functional goals and analgesia vs. adverse effects. Time spent "up front" educating patients as to the limitations of opioid therapy including limitations set by the provider (expectations, duration, "exit strategy," etc.) will also pay dividends for both patient and provider in the long run. This is discussed in greater detail in the next chapter.

Chronic opioid therapy in cancer (and other terminal states) for the treatment of both pain and dyspnea remains prevalent and is much more widely accepted. As with non-cancer pain, the use of opioids should always occur within the context of a multimodal plan.

References

1. American Academy of Pain Medicine. Use of opioids for the treatment of chronic pain: a statement from the American academy of pain medicine. 2013. http://www.painmed.org/files/use-of-opioids-for-the-treatment-of-chronic-pain.pdf
2. Institute of Medicine. Relieving pain in america: a blueprint for transforming prevention, care, education and research. Washington, DC: National Academies Press; 2011.
3. Interagency guideline on prescribing opioids for pain developed by the Washington state agency medical directors' group 3rd Edition, June 2015. http://www.agencymeddirectors.wa.gov/Files/2015AMDGOpioidGuideline.pdf
4. Veterans Administration/Department of Defense. VA/DoD clinical practice guideline for management of opioid therapy for chronic pain. Washington, DC: Veterans Administration; 2010. Available from: http://www.va.gov/painmanagement/docs/cpg_opioidtherapy_fulltext.pdf
5. Centers for Disease Control and Prevention. CDC guideline for prescribing opioids for chronic pain—United States, 2016. MMWR. 2016;65(1):1–49.
6. Strassels SA, McNicol E, Wagner AK, et al. Persistent postoperative pain, health-related quality of life, and functioning 1 month after hospital discharge. Acute Pain. 2004;6:95–104.
7. Sinatra R. Causes and consequences of inadequate management of acute pain. Pain Med. 2010;11:1859–71.
8. McGreevy K, Bottros MM, Raja SN. Preventing chronic pain following acute pain: risk factors, preventive strategies, and their efficacy. Eur J Pain Suppl. 2011;5:365–72.
9. Pogatzki-Zahn EM, Zahn PK. From preemptive to preventive analgesia. Curr Opin Anaesthesiol. 2006;19:551–5.
10. Wood MJ, Kay R, Dworkin RH, Soong SJ, Whitley RJ. Oral acyclovir therapy accelerates pain resolution in patients with herpes zoster: a meta-analysis of placebo-controlled trials. Clin Infect Dis. 1996;22:341–7.
11. American Society of Anesthesiologists Task Force on Acute Pain Management. Practice guidelines for acute pain management in the perioperative setting: an updated report by the american society of anesthesiologists task force on acute pain management. Anesthesiology. 2012;116:248–73.
12. American Academy of Pain Medicine. Acute pain and cancer pain. A position statement from the American academy of pain medicine. 1998. http://www.painmed.org/files/acute-cancer-pain-statement.pdf
13. Thorson D, Biewen P, Bonte B, Epstein H, Haake B, Hansen C, et al. Institute for clinical systems improvement. Acute pain assessment and opioid prescribing protocol. Published January 2014. https://www.icsi.org/_asset/dyp5wm/opioids.pdf
14. Joint Theater Trauma System Management of pain, anxiety, and delirium in injured warfighters. April 2013. www.dvcipm.org/clinical-resources/military-clinical-practice-guidelines.
15. The Management of Postoperative Pain Working Group. VHA/DoD clinical practice guideline for the management of postoperative pain. Version 1.2. http://www.healthquality.va.gov/guidelines/Pain/pop/pop_fulltext.pdf

16. Webster BS, Verma SK, Gatchel RJ. Relationship between early opioid prescribing for acute occupational low back pain and disability duration, medical costs, subsequent surgery and late opioid use. Spine. 2007;32:2127–32.
17. Franklin GM, Stover BD, Turner JA, Fulton-Kehoe D, Wickizer TM. Early opioid prescription and subsequent disability among workers with back injuries: the Disability Risk Identification Study Cohort. Spine. 2008;33:199–204.
18. Huxtable CA, Roberts LJ, Somogyi AA, MacIntyre PE. Acute pain management in opioid-tolerant patients: a growing challenge. Anaesth Intensive Care. 2011;39:804–23.
19. Quinlan J, Carter K. Acute pain management in patients with persistent pain. Curr Opin Support Palliat Care. 2012;6:188–93.
20. Kehlet H, Jensen TS, Woolf CJ. Persistent postsurgical pain: risk factors and prevention. Lancet. 2006;367:1618–25.
21. Johansen A, Romundstad L, Nielsen CS, Schirmer H, Stubhaug A. Persistent postsurgical pain in a general population: prevalence and predictors in the Tromsø study. Pain. 2012;153:1390–6.
22. Haroutiunian S, Nikolajsen L, Finnerup NB, Jensen TS. The neuropathic component in persistent postsurgical pain: a systematic literature review. Pain. 2013;154:95–102.
23. Werner MU, Bischoff JM. Persistent postsurgical pain: evidence from breast cancer surgery, groin hernia repair, and lung cancer surgery. Curr Top Behav Neurosci. 2014;20:3–29.
24. Reddi D, Curran N. Chronic pain after surgery: pathophysiology, risk factors and prevention. Postgrad Med J. 2014;90:222–7.
25. Joshi GP, Ogunnaike BO. Consequences of inadequate postoperative pain relief and chronic persistent postoperative pain. Anesthesiol Clin North Am. 2005;23:21–36.
26. VanDenKerkhof EG, Hopman WM, Goldstein DH, Wilson RA, Towheed TE, Lam M, et al. Impact of perioperative pain intensity, pain qualities, and opioid use on chronic pain after surgery: a prospective cohort study. Reg Anesth Pain Med. 2012;37:19–27.
27. Katz J, Weinrib A, Fashler SR, Katznelzon R, Shah BR, Ladak SS, et al. The Toronto general hospital transitional pain service: development and implementation of a multidisciplinary program to prevent chronic postsurgical pain. J Pain Res. 2015;8:695–702.
28. Kleiman V, Clarke H, Katz J. Sensitivity to pain traumatization: a higher-order factor underlying pain-related anxiety, pain catastrophizing and anxiety sensitivity among patients scheduled for major surgery. Pain Res Manag. 2011;16:169–77.
29. Theunissen M, Peters ML, Bruce J, Gramke HF, Marcus MA. Preoperative anxiety and catastrophizing: a systematic review and meta-analysis of the association with chronic postsurgical pain. Clin J Pain. 2012;28:819–41.
30. Attal N, Masselin-Dubois A, Martinez V, Jayr C, Albi A, Fermanian J, et al. Does cognitive functioning predict chronic pain? Results from a prospective surgical cohort. Brain. 2014;137(Pt 3):904–17.
31. Hoofwijk DM, Fiddelers AA, Peters ML, Stessel B, Kessels AG, Joosten EA, et al. Prevalence and predictive factors of chronic postsurgical pain and poor global recovery one year after outpatient surgery. Clin J Pain. 2015;31(12):1017–25.
32. Wall PD. The prevention of post-operative pain. Pain. 1988;33:289–90.
33. Woolf C, Bromley L. Pre-emptive Analgesia by Opioids. In: Stein C, editor. Opioids in pain control: basic and clinical aspects. Cambridge: Cambridge University Press; 1999. p. 212–33.
34. Clarke JL, Skoufalos A, Scranton R. The american opioid epidemic: population health implications and potential solutions. Report from the national stakeholder panel. Population Health Mgmt. 2016;19(Suppl 1):S1–9.
35. Cullen KA, Hall MJ, Golosinsky A. Ambulatory surgery in the United States, 2006. Natl Health Stat Rep. 2009;11:1–25.
36. Alam A, Gomes T, Zheng H, Mamdami MM, Juurlink DN, Bell CM. Long-term analgesic use after low-risk surgery: a retrospective Cohort study. Arch Intern Med. 2012;172:425–30.
37. Huang A, Azam A, Segal S, Pivovarov K, Katznelson G, Ladak SS, et al. Chronic postsurgical pain and persistent opioid use following surgery: the need for a transitional pain service. Pain Manag. 2016;6(5):435–43.

38. Clarke H, Soneji N, Ko DT, Yun L, Wijeysundera DN. Rates and risk factors for prolonged opioid use after major surgery: population based cohort study. BMJ. 2014;348:g1251. doi:10.1136/bmj.g1251.
39. Carroll I, Barelka P, Wang CK, Wang BM, Gillespie MJ, McCue R. A pilot cohort study of the determinants of longitudinal opioid use after surgery. Anesth Analg. 2012;115:694–702.
40. Hah JM, Sharifzadeh Y, Wang BM, Gillespie MJ, Goodman SB, Mackey SC, et al. Factors Associated with Opioid Use in a Cohort of Patients Presenting for Surgery. Pain Res Treat. 2015;2015:829696. doi:10.1155/2015/829696.
41. Helmerhorst GT, Vranceanu AM, Vrahas M, Smith M, Ring D. Risk factors for continued opioid use one to two months after surgery for musculoskeletal trauma. Bone Joint Surg Am. 2014;96:495–9.
42. Rozet I, Nishio I, Robbertze R, Rotter D, Chansky H, Hernandez AV. Prolonged opioid use after knee arthroscopy in military veterans. Anesth Analg. 2014;119:454–9.
43. Massey GM, Dodds HN, Roberts CS, Servoss TJ, Blondell RD. Toxicology screening in orthopedic trauma patients predicting duration of prescription opioid use. J Addict Dis. 2005;24:31–41.
44. Lawrence JTR, London N, Bohlman HH, Chin KR. Preoperative narcotic use as a predictor of clinical outcome: results following anterior cervical arthrodesis. Spine. 2008;33:2074–8.
45. Armaghani SJ, Lee DS, Bible JE, Archer KR, Shau DN, Kay H, et al. Preoperative opioid use and its association with perioperative opioid demand and postoperative opioid independence in patients undergoing spine surgery. Spine (Phila Pa 1976). 2014;39(25):E1524–30. doi:10.1097/BRS.0000000000000622.
46. Mitra S, Sinatra RS. Perioperative management of acute pain in the opioid-dependent patient. Anesthesiology. 2004;101:212–27.
47. Rozen D, Grass GW. Perioperative and intraoperative pain and anesthetic care of the chronic pain and cancer pain patient receiving chronic opioid therapy. Pain Pract. 2005;5:18–32.
48. De Pinto M, Cahana A. Medical management of acute pain in patients with chronic pain. Expert Rev. Neurother. 2012;12:1325–38.
49. Shah S, Kapoor S, Durkin B. Analgesic management of acute pain in the opioid-tolerant patient. Curr Opin Anaesthesiol. 2015;28:398–402.
50. Franklin PD, Karbassi JA, Li W, Yang W, Ayers DC. Reduction in narcotic use after primary total knee arthroplasty and association with patient pain relief and satisfaction. J Arthroplast. 2010;25:12–6.
51. Zywiel MG, Stroh DA, Lee SY, Bonutti PM, Mont MA. Chronic opioid use prior to total knee arthroplasty. J Bone Joint Surg. 2011;93:1988–93.
52. Pivec R, Issa K, Naziri Q, Kapadia BH, Bonutti PM, Mont MA. Opioid use prior to total hip arthroplasty leads to worse clinical outcomes. Internat Orthol. 2014;38:1159–65.
53. Devin CJ, Lee DS, Armaghani SJ, Bible J, Shau DN, Martin PR, et al. Approach to pain management in chronic opioid users undergoing orthopaedic surgery. J Am Acad Orthop Surg. 2014;22:614–22.
54. Egbert LD, Battit GE, Welch CE, et al. Reduction of postoperative pain by encouragement and instruction of patients—a study of doctor-patient rapport. N Engl J Med. 1964;270:825–7.
55. Suls J, Wan CK. Effects of sensory and procedural information on coping with stressful medical procedures and pain: a meta-analysis. J Consult Clin Psychol. 1989;57:372–9.
56. Powell R, Scott NW, Manyande A, Bruce J, Vögele C, Byrne-Davis LM, et al. Psychological preparation and postoperative outcomes for adults undergoing surgery under general anaesthesia. Cochrane Database Syst Rev. 2016;5:CD008646. doi:10.1002/14651858.CD008646.pub2.
57. Devin CJ, McGirt MJ. Best evidence in multimodal pain management in spine surgery and means of assessing postoperative pain and functional outcomes. J Clin Neurosci. 2015;22:930–8.
58. Gritsenko K, Khelemsky Y, Kaye AD, Vadivelu N, Urman RD. Multimodal therapy in perioperative analgesia. Best Pract Res Clin Anaesthesiol. 2014;28:59–79.

59. http://www.beckershospitalreview.com/quality/cms-proposes-eliminating-pain-management-from-hcahps-payment-score.html
60. Lembke A. Why doctors prescribe opioids to known opioid abusers. NEJM. 2012;367:1580–1.
61. Cowen R, Stasiowska MK, Laycock H, Bantel C. Assessing pain objectively: the use of physiological markers. Anaesthesia. 2015;70:828–47.
62. Chou R, Clark E, Helfand M. Comparative efficacy and safety of long – acting oral opioids for chronic non—cancer pain: a systematic review. J Pain Symptom Manag. 2003;26:1026–48.
63. Kalso E, Edwards J, Moore R, McQuay HJ. Opioids in chronic non-cancer pain: systematic review of efficacy and safety. Pain. 2004;112:372–80.
64. Devulder J, Richarz U, Nataraja SH. Impact of long-term use of opioids on quality of life in patients with chronic, non-malignant pain. Curr Med Res Opin. 2005;21:1555–68.
65. Furlan AD, Sandoval JA, Mailis-Gagnon A, Tunks E. Opioids for chronic non-cancer pain: a meta-analysis of effectiveness and side effects. Can Med Assoc J. 2006;174:1589–94.
66. Martell BA, O'Connor PG, Kerns RD, Becker WC, Morales KH, Kosten TR, et al. Opioid treatment for chronic back pain: prevalence, efficacy, and association with addiction. Ann Intern Med. 2007;146:116–27.
67. Trescot AM, Glaser SE, Hansen H, Benyamin R, Patel S, Manchikanti L. Effectiveness of opioids in the treatment of chronic non-cancer pain. Pain Physician. 2008;11:S181–200.
68. Noble M, Treadwell JR, Tregear SJ, Coates VH, Wiffen PJ, Akafomo C, et al. Long-term opioid management for chronic noncancer pain. Cochrane Database Syst Rev. 2010;1:CD006605. doi:10.1002/14651858.CD006605.pub2.
69. Papaleontiou M, Henderson CR, Turner BJ, Moore AA, Olkhovskaya Y, Amanfo L, et al. Outcomes associated with opioid use in the treatment of chronic non-cancer pain among older adults: a systematic review and meta-analysis. J Am Geriatr Soc. 2010;58:1353–69.
70. Whittle SL, Richards BL, Husni E, Buchbinder R. Opioid therapy for treating rheumatoid arthritis pain. Cochrane Database Syst Rev. 2011;(11):CD003113. doi:10.1002/14651858.CD003113.pub3.
71. Furlan A, Chaparro LE, Irvin E, Mailis-Gagnon A. A comparison between enriched and non-enriched enrollment randomized withdrawal trials of opioids for chronic noncancer pain. Pain Res Manag. 2011;16:337–51.
72. Manchikanti L, Abdi S, Atluri S, Balog CC, Benyamin RM, Boswell MV, et al. American society of interventional pain physicians (ASIPP) guidelines for responsible opioid prescribing in chronic non-cancer pain: Part I--evidence assessment. Pain Physician. 2012;15(3 Suppl):S1–65.
73. Chaparro LE, Furlan AD, Deshpande A, Mailis-Gagnon A, Atlas S, Turk DC. Opioids compared to placebo or other treatments for chronic low-back pain. Cochrane Database Syst Rev. 2013;(8):CD004959. doi:10.1002/14651858.CD004959.pub4.
74. Sehgal N, Colson J, Smith HS. Chronic pain treatment with opioid analgesics – benefits versus harms of long-term therapy. Expert Rev. Neurother. 2013;13:1201–20.
75. DaCosta BR, Nuesch E, Kasteler R. Oral or transdermal opioids for osteoarthritis of the knee or hip. Cochrane Database Syst Rev. 2014;(9):CD003115. doi:10.1002/14651858.CD003115.pub4.
76. Reinecke H, Weber C, Lange K, Simon M, Stein C, Sorgatz H. Analgesic efficacy of opioids in chronic pain: recent meta-analysis. Br J Pharmacol. 2015;172:324–33.
77. Chou R, Deyo R, Devine B, Hansen R, Sullivan S, Jarvik JG, et al. The effectiveness and risks of long-term opioid treatment of chronic pain. Evidence report/technology assessment no. 218. (prepared by the pacific northwest evidence-based practice center under contract no. 290–2012-00014-I.) AHRQ publication no. 14-E005-EF. Rockville, MD: Agency for Healthcare Research and Quality; 2014.
78. Chou R, Turner JA, Devine EB, Hansen RN, Sullivan SD, Blazina I, et al. The effectiveness and risks of long-term opioid therapy for chronic pain: a systematic review for a National Institutes of Health Pathways to Prevention Workshop. Ann Intern Med. 2015;162:276–86.

79. Ballantyne JC, Shin NS. Efficacy of opioids for chronic pain. A review of the evidence. Clin J Pain. 2008;24:469–78.
80. Smith GCS, Pell JP. Parachute use to prevent death and major trauma related to gravitational challenge: systematic review of randomised controlled trials. BMJ. 2003;327:1459.
81. Arnér S, Meyerson BA. Lack of analgesic effect of opioids on neuropathic and idiopathic forms of pain. Pain. 1988;33:11–23.
82. Smith HS. Opioids and neuropathic pain. Pain Physician. 2012;15(3 Suppl):ES93–110.
83. Ballantyne JC, Mao J. Opioid therapy for chronic pain. N Engl J Med. 2003;349:1943–53.
84. Eisenberg E, McNicol ED, Carr DB. Efficacy and safety of opioid agonists in the treatment of neuropathic pain of non-malignant origin: systematic review and meta—analysis of randomized controlled trials. JAMA. 2005;293:3043–52.
85. Hollingshead J, Dühmke RM, Cornblath DR. Tramadol for neuropathic pain. Cochrane Database Syst Rev. 2006;(3):CD003726.
86. McNicol ED, Midbari A, Eisenberg E. Opioids for neuropathic pain. Cochrane Database Syst Rev. 2013;(8):CD006146. doi:10.1002/14651858.CD006146.pub2.
87. Gaskell H, Derry S, Stannard C, Moore RA. Oxycodone for neuropathic pain in adults. Cochrane Database Syst Rev. 2016;(7):CD010692. doi:10.1002/14651858.CD010692.pub3.
88. Stannard C, Gaskell H, Derry S, Aldington D, Cole P, Cooper TE, et al. Hydromorphone for neuropathic pain in adults. Cochrane Database Syst Rev. 2016;(5):CD011604. doi:10.1002/14651858.CD011604.pub2.
89. Schwartz S, Etropolski MS, Shapiro DY, Rauschkolb C, Vinik AI, Lange B, et al. A pooled analysis evaluating the efficacy and tolerability of tapentadol extended release for chronic, painful diabetic peripheral neuropathy. Clin Drug Invest. 2015;35:95–108.
90. Baron R, Likar R, Martin-Mola E, Blanco FJ, Kennes L, Müller M, et al. Effectiveness of tapentadol prolonged release (PR) compared with oxycodone/naloxone PR for the management of severe chronic low back pain with a neuropathic component: a randomized, controlled, open-label, phase 3b/4 study. Pain Pract. 2016;16:580–99.
91. Morley JS, Bridson J, Nash TP, Miles JB, White S, Makin MK. Low-dose methadone has an analgesic effect in neuropathic pain: a double-blind randomized controlled crossover trial. Palliat Med. 2003;17:576–87.
92. Gagnon B, Almahrezi A, Schreier G. Methadone in the treatment of neuropathic pain. Pain Res Manag. 2003;8:149–54.
93. Moulin DE, Palma D, Watling C, Schulz V. Methadone in the management of intractable neuropathic noncancer pain. Can J Neurol Sci. 2005;32:340–3.
94. Mendlik MT, Uritsky TJ. Treatment of neuropathic pain. Curr Treat Options Neurol. 2015;17:50. doi:10.1007/s11940-015-0381-2.
95. Sugiyama Y, Sakamoto N, Ohsawa M, Onizuka M, Ishida K, Murata Y, et al. A retrospective study on the effectiveness of switching to oral methadone for relieving severe cancer-related neuropathic pain and limiting adjuvant analgesic use in Japan. J Palliat Med. 2016;19(10):1051–9.
96. Hans G. Buprenorphine--a review of its role in neuropathic pain. J Opioid Manag. 2007;3:195–206.
97. Pergolizzi J, Aloisi AM, Dahan A, Filitz J, Langford R, Likar R, et al. Current knowledge of buprenorphine and its unique pharmacological profile. Pain Pract. 2010;10:428–50.
98. Leppert W, Kowalski G. Long-term administration of high doses of transdermal buprenorphine in cancer patients with severe neuropathic pain. Onco Targets Ther. 2015;8:3621–7.
99. Simpson RW, Wlodarczyk JH. Transdermal buprenorphine relieves neuropathic pain: a randomized, double-blind, parallel-group, placebo-controlled trial in diabetic peripheral neuropathic pain. Diabetes Care. 2016;39:1493–500.
100. Weiner M, Sarantopoulos C, Gordon E. Transdermal buprenorphine controls central neuropathic pain. J Opioid Manag. 2012;8:414–5.

101. Licina L, Hamsher C, Lautenschager K, Dhanjal S, Williams N, Spevak C. Buprenorphine/naloxone therapy for opioid refractory neuropathic pain following traumatic amputation: a case series. Mil Med. 2013;178(7):e858–61. doi:10.7205/MILMED-D-12-00310.
102. Dworkin RH, O'Connor AB, Backonja M, Farrar JT, Finnerup NB, Jensen TS, et al. Pharmacologic management of neuropathic pain: evidence-based recommendations. Pain. 2007;132:237–51.
103. Attal N, Cruccu G, Baron R, Haanpää M, Hansson P, Jensen TS, et al. EFNS guidelines on the pharmacological treatment of neuropathic pain: 2010 revision. Eur J Neurol. 2010;17:1113–e88. doi:10.1111/j.1468-1331.2010.02999.x.
104. Finnerup NB, Attal N, Haroutounian S, McNicol E, Baron R, Dworkin RH, et al. Pharmacotherapy for neuropathic pain in adults: systematic review, meta-analysis and updated NeuPSIG recommendations. Lancet Neurol. 2015;14:162–73.
105. Chaparro LE, Wiffen PJ, Moore RA, Gilron I. Combination pharmacotherapy for the treatment of neuropathic pain in adults. Cochrane Database Syst Rev. 2012;(7):CD008943. doi:10.1002/14651858.CD008943.pub2.
106. Sengupta JN. Visceral pain: the neurophysiological mechanism. Handb Exp Pharmacol. 2009;194:31–74.
107. Bielefeldt K, Gebhart GF. Visceral pain: basic mechanisms. In: McMahon SB, Koltzenburg M, Tracey I, Turk D, editors. Wall and Melzack's textbook of pain. 6th ed. Philadelphia: Elsevier; 2013. p. 703–17.
108. Mayer EA, Gupta A, Wong HY. A clinical perspective on abdominal pain. In: McMahon SB, Koltzenburg M, Tracey I, Turk D, editors. Wall and Melzack's textbook of pain. 6th ed. Philadelphia: Elsevier; 2013. p. 734–57.
109. Argoff CE, Albrecht P, Irving G, Rice F. Multimodal analgesia for chronic pain: rationale and future directions. Pain Med. 2009;10(Suppl 2):S53–66.
110. Franklin GM. Opioids for chronic noncancer pain: a position paper of the American academy of neurology. Neurology. 2014;83:1277–84.
111. Carville SF, Arendt-Nielsen L, Bliddal H, Blotman F, Branco JC, Buskila D, et al. EULAR evidence-based recommendations for the management of fibromyalgia syndrome. Ann Rheum Dis. 2008;67:536–41.
112. Häuser W, Arnold B, Eich W, Felde E, Flügge C, Henningsen P, et al. Management of fibromyalgia syndrome – an interdisciplinary evidence-based guideline. Ger Med Sci. 2008;6:Doc14.
113. American College of Rheumatology. Fibromyalgia: how is fibromyalgia treated? http://www.rheumatology.org/I-Am-A/Patient-Caregiver/Diseases-Conditions/Fibromyalgia.
114. Hoskin P, Forbes K. Cancer pain: treatment overview. In: McMahon SB, Koltzenburg M, Tracey I, Turk D, editors. Wall and Melzack's textbook of pain. 6th ed. Philadelphia: Elsevier; 2013. p. 1075–91.
115. Mantyh PW. A mechanism-based understanding of bone cancer pain. In: Novartis foundation symposium 261, pathological pain: from molecular to clinical aspects. Chichester: Wiley; 2004. p. 194–219.
116. Zech DF, Grond S, Lynch J, Hertel D, Lehmann KA. Validation of World Health Organization Guidelines for cancer pain relief: a 10-year prospective study. Pain. 1995;63:65–76.
117. Ripamonti CI, Santini D, Maranzano E, Berti M, Roila F, ESMO Guidelines Working Group. Management of cancer pain: ESMO clinical practice guidelines. Ann Oncol. 2012;23(Suppl 7):vii139–54.
118. Caraceni A, Hanks G, Kaasa S, Bennett MI, Brunelli C, Cherny N, et al. Use of opioid analgesics in the treatment of cancer pain: evidence-based recommendations from the EAPC. Lancet Oncol. 2012;13(2):e58–68. doi:10.1016/S1470-2045(12)70040-2.
119. Yamaguchi T, Shima Y, Morita T, Hosoya M, Matoba M, Japanese Society of Palliative Medicine. Clinical guideline for pharmacological management of cancer pain: the Japanese Society of Palliative Medicine recommendations. Jpn J Clin Oncol. 2013;43:896–909.
120. Swarm RA, Abernethy AP, Anghelescu DL, Benedetti C, Buga S, Cleeland C, et al. Adult cancer pain. J Natl Compr Cancer Netw. 2013;11:992–1022.

121. Vargas-Bermúdez A, Cardenal F, Porta-Sales J. Opioids for the management of dyspnea in cancer patients: evidence of the last 15 years--a systematic review. J Pain Palliat Care Pharmacother. 2015;29:341–52.
122. Yamaguchi T, Goya S, Kohara H, Watanabe H, Mori M, Matsuda Y, et al. Treatment recommendations for respiratory symptoms in cancer patients: clinical guidelines from the Japanese society for palliative medicine. J Palliat Med. 2016;19:925–35.
123. Levy MH, Adolph MD, Back A, Block S, Codada SN, Dalal S, et al. Palliative care. J Natl Compr Cancer Netw. 2012;10:1284–309.
124. Kloke M, Cherny N. Treatment of dyspnoea in advanced cancer patients: ESMO Clinical Practice Guidelines. Ann Oncol. 2015;26(Suppl 5):v169–73.

Chapter 8
Best Practices Education, Part III: Regulatory and Advisory Issues Related to Opioid Therapy for Pain

A 55-year-old local small business owner is referred to you by his primary care physician, who is requesting that you provide an epidural steroid injection for subacute low back pain with painful paresthesias into the left calf and foot that began 3 weeks ago, after he was moving equipment into a new office. He denies any weakness or cauda equina symptoms. The pain is worsened by movement of any sort, although spinal flexion, i.e., sitting is the worst provocative maneuver, and his activity has been markedly reduced. Despite his primary physician's admonition not to, he is using ibuprofen, 800 mg to 1600 mg qid and also admits to drinking "one or two drinks" in the evening to try to palliate the pain, ostensibly. He is also using cyclobenzaprine, 10 mg bid. His chiropractor has been unable to help him with this episode.

His history is otherwise notable for hypertension, GERD, and tobacco use. He has had a recent arthroscopic rotator cuff repair and remote right inguinal herniorrhaphy. Medications include lisinopril/HCTZ, omeprazole, and ibuprofen and cyclobenzaprine as above. His only allergy is to penicillin.

Physical exam reveals a mildly overweight male in moderate discomfort who is recumbent on your exam table and resists physical exam. He is dysphoric and admits during exam that he has had suicidal ideation but no plans, due to the financial stress of his company's recent troubles, "downsizing" and move, compounded by the pain. He is hyperalgesic in the left L5 dermatome, but dorsiflexion and hallux extension are preserved, and ankle jerk is 2/4 at both ankles. Ipsilateral supine straight leg raise is markedly positive at 40°.

H.B. McAnally, *Opioid Dependence*, DOI 10.1007/978-3-319-47497-7_8

After discussing his likely pathology with him (suspected annular tear with or without L4/5 paracentral or L5/S1 foraminal intervertebral disc protrusion), you explain to him that in the absence of "red flag" symptoms and signs, advanced imaging is not indicated at this point and furthermore his "payer" requires prior authorization before MRI. They also require that his symptoms persist for longer than 3 months and that he have documented failure of 3 months or more physical therapy for this condition.

You explain that he is at high risk of gastritis, peptic ulcer disease, gastrointestinal bleeding, renal injury, and cardiovascular/cerebrovascular injury with his excessive NSAID use and comorbidities. You instruct him to stop NSAIDs at this point, as well as alcohol use and smoking (after explaining to him the association between smoking and intervertebral disc disease not to mention serious morbidity and mortality) and explain to him that a trial of bupropion is in his best interest for assistance in smoking cessation as well as depressive symptoms (after reviewing the FDA "black box" warning with him) and also potentially for neuropathic pain. After spending some time with him explaining the anatomy and pathophysiology of his suspected condition and necessary postural and ergonomic corrections, you order 6 weeks of physical therapy with avoidance of sit-ups.

After discussing the risks of worsened depression, dependence and addiction, gastrointestinal complications, respiratory complications, especially if he uses alcohol, and giving him instructions not to drive under the sedative effects of the medication, you advise him that you are going to prescribe a limited supply of acetaminophen with codeine (which he has used previously without adverse effects) to be used half an hour prior to physical therapy and in the evening after physical therapy to help facilitate rehabilitation. You explain that this will only be prescribed for the next few weeks while he is getting established with physical therapy and HEP. You also advise that in a week or two, after confirmation of no immediate adverse effects from bupropion, which he is naive to, if the painful paresthesias persist, you will call in a course of gabapentin. You conclude the encounter by reassuring him again that there is no evidence of serious pathology and that he has a greater than 2/3 likelihood of this situation resolving in the next few months without any complication including chronification if he stops smoking and corrects his posture/ergonomics and is diligent with physical rehabilitation. You plan on reevaluation in 6 weeks or sooner if his condition worsens and assure him once again that there is no indication for surgery here, but if his condition persists or worsens, then the issue of advanced imaging and possible interventional care (i.e., epidural steroids) can be revisited.

Introduction

In the previous chapter, we began exploring the role that opioids play within the context of treating both acute and chronic pain and examined *why* and *when* the practitioner might consider prescribing opioids. In this chapter, we cover both regulatory and advisory (including recent consensus guidelines) aspects of *how* opioids can and should be prescribed, which as the past 2 decades have taught us, is more fraught with difficulties and negative consequences than was appreciated at the outset of the opioid epidemic.

The focus of this chapter is to improve prescription patterns; evidence of widespread flaws in opioid-prescribing practice confronts us every day in the news. These flaws need to be exposed systematically and corrected accordingly; at a "big picture" level, they can be categorized roughly into:

- (*Fairly rare*) ignorance of federal and state laws applicable to opioid prescription
- (*Fairly common*) ignorance of state medical board rules and policies applicable to opioid prescription
- (*Fairly common*) ignorance of best practices to reduce diversion of prescription opioids
- (*Rampant*) ignorance of best practices to optimize overall patient benefit (analgesia, improved function and quality of life): risk (physiologic, psychological, functional, relational, societal) ratio from opioid prescription

The first category is addressed briefly in the initial "regulatory" section; the prescriber however is referred to the US Drug Enforcement Administration (DEA) *Practitioner's Manual* [1] for definitive instruction. The latter three categories are addressed in the "Advisory" section which follows. "How to" start and trial patients on opioids is introduced in this section; the subject of weaning and discontinuing opioid therapy is dealt with primarily in Chap. 11.

Finally, a brief overview of current recommendations for the use of opioids in treating cancer pain is provided.

How to Prescribe Opioids: Regulatory Issues

Regulations (and guidelines, discussed below) regarding opioid prescription evidence quandaries and difficulties unique among medication classes. While other controlled substances are subject to regulations, none of them carry indications associated with the same degree of emotional urgency experienced and communicated by most patients in pain and felt by providers. In many cases, there are no viable alternatives to the prescription of opioids if severe pain is to be treated efficaciously, and "undertreated pain" is a real issue. Conversely, overtreated pain is a real issue as well, at the level of the individual patient and also at a societal level, with adverse effects and diversion comprising the two chief concerns.

As the opioid crisis in this country has grown over the past 20 years, so has scrutiny of prescriber behavior by both the medical and legal communities. In 1980, the American Medical Association (AMA) proposed a framework for categorizing prescribers who are knowingly or unknowingly complicit with prescription opioid misusers, abusers, and diverters [2]. Referred to as the "4D" model, this framework has been widely discussed by policymakers and authorities for the past few decades as a means of attempting to assist in stratifying the culpability of providers involved in overprescription/misprescription, and in guiding disciplinary measures. The 4D model is presented in a more recent iteration borrowed from the American College of Preventive Medicine in Table 8.1.

More recently, a "3C" model (Careless, Corrupt, Compromised) has been proposed that attempts to remove patient factors from the equation and in essence collapses the first two categories of "Dated" and "Duped" into the category of "Careless" [4]. While no effective (or appropriate) remedy aside from prosecution and sanction, respectively, exists for the latter two "C" categories in this author's opinion, prevention of misdeeds attributable to carelessness begins with (but is by no means limited to) understanding the laws (acts and regulations) pertaining to opioid prescribing.

Table 8.1 The 4Ds of prescriber involvement in prescription abuse [3]

Deficient (dated)	Duped
• Unaware of federal and state laws regarding opioid prescription • Unaware of multimodal treatment options • Unaware of signs and symptoms of addiction • Too busy (or disinterested) to keep up with CME; education comes primarily from pharmaceutical companies • Isolated from peers, medical community, and ignorant of standards of care	• Fails to exercise "due diligence" in assessing patient's risk of abuse and diversion; trusts but does not verify • Fails to secure prescription pads or use tamper-proof prescription means • Fails to direct care appropriately and allows patient to dictate care ("OK, here's a script for your "percs") • Fails to exercise boundaries regarding aberrant behavior (early refill requests, dose escalation, etc.)
Deliberate (dealing)	**Drug dependent**
• Deliberately/knowingly prescribes opioids for nonmedical purposes, e.g., recreational use/abuse and diversion • Trades prescriptions for money, sex, street drugs, etc. • "Pill-mill"	• Forges prescriptions from other providers • Prescribes to others, real or fictitious, and intercepts prescriptions

History of (Federal) Opioid Prescribing Legislation

The quandary of opioid misuse and prescription negligence has long been recognized by the government, and federal regulation has evolved over the past century. Despite widespread claims (especially in the 1990s) that dependence and addiction are exceedingly rare sequelae of opioid therapy, it has been evident to elected leadership that from a public health perspective at least, opioid addiction is a significant societal burden closely intertwined with the medical profession. While early legislation focused more on consumer safety, the issues of psycho-/behavioral effects of mind-altering substances including opium and dependence/addiction have been more than implicit in local, state, and federal governmental policy for over a century. Virtually, all legislation for the past 50 years having to do with opioids has been written to address abuse liability and frank addiction management.

The first major legislative effort by Congress to control opioid distribution was the Harrison Narcotics Tax Act of 1914, which dealt primarily with commercial registration and taxation issues pertaining to "opium or coca leaves, their salts, derivatives, or preparations" but also introduced legal requirement for recordkeeping of prescriptions for these substances. Five years later, in *Webb* vs. *United States*, the US Supreme Court ruled that physicians could not prescribe opioids solely for maintenance of addiction.

In 1924, the Heroin Act rendered manufacture or importation and possession of heroin illegal for all purposes. In 1932, the Uniform State Narcotic Act called for states to pass legislation in line with federal legislation (the Narcotic Drug Import and Export Act). The Food, Drug, and Cosmetic Act in 1938 brought the determination of safety of these substances under the control of the *Food and Drug Administration (FDA)*, mandating new drug approval by that agency prior to marketing, and also required safe use instruction labeling. The Durham-Humphrey Amendment of 1951 further established the classification of certain drugs, especially those that are "habit-forming" as prescription only.

The *Controlled Substance Act (CSA) of 1970* reorganized and consolidated several previous laws regulating drugs and substances with high abuse potential. Five "Schedules" were created, based primarily upon abuse and addiction potential, with Schedule I containing drugs with no recognized legitimate medical use (e.g., heroin, LSD, marijuana) and Schedules II through V containing drugs such as opioids, sedatives, stimulants, and others in tiers of decreasing risk.

The *Narcotic Addict Treatment Act of 1974* amended the CSA to provide for the federally supervised treatment of opioid dependence by either maintenance of dependence using prescription opioids for longer than 21 days or detoxification using a weaning schedule of 21 days or less. This provided the legal basis for methadone maintenance therapy.

The *Drug Addiction Treatment Act of 2000* (DATA 2000) established office-based treatment (OBT) of opioid dependence using FDA-approved Schedule III–V opioids (the only one currently approved is buprenorphine). Physicians must obtain a special DEA number ("waiver" or "X-number") in order to prescribe buprenorphine for OBT; requirements for waiver include:

- Board certification in addiction psychiatry
- Certification in addiction medicine by the American Society of Addiction Medicine (at the time of this writing responsibility for this certification has been transferred to the American Board of Preventive Medicine)
- Certified in Addiction Medicine by American Osteopathic Association (AOA)
- Investigator in buprenorphine clinical trials
- Completion of 8 h of CME provided by American Psychiatric Association, American Academy of Addiction Psychiatry, ASAM, American Medical Association, AOA, (or other organizations designated by Health and Human Services)

Subsequent amendments in 2005, 2006, and 2016 have sequentially increased the limit or "cap" on how many patients may be treated with OBT per qualifying physician.

The *Comprehensive Addiction and Recovery Act of 2016* (CARA 2016) represents the first major piece of legislation attempting to comprehensively address the opioid epidemic, with components including prevention, treatment, recovery, law enforcement, criminal justice reform, and overdose reversal. Among other initiatives, an interagency group (comprising HHS, VA, DEA, CDC, other federal agencies, addiction treatment organizations, and other stakeholder communities) have been tasked with the development of best practices for opioid prescription. Mandatory prescriber education recommendations have been assigned to the Secretary of Health and Human Services (HHS). Among the vast scope and provisions of CARA 2016, one of the more striking decisions is the amendment of the CSA to allow mid-level practitioners to become eligible to prescribe buprenorphine for the treatment of opioid use disorder.

Federal Regulations for Opioid Prescribing

The CSA and Title 21 of the Code of Federal Regulations 1300–1316 (the "DEA Regulations") allow, inform, and direct legal prescription of opioids, including:

- Providing the legal basis for prescribing opioids (21 CFR 1306.07— "May administer, prescribe or dispense a Schedule II controlled substance to a person with intractable pain, in which no relief or cure is possible or none has been found after a reasonable effort"

- Delineating which opioids (and other controlled substances) can be prescribed
- Delineating who can prescribe them
- Regulating how they can be prescribed (e.g., means of prescribing, whether or not they may be refilled, etc.)

Regulatory and enforcement authority is delegated primarily to the FDA and the DEA. The FDA's "scope of practice" pertinent to prescription opioids is to ensure public safety by determining the safety of the drug, recommending scheduling within the five CSA schedules, and recommending indications for use. The DEA is ultimately responsible for the scheduling of controlled substances and is also tasked with enforcing the CSA.

The CSA and DEA regulations are summarized for providers within the *DEA's Practitioner's Manual*, available online at https://www.deadiversion.usdoj.gov/pubs/manuals/pract/index.html; a cursory review of highlights follows below.

Opioids (with the exception of heroin, which is classified as Schedule I, i.e., no medical use) fall within Schedules II through V as shown in Table 8.2, with the majority classified as Schedule II, the most stringently controlled category. Considerable differences in prescriptive regulation exist between Schedule II and lower categories and are highlighted in Table 8.2. All controlled substances,

Table 8.2 Oral, sublingual, and transdermal opioids by controlled substance schedule

Schedule	Commonly prescribed opioids (excluding intravenous forms)	Legal means of prescribing	Refills
II	Codeine (≥ 90 mg) Fentanyl Hydrocodone (including combination products) Hydromorphone Levorphanol Meperidine Methadone Morphine Oxycodone (including combination products) Oxymorphone Tapentadol	Electronic or written prescription only* **a telephoned emergency prescription not exceeding three (3) days' supply may be prescribed so long as a written copy follows within 7 days* *Schedule II prescriptions for residents of long-term care facilities or those enrolled in a hospice program may be FAXed to the dispensing pharmacy*	Not allowed
III	Buprenorphine Codeine combination products	Electronic, written, FAXed, or telephoned prescription	≤five (5) refills within six mo.
IV	Butorphanol Pentazocine Tramadol (including combination products)	Electronic, written, FAXed, or telephoned prescription	≤five (5) refills within six mo.
V	Codeine cough syrups ≤200 mg/100 mL or 100 g	Electronic, written, FAXed, or telephoned prescription	Not limited by federal law

however, by law must be prescribed only for "legitimate medical purpose by a practitioner acting in the usual course of professional practice" [1].

Federal law restricts opioid prescription privileges to practitioners who are registered with the DEA to prescribe controlled substances within Schedules II through V and then assigned a registration number ("DEA number"). Practitioners in training, or who work solely as employees of a hospital may use the hospital's DEA registration, and federal government practitioners (e.g., armed services or US Public Health Services or Prison Bureau practitioners) receive a waiver of this requirement.

Strict legal requirements concerning the security and accounting of stored and administered or dispensed controlled substances do not apply to most practitioners. Security of prescriptions however are the responsibility of all prescribers and tamper-resistant prescription pads or paper are advised by the DEA (and mandated by several states). In addition, by federal law, controlled prescriptions require notation of the patient's address as well as name and date of birth. The drug name, dosage form, strength, quantity, and directions for use, and of course the name, address, and registration number of the prescriber must also be on the prescription. Until recently, when electronic prescription of Schedules II through V substances was allowed, Schedule II substances required hard copy/paper prescription with a manual signature (no stamps).

Recordkeeping of controlled substances prescribed (not administered/dispensed) is not mandatory unless said prescriptions are for maintenance or detoxification purposes.

State Regulations for Opioid Prescribing

In 1970, after the CSA was enacted, the states commissioned a Uniform Controlled Substances Act (UCSA) as a model for individual states to consider when updating and revising their own drug laws, with the intent of promoting uniformity and a means of achieving consistent and more effective control of the possession, use, sale, distribution, and manufacture of controlled substances. The most recent revision took place in 1994 and may be accessed at (http://www.uniformlaws.org/shared/docs/controlled%20substances/UCSA_final%20_94%20with%2095amends.pdf).

The diversity of state-specific statutes concerning controlled substances is complex to the point that a comprehensive presentation of these laws state-by-state is prohibitive. Every prescriber should be aware of their own state's legislation concerning the prescription of controlled substances, and the internet has rendered that task a relatively simple one. For those interested in an overview of state regulations, the National Criminal Justice Association created a Guide to State Controlled Substances Acts in 1988 that presents a thorough albeit currently dated compilation of state-specific regulations [5]. At present, the National Association of State Controlled Substances Authorities provides an easily navigable website (http://

www.nascsa.org/stateprofiles.htm) with links to each state's statutes and rules pertinent to controlled substances, current authorities, and other pertinent deviations from federal regulations/scheduling.

Despite recent confusion (and frank violation of national law) surrounding the marijuana controversy in several states, the states may not enact controlled substance schedules less stringent than the national schedule determined by the DEA. Some states have historically classified some controlled substances more restrictively than the national schedule; for example, codeine cough syrups are assigned a category more restricted than Schedule V in several states, and many states controlled tramadol prior to federal categorization as a controlled substance in 2014. The state of Massachusetts recently passed legislation restricting initial opioid prescriptions for adults (and all opioid prescriptions for minors) to a seven-day prescription; this is to date the most stringent limitation on prescription duration in this nation.

At the time of this writing, 22 states, the District of Columbia, Puerto Rico, and Guam also require a state (or territory)-specific controlled substance prescription registration as well. While most states currently allow mid-level practitioners (e.g., physician assistants and nurse practitioners) to prescribe most controlled substances, there are several that restrict Schedule II drugs to the order of a physician only, and some states do not allow controlled substance prescribing at all by mid-levels. The question of whether or not opioids should be prescribed by physicians or mid-level practitioners who have not been adequately trained to do so is a "hot-bed issue" enjoying discussion in many circles and at various levels of governance. There is no easy answer to this question, and in many cases there are no providers available who have undergone formal residency or fellowship-level training in opioid prescription. This will always remain impractical for many communities, and regarding these situations where nonspecialists are responsible for the pain management component of the health and well-being of their communities, the question should not be so much "should they be prescribing?" but rather "how can we best educate them and provide guidance?" This book is one such attempt to answer that question, and a significant amount of continuing medical education has become available over the past several years in order to assist with this endeavor as well. In many states, it is now becoming mandatory for prescribers to undergo opioid-related continuing medical education (CME), in some cases once in a lifetime and in others on an ongoing basis. At the time of this writing:

- Florida mandates controlled substances CME on a regular basis for allopathic physicians working in a pain clinic.
- Kentucky mandates regular CME related to pain management, addiction disorders, and the use of their PDMP.
- Maryland requires regular opioid prescribing CME.
- Massachusetts requires regular opioid prescribing CME.
- New Mexico mandates controlled substances CME on a regular basis for allopathic physicians with a DEA number.

Table 8.3 State requirements regarding use of prescription drug monitoring programs prior to prescribing controlled substances

State	Bill	Provisions
Alaska	SB 74	PDMP to be checked before prescribing or dispensing Schedule II–III controlled substance with exceptions
Arizona	SB 1283	PDMP to be checked before prescribing a Schedule II–IV opioid or benzodiazepine for a new course of treatment. Subsequent check at least quarterly while the substances remains part of the treatment. Exceptions may apply
California	SB 482	PDMP to be checked before first-time prescribing, ordering, administering, or furnishing of a Schedule II–IV controlled substance except for veterinarians, pharmacists, and other specified exemptions; check shall not be earlier than 24 h or the previous business day prior to first-time prescribing, ordering, administering, or furnishing. Subsequent check every 4 months if the substance remains part of the treatment
Connecticut	HB 5053	PDMP to be checked before prescribing more than a 72 h supply of a controlled substance. Check required at least every 90 days when prescribing other than a Schedule V non-narcotic controlled substance for continuous or prolonged treatment. Prescribing a Schedule V non-narcotic controlled substance for continuous or prolonged treatment requires a PMP check not less than annually. Exceptions may apply
Indiana	SEA 297	Appropriate state agency shall develop best practices for opioid treatment by an opioid treatment provider that shall include a review of a patient's INSPECT report
Maine	LD 1646	PDMP to be checked before initial prescribing of a benzodiazepine or an opioid. Subsequent check every 90 days as long as substance is renewed as part of treatment. Exceptions may apply
Maryland	HB 437	PDMP to be checked before initiating course of treatment that includes prescribing or dispensing an opioid or benzodiazepine. Subsequent check every 90 days if treatment continues with the opioid or benzodiazepine. Exceptions may apply
Massachusetts	HB 4056	Department of Health shall issue rules that requires a registered participant to check the PMP each time the participant issues a schedule II–III narcotics prescription
New Hampshire	SB 576-FN-A	PDMP to be checked before prescribing a schedule II–IV opioid for the treatment of pain, with subsequent check at least twice a year. Exceptions may apply
New Mexico	SB 263	PDMP to be checked before prescribing/dispensing for the first time more than a 4-day supply of an opioid. Check required at least every 3 months during the continuing prescribing/dispensing of an opioid

(continued)

Table 8.3 (continued)

State	Bill	Provisions
Pennsylvania	SB 1202	A dispenser shall query the PMP before dispensing an opioid drug product or a benzodiazepine in specified circumstances. A prescriber shall query the PMP each time a patient is prescribed an opioid drug product or a benzodiazepine. Exception applies
Rhode Island	SB2823A	PDMP to be checked before starting an opioid and before refilling or initiating opioid therapy with an intrathecal pump. Check required every 3 months during continuous opioid therapy for pain for 3 months or longer. Exceptions may apply
Utah	HB 375	Prescriber/dispenser of opioid for outpatient use shall determine when PDMP check is necessary in his/her professional judgment to prevent opioid abuse
Virginia	HB 293	PDMP to be checked before initiating a new course of treatment that includes prescribing of opioids anticipated at outset to last more than 14 consecutive days. Exceptions may apply
West Virginia	SB 454	Before prescribing/dispensing medication assisted treatment, PDMP check required to ensure the patient is not seeking controlled substances from multiple sources and to assess potential adverse drug interactions. Exceptions may apply
Wisconsin	AB 364	PDMP to be checked before practitioner issues a controlled prescription order for the patient. Exceptions may apply

- Ohio requires physician owner/operators of pain management clinics to complete regular CME in pain medicine every 2 years, to include one or more courses addressing the potential for addiction.
- Oklahoma requires regular CME on controlled substances prescribing for osteopathic physicians.
- South Carolina requires regular CME on controlled substances prescribing for physicians.
- Texas mandates controlled substances CME on a regular basis for physicians working in a pain clinic.
- Vermont mandates controlled substances CME on a regular basis for allopathic physicians with a DEA number.
- West Virginia requires regular CME on controlled substances prescribing and diversion prevention for physicians.

Several other states require pain management CME on a regular basis without specifying a requirement for controlled substances/opioid education.

State *Prescription Drug Monitoring Programs/Databases (PDMPs)* have become a ubiquitous tool in the monitoring of controlled substance prescriptions and serve a valuable role in diversion prevention. At the time of this writing, all but one state (Missouri) have adopted legislation requiring creation of a PDMP, and many states have been using them for several years now. At the time of this writing, 16 states require checking the State Prescription Drug Monitoring Program prior to issuing controlled substance prescriptions [6]. (Interestingly only 11 states, not all of which are represented in the 16 mentioned above require registering with the PDMP.) These requirements are summarized in Table 8.3.

State Medical and Nursing Board Rules for Opioid Prescribing

State medical boards (and nursing boards) have a supervisory role over members of their professions, with authority generally delegated by the state's legislation to enact and enforce rules and standards that govern the practices of the profession. It is within the purview of these boards to grant (and renew) professional licensure and thus to protect both individuals and the health of the public by ensuring competence and ethical practice. As with individual state governments, the degree of oversight both general and specific to prescribing practices varies widely.

State medical (and nursing) boards generally address issues pertaining to the prescription of controlled substances by rules based on the national Federation of State Medical Boards' "Model Policy" (discussed more later). While not usually carrying the force of law in their own right, the boards do wield substantial authority in the arenas of sanction/discipline and may suspend or revoke licenses altogether if in their judgment a practitioner is not exercising competent and ethical practice; an increasing number of these cases involve controlled substances.

How to Prescribe Opioids: Advisory Issues

Again, while not carrying the force of law, numerous recent guidelines on opioid prescribing have been proliferated that influence and affect professional standards of care, which in turn may exert significant impact on licensure and other professional privileges. Sources include both governmental agencies (e.g., Veterans' Administration, US Centers for Disease Control, Washington State Agency Medical Directors' Group) and also professional organizations (e.g., Federation of State Medical Boards, American Academy of Pain Medicine, American Society of Interventional Pain Physicians). Guidelines specific to the prescription of methadone and buprenorphine in the context of opioid dependence have also been put forth by both governmental and professional entities and are discussed in Chap. 11.

The *Federation of State Medical Boards' (FSMB) "Model Policy"* was first published in 1998 and subsequently revised in both 2004 and then again in 2013. Its explicit purpose is:

> To provide a resource for use by state medical boards in educating their licensees about cautious and responsible prescribing of controlled substances while alleviating fears of

> regulatory scrutiny... to provide a framework for the legitimate medical use of opioid analgesics for the treatment of pain while emphasizing the need to safeguard against their misuse and diversion. [7]

The model policy has been adopted either in its entirety or in part by most state medical boards as part of their individual policies and as such deserves attention by all practitioners due to its widespread adoption as defining standard of care. While ostensibly aimed at providing guidelines for managing pain (with encouragement to understand pain physiology and pathophysiology and exhaust non-opioid methods prior to opioid trial), it is addressed primarily to non-pain specialists whose treatment arsenal is more limited, and as such it focuses primarily on opioid pain management best practices. Recommendations from the model policy, with some additional input from other guidelines including those from the CDC [8], Canadian National Guidelines [9], Veterans Affairs/Department of Defense [10], Washington State Agency Medical Directors' Group [11], American Pain Society/American Academy of Pain Medicine [12], and the American Society of Interventional Pain Physicians [13] are summarized below with brief commentary.

Legal Compliance

Not in contradiction to the long-standing commitment of the federal government to avoid "meddling" in the direct practice of medicine, controlled substance laws and regulations are criminal laws created to protect society. Every prescriber has a legal as well as ethical and professional mandate to understand and comply with them.

Understanding Pain

From a basic grasp of nociceptive and non-nociceptive processes to recognition of life-threatening visceral rupture or aortic dissection, adequate understanding of pain's genesis and perpetuation is essential for safe and optimal treatment of those who entrust their well-being to us. Chapter 6 addresses this.

Thorough Evaluation and Risk Stratification

Good history taking (not limited to the chief complaint and current/prior treatment, but including adequate assessment of past medical history, social and family history, review of systems) and physical examination are necessary prior to any consideration of opioid prescription, and documentation of such is required by virtually all oversight bodies, e.g., state medical boards. Indeed, it is hard to imagine trying to prove "legitimate medical purpose by a practitioner acting in the usual course of professional practice" without these basic elements. In addition, appropriate ancillary tests (e.g., laboratory studies, imaging, electrodiagnostics, etc.) are necessary not only to clarify diagnoses but also inform treatment decisions based on physiologic risks (e.g., renal or hepatic dysfunction). Corroboration of patient report by other providers' records, imaging and laboratory review, prescription drug monitoring program (PDMP), etc., comprises due diligence and is only in the patient's best interest.

Evaluation of possible pregnant state by history and point-of-care urine hCG testing is more than reasonable in any woman of childbearing age.

Risk stratification for prescription opioid misuse/abuse is as important as evaluating for adverse physical effects, and assessment of psychosocial factors both past and present are necessary to gauge misuse/abuse liability whenever considering opioid prescription. Due to more stringent confidentiality requirements, obtaining behavioral health records can be a difficult if not impossible task but may be essential for optimal care. Basic/brief mental health screening tools are readily available to help clarify where a patient may currently be on the spectrum of various common psychiatric dysfunctions such as depression (e.g., Patient Health Questionnaire-9 [PHQ-9], Beck Depression Inventory-Short Form [BDI-SF]) and substance abuse (e.g., Screener and Opioid Assessment for Patients with Pain-Revised [SOAPP-R], Opioid Risk Tool [ORT]). Oftentimes, the higher the psychiatric dysfunction quotient (including substance abuse disorders), the more pressure the patient exerts for "urgent" opioid therapy, and this can be obviated a priori by establishing policies and procedures such as no opioid prescriptions on initial visit. More readily, available information indicating potential aberrancy or opioid use disorder may be determined virtually instantly these days using prescription drug monitoring programs (PDMP) to screen for "red flags" such as "doctor-shopping," or multiple addresses or names, or gross inconsistencies between patient report and documented dispensation. Criminal records are a matter of public record as well, and a "Courtview" online search may reveal a history of illegal possession or distribution of controlled substances, convictions for driving under the influence of alcohol or other substances, etc. Many guidelines recommend initial urine drug screening (UDS) to establish a baseline measure of risk.

Social stability (e.g., family or other support infrastructure, employment status, litigation issues from auto accidents, and workers' compensation claims) or lack thereof may correlate with misuse and abuse risk and should always be assessed to the extent possible.

Clear Functional and Analgesic Treatment Goals and Plan

Clearly delineated expectations and goals pertaining to functional improvement as well as analgesia (e.g., "we will attempt to achieve 30% reduction in your pain with multimodal pharmacotherapy, physical therapy, counseling, and interventional procedures as indicated; we also expect to see ongoing progress in tobacco cessation, sleep normalization, work capacity, and quality) provide reassuring boundaries for both patient and provider.

Crafting a plan focused on functional goals carries several advantages including providing objective/verifiable outcome measures, and multiaxial and more robust dataset to evaluate either benefit or harm of therapy. As Dr. Scott Fishman states in his handbook *Responsible Opioid Prescribing* [14]:

> Simply "feeling better" without measurably improving functioning in some aspect of a patient's life is an insufficient outcome. Framing the treatment goal solely around "feeling better" also leaves the clinician with no objective evidence by which to gauge the efficacy of therapy and justify potential risks associated with the treatment… It can be difficult to navigate the clinical landscape when a patient's subjective report of improvements in pain intensity are weighed against objective evidence that functional gains have not been achieved—or, worse, that actual harm is taking place. But clinicians frequently encounter analogous situations in other areas of medical practice. For example, if a diabetic also has problems with chronic vasculitis, corticosteroids may effectively ease some of his or her symptoms… [but not without] serious consequences.

Some functional improvement goals are more readily objectively verified than others (e.g., weight loss, return to work), while others may be more difficult if not impossible to verify beyond doubt (e.g., improved stress management, relationships, household chores) but with a little collaborative effort from both parties a simple tailored plan should be achievable. This also carries the advantage of internalizing some control for the patient and providing objective feedback to them of their gains.

Informed Consent and Treatment Agreement ("Opioid Contract")

Patients must be educated about risks (discussed in Chap. 3), potential benefits (Chap. 7), and alternatives (Chap. 6) even if they have been using opioids for long term. Informed consent is a basic principle of ethical medical care, and its importance increases commensurate with the risks involved, which in the case of opioid therapy is very high. The majority of patients we counsel as part of initiation of an opioid therapy trial express unfamiliarity with many of the basic adverse effects (let alone more recently appreciated risks such as endocrinopathy and hyperalgesia) even though they may have been using opioids for many years. Proper documentation of the discussion in a standardized consent form signed by the patient is minimally time-consuming and may protect the prescriber from potential future allegations of failure to inform. Effective documentation of risk management goes beyond a standardized consent, of course, and should be on the mind of every clinician in today's medicolegal climate. To quote Dr. Fishman again, "both treating and not treating involve risks, so prescribers cannot avoid managing risks" [14].

Treatment agreements or opioid contracts should include language clearly indicating the responsibilities of the patient to comply with prescription instructions, to refrain from seeking opioid or other controlled substance prescriptions from other providers unless explicitly authorized, and in some cases to only use one pharmacy for controlled substances. Other issues such as cautions against driving under the sedative effects of medications, instruction on safe storage and disposal of medications, the clinic's policies on replacing lost medications or prescriptions, requests for early refills, random urine drug screening and pill counts, etc. should of course be included. It is advisable that at least generic language related to opioid trial period duration, functional goal assessment, and likelihood of eventual discontinuation of opioid therapy (with reasons for accelerated discontinuation spelled out) be included as well.

Initiating (or Continuing) a Trial of Opioid Therapy

Opioid therapy should always be initiated only if benefit is deemed to outweigh the risk, and if less dangerous methods are contraindicated or have failed. Opioid therapy should also always be considered a trial with ongoing evaluation of benefit/achievement of treatment goals vs. adverse effects. More often than not for the pain specialist (but increasingly common in primary care these days as well), the patient presenting to you for the first time may be a chronic user of opioids/tolerant/dependent, and thus, while not opioid-naïve may be at even higher risk of certain cumulative adverse effects such as depression, dependence, endocrinopathy, and hyperalgesia. A defined trial period (e.g., 6–12 weeks) should be clearly delineated and documented, and if the plan is a priori to begin weaning/eliminating opioids in a gradual fashion, that should also be made clear.

It is fairly universally recommended that initiation of an opioid trial begin with short-acting/immediate-release opioids rather than extended-release/long-acting (ER/LA) agents. The CDC guidelines [8] advise against the prescription of ER/LA opioids if a patient has not received regular immediate-release opioids for at least a week prior; all of the guidelines referenced above advise initiating treatment with the lowest possible dose and adopting a slow titrated increase policy if at all, with continuous assessment of benefit versus harm. Doses in the range of 50 mg–90 morphine milligram equivalents (MME) have been shown to confer statistically significantly increased risk of harms including overdose [8] and should be prescribed with careful risk-benefit ratio analysis and documentation; it is recommended that overdose education and consideration of naloxone prescription ensue beyond the 50 MME threshold. Doses in excess of this carry exponentially increasing risk and should be viewed with extreme caution, possible consultation or referral to a pain specialist, and/or addictionologist, and the patient should be counseled about the marked risk they (and the prescriber) are assuming.

Efficacy/Harm Monitoring and Treatment Plan Adaptation

Well-publicized outcome measures such as *4As* (analgesia, activity, adverse effects, and aberrancy) should be regularly assessed throughout the trial, with modification, continuation, or termination always deliberated.

Compliance Monitoring

Periodic random urine drug testing and pill counts assist in assuring the provider of compliance with therapy and lack of diversion. PDMP surveillance is another high-yield means of screening for aberrancy. As discussed above, consequences for non-compliance/contract violation should be spelled out clearly at the outset of the therapeutic trial.

Consultation and Referral

The care of patients with chronic pain generally requires a collaborative effort between multiple disciplines, and the physician prescribing opioids should always seek appropriate consultation from areas they are not expert in (e.g., pain management, psychiatry, addictionology, surgery). The guidelines referenced herein recommend specialty consultation when the MME exceeds 90–200 mg.

The most notable governmental oversight to date related to the referral of patients to specialists is the state of Washington's Engrossed Substitute House Bill 2876, passed in 2010, which among many other provisions requires a consultation from a pain management specialist for a patient with chronic non-cancer pain whose daily opioid dose exceeds a threshold dose (currently 120 mg MME).

Prescribing Methadone for Pain

The use of methadone for the treatment of chronic non-cancer pain saw a significant upswing (along with other opioid agents) in the 1990s and 2000s due to its low cost, good efficacy, long half-life, and perceived low abuse liability. Beginning in the mid-2000s, it began to be apparent that this agent is exceptionally dangerous, with disproportionate mortality compared to other opioids (some data showing as much as 1/3 of all opioid-related mortality); this is described in greater detail in Chap. 3. The guidelines almost universally recommend extra caution with the use of methadone and most recommend that this agent be prescribed only by clinicians trained in its use and very familiar with it. Some basic recommendations from the American Academy of Pain Medicine [15] include:

- Screen for OSA and additional respiratory depressant risk factors and don't prescribe methadone for patients with known sleep disordered breathing who are noncompliant with their respiratory assistive devices.
- Assess patient's risk for developing a prolonged QT interval and provide appropriate surveillance of ECG. For example, patients with cardiac disease taking other QT interval prolonging drugs, patients with electrolyte abnormalities (renal insufficiency/diuretic therapy/hemodialysis), patients with poorly controlled DM, or patients taking 60–100 mg or more of methadone a day. Repeat ECG following dose increases in these high-risk patients. Decrease methadone dose or discontinue therapy if QT interval exceeds 470 ms in men or 480 ms in women.
- Initiate methadone therapy at 15 mg or less per day in divided doses; lower doses are recommended for older patients, frail patients, or individuals with at-risk comorbidities (e.g., COPD).
- Increase methadone dose no more often than once per week, with total daily dose increases not to exceed 5–10 mg per week.
- Communicate with patient the critical importance of not using more methadone than directed even if the pain is not well controlled.

Discontinuing Opioid Therapy

Reasons for discontinuing opioid therapy include resolution of the underlying painful condition, emergence of intolerable side effects, inadequate analgesic effect, and failure to improve the patient's quality of life despite reasonable titration, deteriorating function, or significant aberrant medication use. If opioid therapy is discontinued, the patient who has become physically dependent should be provided with a safely structured tapering regimen. In general, a target wean of 10–15% per week is recommended. Withdrawal can be managed either by the prescribing physician or by referring the patient to an addiction specialist. The termination of opioid therapy should not mark the end of treatment, which should continue with other modalities, either through direct care or referral to other healthcare specialists, as appropriate.

These recommendations are summarized in Table 8.4. Documentation of all of the above in the medical record, as well as strict compliance with privacy/confidentiality laws are mandatory.

Guidelines on Opioid Prescribing for Cancer Pain

As discussed in the previous chapter, the use of opioids in treating moderate to severe cancer pain is virtually axiomatic. The use of the World Health Organization's (WHO) analgesic ladder (see Fig. 7.1) has been the de facto blueprint for clinical practice, and most recent guidelines and protocols, some of which are presented below. While providing a useful concept (stepwise care tailored to pain severity) the

Table 8.4 Consensus recommendations for initiating and continuing opioid therapy

• Conduct a thorough history and physical exam, including assessments of patient's psychosocial state/milieu, and obtain pertinent objective ancillary studies (e.g., imaging, labs) prior to considering opioid therapy
• Risk-stratify the patient along the axes of physical risks (e.g., cardiopulmonary, renal, hepatic dysfunction) and also psychological risks (e.g., depression, abuse/dependence liability). Assessment of diversion risk is mandatory as well. Prescription drug monitoring program use is advised. Baseline urine drug screen recommended by many organizations
• Initiate opioid therapy on a trial basis, with the lowest possible dose and for the shortest possible duration, if benefits are deemed to outweigh the risks and if more appropriate and conservative treatment options have failed or are contraindicated
• Initiation of opioid therapy should commence with immediate-release agents, and extended- and immediate-release agents should not be used simultaneously if possible. Methadone should be used only by clinicians trained in and well-versed with its dangers
• Multimodal pain management (including heavy emphasis on behavioral health) is essential for good outcomes and must be stressed at every encounter
• Ongoing assessment of outcomes (e.g., "4As—analgesia, activity, adverse effects, and aberrancy) must guide therapy. Frequent assessment of functional improvements should contribute the greatest weight of data toward the decision to continue or abandon ongoing opioid therapy trial
• A "ceiling dose" between 50 and 90 morphine milligram equivalents (MME) should be targeted, and escalation beyond this threshold should probably be undertaken under the supervision of a pain management specialist
• Frequent compliance monitoring (PDMP use, urine drug screening, random pill counts, etc.) are recommended and should be tailored to initial risk stratification as well as ongoing assessment for aberrancy. Aberrancy and especially suspected diversion must be addressed immediately
• Discontinuation of therapy for resolution of painful condition, adverse effects, inadequate analgesic effect, lack of functional improvement or deteriorating function, or significant aberrancy should be carried out in a supportive and nonjudgmental fashion but with decisiveness if indicated. Alternatively referral to pain specialist and/or addictionologist is an option

ladder represents only one small aspect of providing safe and effective analgesia, and some more basic guidelines in treating cancer pain include the following [16]:

- Comprehensive assessment of pain complaints; underlying non-tumor pathology or reversible pathologic effects of tumor should not be overlooked and simply palliated by medications.
- Multimodal therapy including both pharmacologic and nonpharmacologic approaches should always be used.
- Opioid agents (and adjuvant agents) should always be selected with comorbidities (e.g., renal failure) in mind.
- Continuous pain should be treated with around-the-clock dosing.
- *Breakthrough pain* is defined as an increase in VAS rating of two or more points. It may be spontaneous or activity-associated. Recurrent spontaneous pain occurring toward the previous opioid dose's expected end of pharmacologic activity is not considered breakthrough pain but rather an indicator of inadequate baseline analgesia.

- Inadequate baseline analgesia should be treated by increasing the baseline regimen. Breakthrough pain should be treated with *rescue doses* of opioids in addition to the baseline regimen.

Numerous national organizations have put forth clinical practice guidelines (CPG) for the treatment of cancer pain; they are informed by a range of input from randomized controlled trial data and meta-analyses to expert opinion.

The United States' *National Comprehensive Cancer Network* 2013 CPG in Oncology [17] advocates thorough assessment of pain complaints at every visit, and multimodal treatment tailored to the severity of pain, appropriateness of varied interventions, and also opioid tolerance. The principle of autonomy underlies the recommendations, with the patient's goals and quality of life driving the process, and the guidance of the physician in providing ongoing assessment both for areas of potential improvement (e.g., dose increases, agent rotation, or adjuvant therapies) and harm reduction. This includes vigilance for physiologic adverse effects (e.g., constipation, nausea, pruritus) as well as psychological adverse effects (e.g., aberrant behaviors and misuse). When using opioids, round-the-clock dosing is recommended as a general rule, titrated to patient requirements.

For opioid-naive patients, defined as those not chronically receiving opioid analgesics and without tolerance (with suggested criteria of morphine 60 mg, oxycodone 30 mg, or hydromorphone 8 mg daily for a week or longer), stratification by pain scale rating and titration of short-acting opioids are recommended along with adjuvant therapy and bowel regimen. Oral therapy recommendations are to start with 5–15 mg of immediate-release morphine (or equivalent), reassess in an hour and titrate to effect, essentially, with dose increase of 50–100% if necessary for unremitting or increasing pain.

For opioid-tolerant patients, it is recommended that the previous 24 h total dose be maintained (either by immediate-release or if appropriate and safe, extended-release agent) and "breakthrough" or "rescue" dose of 10–20% of the previous 24 h total dose be made available every hour as needed, again titrating to effect with rescue dose increases up to 50–100% (of rescue dose) if necessary. Rotation is recommended in case of intolerable/untreatable adverse effects.

The *Japanese Society of Palliative Medicine* 2013 CPG [18] also recommends comprehensive assessment of pain complaints, and a stepwise approach to analgesics, with opioids considered first line for moderate to severe pain. For severe or "unstable" pain, immediate-release agents are recommended; for "stable" pain extended-release agents are considered. Multimodal therapy and vigilance for/prophylaxis against common adverse effects (e.g., constipation, nausea) are advised.

Dose increase (by 30–50% of previous daily dose) or opioid rotation is advised in case of tolerance/tachyphylaxis or other agent failure. In case of breakthrough pain, a "rescue dose" beginning at 10–20% of the total daily dose is recommended.

The *European Association for Palliative Care* 2012 CPG [19] presents the WHO ladder and recommends generally accepted consensus principles such as rotation in terms of failure, reducing the dose from "equianalgesic" conversions when rotating, and consideration of alternative routes (e.g., rectal, subcutaneous, transdermal) if adverse effects prohibit oral dosing. Rescue agents for breakthrough pain and monitoring for/treatment of adverse effects are recommended.

The *European Society for Medical Oncology* 2010 CPG [20] recommends thorough assessment of pain complaints at every visit, and multimodal treatment tailored to the severity of pain, appropriateness of varied interventions, and also opioid tolerance. The WHO analgesic ladder is invoked, and opioids are recommended only for moderate to severe pain. Initial oral dosing suggested for the opioid-naïve patient includes immediate-release morphine 20–40 mg, oxycodone 20 mg, or hydromorphone 8 mg. Round-the-clock dosing is recommended, with consideration of extended-release formulations for baseline analgesia and "breakthrough" doses of 10–15% of the total daily dose recommended up to four times per day before alteration of the baseline regimen is required. Rotation is recommended in case of intolerable/untreatable adverse effects.

Other Recommendations

Specific Precautions

While discussed in greater detail in both Chaps. 3 and 4, it bears repeating that mu-receptor agonism carries a high risk of multiple adverse effects including respiratory depression/apnea, and when considering opioid prescription, the physician must always be mindful of comorbid conditions such as pre-existing airway or pulmonary compromise, as well as co-prescribed central nervous system depressants that might confer synergistic risk of apnea. In addition, as with any medication prescribed, the physician must be aware of renal or hepatic dysfunction and the effect that metabolic compromise might have on the pharmacodynamics of the drug(s) prescribed. As pharmacogenetic testing becomes more common, awareness of cytochrome P450 system allelic variation, which may influence metabolism/elimination, may become "standard of care."

Driving Precautions

The issue of driving while using opioid medications is one that affects the individual as well as public health, and the prescriber is certainly "part of the equation." It is clear that a substantial number of drivers operate motor vehicles or other heavy machinery with potentially impairing substances (including but not limited to opioids)—the 2014 National Survey on Drug Use and Health reports 10 million people driving under the influence of illicit drugs during the year prior to being surveyed [21]. What is less clear is the degree of increased risk of harm to self or others is assumed by driving while using prescription opioids; while outcome variables (MVA, fatalities) are relatively easy to measure, predictor variables (serum opioid levels, degree of cognitive compromise) are much more difficult to assess. In fact, the question is to some degree without answer due to the spectrum of impairment based upon dose, drug naivete and other confounding factors such as other medications, sleep deprivation, and distractions including electronic devices or passenger conversation and even including pain itself.

Fishbain et al. [22] performed a review of 22 studies examining the effects of opioids on psychomotor function and attempted to extrapolate the results of these largely non-real-life investigations to driving safety. While reporting that overall there appears to be no consistent evidence for impairment of psychomotor abilities or cognitive function of opioid-maintained patients and no evidence for greater incidence in motor vehicle violations/motor vehicle accidents for opioid-maintained patients versus comparable controls, they do admit that the evidence is inconsistent and recommend further well-controlled studies.

The most commonly cited prospective evaluation to date is that of Galski [23] who compared 16 chronic prescription opioid users against a group of 327 other "cerebrally compromised patients" in a battery of simulated driving skills assessment. There were no statistically significant differences between the groups. Limitations of this study of course include the very small case number and the generalizability of the control populace.

Nearly 1 million drivers were involved in fatal crashes from 1993 to 2010; only 29.2% of these were known to have undergone testing for drugs; the testing status of 13% is unknown [24]. Of those tested for drugs, 35.8% tested positive, and of those 58.7% had an identifiable drug reported. Schedule II–V prescription drugs represented the majority (roughly 40%) of all drugs identified, with marijuana, and stimulants (cocaine and methamphetamines) representing roughly another third each. In subanalysis of 2010 data, opioids represented the most commonly identified drug (with hydrocodone and oxycodone representing 21.3% of all detected drugs, with benzodiazepines comprising 20.5%).

In 2008, the Department of Transportation reported data derived from over 33,000 MVAs; among other analyses, a case-control analysis was performed to evaluate the potential contributions of various commonly prescribed medications to crashes [25]. Fifteen drug classes (including NSAIDs and hypoglycemic agents) were shown to confer statistically significant increased risk of MVA, and opioids placed fourth in the rankings, with an odds ratio (OR) of 2.22. (Barbiturates ranked first at OR 7.5, and antihistamines and non-narcotic antitussives also had an OR greater than that of opioids. Opioids however conferred greater risk than anxiolytics and anticonvulsants.)

State laws addressing the issue of driving under the influence of opioids (or other nonalcoholic sedatives) vary tremendously and are beyond the scope of this book to address. For greater detail, the reader is referred to the National Highway Traffic Safety Administration's 2009 report [26] on *driving under the influence of drugs (DUID)*. In general, laws addressing DUID can be categorized as those that:

- Require proof that drugs rendered a driver "incapable" of driving safely for conviction.

- Require proof that the drug impaired the driver's ability to operate the vehicle safely for conviction. These statutes generally carry language along the lines of "under the influence of" or "affected by" an intoxicating drug.
- Require only proof of a drug or metabolite in one's body/body fluids while operating a motor vehicle for conviction. These statutes, also known as "Zero tolerance" or "Per se" statutes exist in 17 states, covering 40% of all drivers in the United States.

Five states (California, Colorado, Idaho, Kansas, and West Virginia) make it illegal for any drug addict or habitual user of drugs to drive a vehicle in their States.

The Office of National Drug Control Policy and the Governors' Highway Safety Association have stated that they will encourage states to adopt "Zero tolerance/Per se" statutes [27], which would almost certainly result in increasing convictions and likely reduce the number of opioid-related MVAs, although this opinion is contested by those who appeal to the data suggesting no significant impairment from appropriately used opioid prescriptions in tolerant individuals. In opposition to this stance also are those who feel strongly that patients using opioids for legitimate chronic pain reasons are at risk of having substantial personal liberties and functionality/productivity compromised.

The proverbial "rock and hard place" of opioid prescribing may pose no greater dilemma than that of this arena, where personal liberties and frequently necessary transportation must be balanced with public (and individual) safety. Barring clear evidence of intoxication/impairment at an encounter (or perhaps by third-party report), the prescriber is not generally in a position to render judgment on a patient's capacity to safely operate a vehicle (or other machinery). The prescriber, however, like it or not, is the best authority on the pharmacokinetics and pharmacodynamics of the drug prescribed as well as the salient risk factors of the patient (e.g., underlying cognitive deficit, sleep architecture disruption, concurrent medications). Sparse and conflicting data aside, the prescriber must in every situation first advise the patient that opioids are generally pro-somnolent, may impair reflexes and judgment, may decrease concentration, etc. All patients receiving an opioid prescription should be counseled:

- Not to drive under the sedative effects of the opioid prescribed, nor any other substance. In general, it is advisable to refrain from driving for at least 3–5 days while adjusting to a new drug or dosage.
- Not to use any other CNS depressants (including alcohol, marijuana, antihistamines, etc.) without the express authorization of the physician.
- To immediately report whether they are experiencing sedation/unsteadiness/cognitive decline, so that urgent workup and/or a reduction/modification in dosage can be initiated.

Second, while not ultimately responsible for the actions of the patient, the prescriber is responsible for the prescription and must determine when opioid prescription harms outweigh benefit—bearing in mind no greater potential harm exists than that of an impaired vehicle operator. A corollary to this principle is the moral and ethical (and increasingly legal) duty of the physician to report potentially impaired drivers. The American Medical Association's Code of Medical Ethics clearly documents the physician's responsibility "to recognize impairments in patients' driving ability that pose a strong threat to public safety and which ultimately may need to be reported to the Department of Motor Vehicles" [28], and case law in many courts has upheld the physician's "duty to protect" [29]. Many states have mandatory reporting laws requiring physicians to report either specific medical conditions (e.g., epilepsy, dementia) or other factors that may impair driving to the Department of Motor Vehicles. Physicians have been held liable for civil damages for failing to disclose this information, and on the other hand, concerns exist for allegations of breach of confidentiality. In general, legal immunity for reporting applies, but the onus of keeping abreast of these rapidly changing issues falls on the prescriber. The AMA and NHTSA have provided a resource for exploring these requirements state-by-state [30], and prescribers may also inquire with their specific state agency.

Eugeroics and Stimulants

Some providers favor the use of wakefulness-promoting agents (e.g., modafinil, armodafinil, or traditional psychostimulants) to counteract the sedative effects of opioids. At present, there are no policies nor guidelines addressing this issue. Outside the context of palliative care, it is the author's opinion that excess sedation caused (or contributed to) by opioids is best addressed by careful evaluation for other potential contributors (e.g., sleep deprivation from poor sleep hygiene, obstructive sleep apnea) and by reducing opioid burden.

Bowel Hygiene Agents

Given the ubiquitous complication/adverse effect of constipation, bowel hygiene should always be addressed with the patient. Plentiful hydration and a diet rich in fiber should be encouraged; many patients are unaware of the importance of these basic measures and their importance for overall health. Stool softeners (e.g., docusate) and/or osmotic agents such as polyethylene glycol are first-line agents to prevent or treat constipation. Magnesium compounds are often an effective and benign means of treating constipation and carry the additional benefit of analgesic efficacy for many neuropathic conditions. Stimulant laxatives are generally not advisable, certainly not for prolonged use. Newer prescription agents (e.g., lubiprostone, peripheral mu-receptor antagonists) are discussed in greater detail in Chap. 3.

Naloxone Prescription

The idea of prescription of *naloxone* for opioid overdose prophylaxis (*bystander Narcan*) has been a recent and contentious development in our society but appears to be gaining political and professional traction with widespread adoption over the past few years. Proponents offer the plausible argument that a simple and inexpensive naloxone delivery mechanism (whether nasal spray or auto-injector) may save a life. Indeed, a considerable and growing body of case reports around the country and the world supports this position [31, 32]. Opponents claim that similar to "clean needle programs," Community Narcan programs/publicity and naloxone prescription will result in reduced caution among opioid users and only lead to greater dependence and abuse issues. Regardless of the personal opinion of the prescriber on the matter, it appears that the co-prescription of naloxone with moderate to high-dose opioid therapy (or in cases of heroin addiction) is here to stay, and the recent CDC guidelines [8] recommend prescription of naloxone whenever opioid prescription exceeds 50MME.

Rotation and Holidays

Various strategies exist to combat tolerance to analgesic effects from chronic opioid use, including dose escalation, rotation of agents, and holidays. In the author's opinion, the current twin epidemics of chronic pain and opioid misuse/abuse/dependence bear witness to the failure of the former approach.

Rotation is a time-honored concept and strategy in attempting to optimize the efficacy of opioid therapy and also reduce dose escalation and adverse effects. While the mechanisms underlying the purported benefit of this technique are not yet fully elucidated (and may never be), factors that may explain the apparent benefit include [33]:

- Incomplete cross-tolerance
- Pharmacogenetic variation
- Drug-drug interactions

These same factors may also confer increased risk/harm when rotating opioid agents.

Equianalgesic tables have been widely published over the past 2 decades in an attempt to help clinicians determine safe and effective comparable doses of various opioid agents. They are limited by highly variable data, likely owing in part to inter-subject variations in pharmacogenetics and P450 interactions, and tolerance and as such must be interpreted with caution. A general rule of thumb when rotating agents is to reduce the "equianalgesic dose" by 25% to 50% upon initial conversion. Other considerations include age and organ dysfunction on varying mechanisms of metabolism and clearance, cardiopulmonary vulnerabilities, and predisposition to abuse and addiction [34].

Intermittent *holidays* serve to reduce tolerance and also potentially reduce an opioid-hyperalgesic state. Opioid *weaning* accomplishes the same benefits in many cases. In the author's experience, taking a few minutes to explain the phenomena of tolerance and hyperalgesia, and the goal of restricting consumption to "recalibrate the brain" and improve pain control is almost always well received.

Summary

The past two decades have taught us that opioid prescription is more fraught with difficulties and negative consequences than was appreciated at the outset of the opioid epidemic. Failure on the part of physicians and mid-level practitioners to follow best practices (and in some cases the law) is unarguably a significant contributor to this crisis. Opioid prescription is governed at a professional level by guidelines and standards of care established to protect individual patients. At a societal level, both state and federal government have developed laws regarding opioid prescription to minimize the risk of diversion while preserving the physician's privilege of providing these powerful medications to the right patients in the right manner. Knowledge of, and compliance with federal and state law, and state medical board rules is mandatory for anyone authorized by the Drug Enforcement Administration to prescribe controlled substances, and standards of care for opioid prescription are being increasingly influenced by national guidelines from professional societies and agencies of the government.

The prescription of opioids for pain, whether acute or chronic, cancer or non-cancer related, should always follow thorough evaluation of pain complaints and comprise part of a comprehensive treatment plan involving other primary modalities as applicable, with opioids as the adjunctive therapy. Opioid prescription should always be considered a trial, with continuous assessment of efficacy in facilitating functional goals and analgesia vs. adverse effects. This tentative approach of constant reevaluation is necessitated by the low therapeutic window of these agents, with increasing evidence of cumulative harms with long-term use as discussed in previous chapters. A treatment agreement/opioid contract should be entered into, with clear instructions as to patient responsibility for exclusive prescription by one provider, compliance with the prescription and other clinic policies, safe use including driving restrictions, safe storage, non-diversion, etc. Compliance and harms monitoring should be observed, with random urine drug screens, pill counts, etc. explained to the patient as a universal protocol for their safety and that of society. An "exit strategy" should be discussed a priori. When harms outweigh benefits, or if concern for diversion exists, discontinuing opioid therapy is necessary. Consideration of referral to a board-certified pain specialist and/or an addictionologist may be warranted.

The use of opioids in treating cancer pain is universally accepted and follows similar principles, with aggressive monitoring for and treatment of pain complaints recommended.

Finally, numerous other medicolegal issues surround the prescription of opioids and are likely to increase in number and profile as public awareness of the opioid epidemic grows. The issue of driving under the influence of opioids (and other prescription medications) involves prescribers, like it or not, and places a significant and sobering responsibility upon the physician/mid-level provider to exercise due diligence in protecting the patient and society from impaired drivers. Recently, the practice of prophylactic naloxone ("Community Narcan") prescription has gained momentum has been recommended by the CDC in their recent guidelines.

References

1. United States Department of Justice, Drug Enforcement Administration, Office of Diversion Control. Practitioner's manual: an informational outline of the controlled substances act. 2006. Available from: https://www.deadiversion.usdoj.gov/pubs/manuals/pract/. Accessed 20 Nov 2016.
2. Smith DE, Seymore RB. Prescribing practices: the educational alternative for the misprescriber. Proceedings of the White House Conference on Prescription Drug Abuse, Washington, DC; 1980.
3. The American College of Preventive Medicine. Use, abuse, misuse & disposal of prescription pain medication clinical reference. 2011. http://www.acpm.org/?UseAbuseRxClinRef. Accessed 20 Nov 2016.
4. Dineen KK, Dubois JM. Between a rock and a hard place: can physicians prescribe opioids to treat pain adequately while avoiding legal sanction? Am J Law Med. 2016;42:7–52.
5. Holden GA, Wakefield P, Brown AB, Talbot RW, Brasher L. A guide to state controlled substances acts. Washington, DC: National Criminal Justice Association; 1988.
6. National Alliance for Model State Drug Laws (NAMSDL), Sherry L. Green & Associates, LLC (SLGA). Highlights 2016 state prescription drug monitoring program (PMP) bills. http://www.namsdl.org/library/73FC8E48-B877-B246-8B1F3EEB329C45BF/. Accessed 23 Nov 2016.
7. Federation of State Medical Boards of the United States, Inc. Model policy on the use of opioid analgesics in the treatment of chronic pain. Available from: http://www.fsmb.org/Media/Default/PDF/FSMB/Advocacy/pain_policy_july2013.pdf. Accessed 20 Nov 2016.
8. Dowell D, Haegerich TM, Chou R. CDC guideline for prescribing opioids for chronic pain – United States, 2016. MMWR. 2016;65:1–49.
9. Canadian guideline for safe and effective use of opioids for chronic non-cancer pain. Canada: National Opioid Use Guideline Group (NOUGG); 2010. Available from: http://nationalpaincentre.mcmaster.ca/opioid/
10. Veterans' Administration/Department of Defense. VA/DoD clinical practice guidelines for management of opioid therapy for chronic pain. Washington, D.C.: Veterans' Administration; 2010. Available from: http://www.va.gov/painmanagement/docs/cpg_opioidtherapy_fulltext.pdf
11. Washington Agency Medical Directors Group. Interagency guideline on opioid dosing for chronic non-cancer pain. 2010. Available from: http://www.agencymedicaldirectors.wa.gov/Files/OpioidGdline.pdf

12. Chou R, Fanciullo GP, Fine PG, Adler JA, Ballantyne JC, Davies P, et al. Clinical guidelines for the use of chronic opioid therapy in chronic noncancer pain. J Pain. 2009;10:113–30.
13. Manchikanti L, Kaye AM, Knezevic NN, McAnally H, Slavin K, Trescot AM, et al. Responsible, safe, and effective prescription of opioids for chronic non-cancer pain: American society of interventional pain physicians (ASIPP) guidelines. Pain Physician. 2017;20(2S):S3–S92.
14. Fishman SM. Responsible opioid prescribing, chapter 1. Washington, D.C.: Waterford Life Sciences; 2014. p. 9.
15. American Academy of Pain Medicine. Methadone for pain management: improving clinical decision making. 2016. Available from: http://www.painmed.org/files/methadone-for-pain-management-improving-clinical-decision-making.pdf. Accessed 23 Nov 2016.
16. Davis MP, Smith HS. Opioid therapy for cancer pain. In: Smith HS, editor. Opioid therapy in the twenty-first century. New York: Oxford University Press; 2013.
17. Swarm RA, Abernethy AP, Anghelescu DL, Benedetti C, Buga S, Cleeland C, et al. Adult cancer pain. J Natl Compr Cancer Netw. 2013;11:992–1022.
18. Yamaguchi T, Shima Y, Morita T, Hosoya M, Matoba M, Japanese Society of Palliative Medicine. Clinical guideline for pharmacological management of cancer pain: the Japanese society of palliative medicine recommendations. Jpn J Clin Oncol. 2013;43:896–909.
19. Caraceni A, Hanks G, Kaasa S, Bennett MI, Brunelli C, Cherny N, et al. Use of opioid analgesics in the treatment of cancer pain: evidence-based recommendations from the EAPC. Lancet Oncol. 2012 Feb;13(2):e58–68. doi:10.1016/S1470-2045(12)70040-2.
20. Ripamonti CI, Santini D, Maranzano E, Berti M, Roila F, ESMO Guidelines Working Group. Management of cancer pain: ESMO clinical practice guidelines. Ann Oncol. 2012;23(Suppl 7):vii139–54.
21. Center for Behavioral Health Statistics and Quality (CBHSQ). Behavioral health trends in the United States: results from the 2014 national survey on drug use and health. Rockville, MD: Substance Abuse and Mental Health Services Administration; 2015. HHS Publication No. SMA 15-4927, NSDUH Series H-50
22. Fishbain DA, Cutler RB, Rosomoff HL, Rosomoff RS. Are opioid-dependent/tolerant patients impaired in driving-related skills? A structured evidence-based review. J Pain Symptom Manag. 2003;25:559–77.
23. Galski T, Williams JB, Ehle HT. Effects of opioids on driving ability. J Pain Symptom Manag. 2000;19:200–8.
24. Wilson FA, Stimpson JP, Pagán JA. Fatal crashes from drivers testing positive for drugs in the U.S., 1993–2010. Public Health Rep. 2014;129(4):342–50.
25. LeRoy AA, Morse ML. Department of Transportation. HS 810 858. Multiple medications and vehicle crashes: analysis of databases. 2008. Available from: http://www.nhtsa.gov/DOT/NHTSA/Traffic%20Injury%20Control/Articles/Associated%20Files/810858.pdf. Accessed 24 Nov 2016.
26. Walsh JM. A state-by-state analysis of laws dealing with driving under the influence of drugs. U.S. Department of Transportation, National Highway Traffic Safety Administration. Washington, D.C. 2009. Available from: www.nhtsa.gov/staticfiles/nti/pdf/811236.pdf. Accessed 24 Nov 2016.
27. Office of National Drug Control Policy. National Drug Control Strategy 2014. Washington, D.C; 2014. https://www.whitehouse.gov/sites/default/files/ondcp/policy-and-research/ndcs_2014.pdf
28. American Medical Association. Opinion 8.2 impaired drivers and their physicians. AMA Code of Medical Ethics. Chicago, IL: American Medical Association; 2016. Available from: https://www.ama-assn.org/sites/default/files/media-browser/code-of-medical-ethics-chapter-8.pdf. Accessed 25 Nov 2016.
29. Black L. Physicians' legal responsibility to report impaired drivers. Virtual Mentor. 2008;10:393–6.

30. National Highway Traffic Safety Administration. State licensing requirements and reporting laws. In Physician's guide to assessing and counseling older drivers, 2nd ed. 2010. Available from: http://www.nhtsa.gov/people/injury/olddrive/OlderDriversBook/pages/Chapter8.html. Accessed 25 Nov 2016.
31. Giglio RE, Li G, DiMaggio CJ. Effectiveness of bystander naloxone administration and overdose education programs: a meta-analysis. Inj Epidemiol. 2015;2(1):10. doi:10.1186/s40621-015-0041-8.
32. McDonald R, Strang J. Are take-home naloxone programmes effective? Systematic review utilizing application of the Bradford Hill criteria. Addiction. 2016;111(7):1177–87. doi:10.1111/add.13326.
33. Smith HS, McCarberg BH. Optimizing pharmacologic outcomes: principles of opioid rotation. In: Smith HS, editor. Opioid therapy in the twenty-first century. Oxford: Oxford University Press; 2013. p. 121–33.
34. Smith HS, Peppin JF. Toward a systematic approach to opioid rotation. J Pain Res. 2014;7:589–608.

Part IV
Focusing on the Host

"For that which I do I allow not: for what I would, that do I not; but what I hate, that do I… for to will is present with me; but *how* to perform that which is good I find not… For the good that I would I do not; but the evil which I would not, that I do."

"Brethren, if a man be overtaken in a fault, ye which are spiritual, restore such an one in the spirit of meekness; considering thyself, lest thou also be tempted."

St. Paul, *Letter to the Romans, Letter to the Galatians*

Chapter 9
Addressing Host Factors: Overview of Dependence and Addiction

A 26-year-old male presents to your practice with a complaint of low back pain that he states has been troubling him for 8 years and which he attributes to manual labor as a roofer and also a history of multiple motor vehicle accidents. There are no radicular nor cauda equina symptoms. He states that physical therapy has failed to benefit him as have NSAIDs and tramadol. He reports that he has been using hydrocodone-acetaminophen products for the past 5 years, currently using eight 10/325 tablets daily and that this is the only therapy that "works for him" and allows him to remain functional as a roofer. He is a smoker and admits to two to three beers per evening. Upon further questioning he admits to regular use of marijuana as well. Family history is remarkable for a "bad back" in his father, who underwent several spine operations in his 40s and 50s. Review of systems is positive for insomnia and constipation. Review of the PDMP shows multiple hydrocodone prescriptions by various providers, mostly emergency room physicians, filled at various pharmacies.

On exam he is well-developed, well-nourished, alert, and oriented x4. Vital signs are T99.5, HR 108, BP 166/98, RR 18. Pupils are 8 mm. There are no fresh punctate wounds nor tracks, and he exhibits no stereotypic stimulant behaviors. He is without any obvious neurologic deficits. His lumbar spine ROM is limited in flexion and extension by pain, and there is obvious thoracolumbar myospasm. Straight leg raise is negative bilaterally, as are Kemp's and Patrick's maneuvers.

He requests that you prescribe him "240 'hydros' for the month."

H.B. McAnally, *Opioid Dependence*, DOI 10.1007/978-3-319-47497-7_9

Introduction

We turn our analysis now to the final component of the classic epidemiologic triangle, and that which is arguably the most complex, as well as the most important: the *host*. In the arena of infectious disease epidemiology and public health efforts, attempts to intervene upon the *agent* itself are generally of very limited utility; similarly, while alteration of opioid agents (the subject of Chap. 5) has shifted abuse patterns, we have not seen concomitant decrease in consumption, misuse/abuse, or adverse consequences. *Vector* modification (e.g., reduction of mosquito populations) has borne some success in certain disease reduction efforts; similarly, modification of prescriber practices may be fruitful by certain metrics (e.g., reduced methadone overdose). The overall data however are not as encouraging; opioid death rates increased by 15.6% from 2014 to 2015 and surpassed 33,000 deaths in 2015 [1]. While "street drugs" (heroin and illicitly manufactured fentanyl) were responsible for most of the increase, abuse of prescription opioids has not declined significantly (with possible increase over the past year) and furthermore continues to elicit concern as a "gateway" to heroin, etc. (Fig. 9.1).

Regardless of the source and structure of the opioid involved, it is clear that efforts to date (e.g., nearly $29 billion federal monies spent in 2015, with $31 billion earmarked in 2017 [2]) have not yet been sufficient to turn the tide.

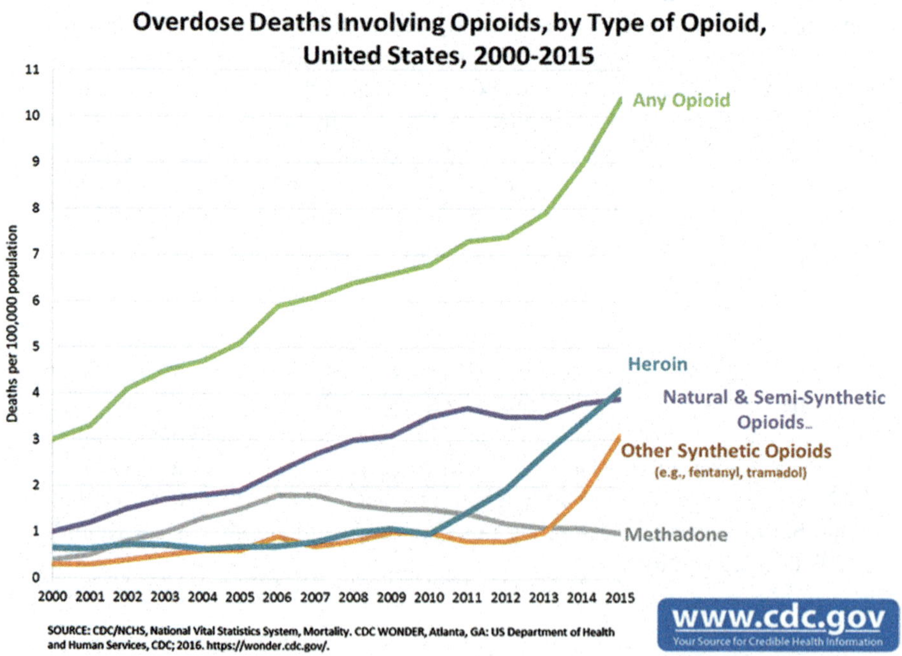

Fig. 9.1 US opioid deaths, 2000–2015. Source: CDC/NCHS, National Vital Statistics System, Mortality. CDC WONDER, Atlanta, GA: US Department of Health and Human Services, CDC; 2016. https://wonder.cdc.gov

It is the author's contention that, as with other historically significant epidemics, success in reversing the grim and rising toll of opioid morbidity and mortality will come only with alteration of host factors including vulnerability and exposure behaviors. Despite modern-era elucidation of agent factors (e.g., mutations in influenza strains rendering them exponentially more capable of ravaging vulnerable populations) as key determinants of infectious organism pathogenicity/virulence, current evidence suggests that exclusive focus on the agent is antiquated and reductionist. Our understanding of the complex interactions between host and agent has grown to include an appreciation for the commensal if not even symbiotic relationship between many microorganisms and human beings, and diminution of host resistance is known to be a key element in the balance between health and disease.

In the area of opioid misuse and abuse, host vulnerability to the agent rather than agent virulence may represent the more important area of focus given that we remain largely reliant upon (appropriate) therapeutic opioid use for the control of much severe and acute pain. Dr. Sydenham's recently often-quoted applause of opiates:

> And here I cannot but break out in praise of the great God, the Giver of all good things, who hath granted to the human race, as a comfort in their afflictions, no medicine of the value of opium, either in regard to the number of diseases that it can control, or its efficiency in extirpating them. [3]

remains admissible today. Until safer means analgesic means of similar potency (and broad spectrum) become widely available, the judicious application of mu-agonists remains inevitable for the effective treatment of acute pain. As such, adaptation of the host to enable containment and control of the agent is of the essence (Fig. 9.2).

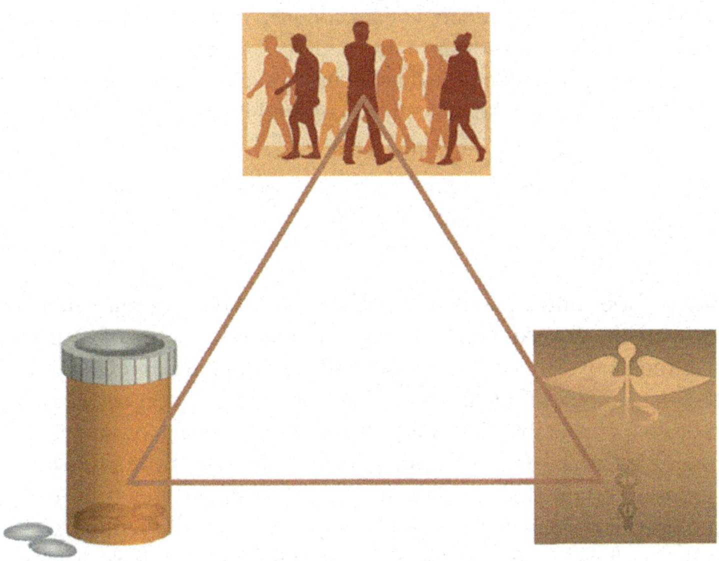

Fig. 9.2 Epidemiologic triangle

The propagation of an infectious epidemic is retarded when exposure of vulnerable hosts to the agent falls below a certain threshold rate, and the epidemic itself is eliminated with the eventual development of resistance or immunity within the population. Historically the pressures of natural selection within these dynamics have been the sole mediator of adaptation and survival; more recently within human history, we have been able to engineer immunity with vaccinations, etc. While immunity in the form of long-term mu-opioid receptor blockade by depot naltrexone (or occupancy by buprenorphine) is currently state-of-the-art prevention, the development of a literal "vaccine" for opioids has been contemplated and even explored [4]. Such measures however are not without their disadvantages, as might be expected from disruption of natural processes with the complexity/ubiquity of the endogenous opioid system. One of the more immediate and obvious consequences of such a strategy, well known now to trauma and perioperative practitioners is the marked difficulty conferred by such pharmacologic constraints upon acute pain control. Furthermore, as suggested by the apparent trend away from prescription opioids to heroin attributed to agent/vector modification, restriction of mu-agonist efficacy may only serve to drive a shift in "drug of choice" away from opioids to other substances capable of eliciting similar reward-seeking behavior.

Cultivating control and containment over perceived "appropriate requirement" for opioid analgesia, i.e., pain, (and certainly over inappropriate euphoric or other mood-affecting properties) is critical to overcoming dependence and addiction individually and arguably at a societal level as well. This effort is arguably also the most salient (and collectively overlooked) province toward which medical and public health endeavor should be directed. As discussed in Chap. 1, a critical and assumed ingredient in a population's effort to end an epidemic is the inherent desire of the vulnerable population to avoid the agent. Unfortunately in the case of addiction, rational self-preservation instincts are surrendered or are conquered by the overwhelming compulsion to seek the addictive substance (or activity) regardless of the results. What renders some hosts more vulnerable than others to such compulsion for inappropriate or even uncontrolled use is a key question, explored in greater detail in Chap. 10.

Outcome Definitions

The attention of the nation, and that of policymakers both governmental and professional, has been upon overdoses. Defining outcome variables is of course important in any scientific analysis, and failure to clearly delineate such renders investigation and conclusions empirical. Quantifiable metrics such as emergency room overdose visits and deaths attributable to opioids provide some means of attempting to track the efficacy of interventions, but comprise only the tip of the proverbial iceberg. While overdoses certainly occur in the opioid-naïve, underlying these outcomes is a much more prevalent problem of opioid dependence and addiction that is not only driving mortality figures but also confers tremendous morbidity physically, psychologically, spiritually, relationally, and societally.

There are significant difficulties involved in attempting to investigate dependence and addiction. Descriptive statistics, let alone analyses are hampered by the challenges of a broad spectrum of "subclinical" illness, lack of criteria consensus, and insensitive instruments for identifying the conditions, to name a few.

As discussed in Chap. 3, by most commonly accepted definitions, the state described as opioid *dependence* involves recurrent use, withdrawal phenomena, and behavioral components including desire/unsuccessful attempts to quit, effort expended in pursuit of opioids, etc. *Addiction* is a term currently again deliberately avoided by the American Psychiatric Association (and the World Health Organization) yet commonly used in the scientific community (e.g., NIDA) to describe "compulsive drug seeking despite negative consequences." As discussed previously, the trend is currently away from the attempted specificity of categorical variables and toward the sensitivity of a continuum, and the DSM-5 has recently described a spectrum of *opioid use disorder (OUD)* that "includes signs and symptoms that reflect compulsive, prolonged self-administration of opioid substances that are used for no legitimate medical purpose or, if another medical condition is present that requires opioid treatment, that are used in doses greatly in excess of the amount needed for that medical condition" [5]. Four main "symptom clusters" within the current substance use disorder framework include impaired control, risky use, social problems, and physical effects such as tolerance and withdrawal.

Pseudoaddiction is a concept/term not considered previously in this book, which was originally coined in 1989 [6] and gathered some support within the pain management community while failing to gain recognition and acceptance by the greater medical and psychiatric communities. The concept proposes in essence that inadequately treated pain can cause individuals to escalate pain behaviors in order to acquire more opioids. The only real distinction between pseudoaddiction and true addiction in this paradigm is whether the patient cites pain or euphoria-seeking as the reason for opioid-seeking and whether they correspondingly attribute cessation of aberrant drug-related behaviors and opioid misuse after subjective report of pain relief. The difficulties in this theoretical construct (including lack of any scientific basis, plentiful pharmacologic industry support for the reports) have been objectively criticized in recent publications [7–9].

Common to this continuum (dependence, "pseudoaddiction," addiction) is the disordered behavioral state the American Psychiatric Association describes as "compulsive, prolonged self-administration." Whether the primary underlying motivation is a relief from physical or mental suffering or merely pleasure-seeking, failure to exercise control over powerful impulses and desires characterizes OUD. Regardless of the outcome variable chosen, at the heart of the opioid epidemic lies loss of control. This final section of the book is concerned with preventing that loss of control or reinstating lost control to the habituated user. While addictionology comprises a very small part if any of the most clinicians' practices, growing appreciation of the hitherto unrecognized prevalence (and incidence) of substance use disorders should motivate physicians in all fields to, at the very least, familiarize themselves with the basic issues at hand, especially in the era of heavy-handed pharmacotherapy. Certain fields more than others share overlap with the domain of addictionology and also carry increased liability for iatrogenic facilitation of addiction. It is assumed that the self-selected audience of this book falls within this latter category, and as such, this entire chapter is devoted to presenting a hopefully comprehensive yet concise clinical framework of addiction theory.

Overview of Addiction

West and Brown [10] define addiction as "a chronic condition in which there is a repeated powerful motivation to engage in a rewarding behavior, acquired as a result of engaging in that behavior, that has significant potential for unintended harm." This elegant definition has shed some of the conventional thought and language concerning addiction (e.g., unsuccessful desire to disengage from the behavior, which may or may not be present; use despite significant harm and loss, which may or may not occur) and as such is more applicable to the spectrum of OUD that has traditionally fallen outside that rubric. As mentioned above, we will use the language of addictionology within the brief survey presented below to encompass this expanded scope and hopefully inform better care across the spectrum of severity. At the outset of this discussion, we will present some commonly observed cardinal features/characteristics of addiction pertinent to both preventive and therapeutic efforts, followed by some basic clinical and public health questions framed around these and related phenomena.

Finally, a survey of addiction theories and models is presented. Most of these theories and models generally exhibit fairly unidimensional foci (e.g., moral failure, genetic predisposition, dysregulation of mesolimbic dopaminergic activity, social learning). While many do not lend themselves well to a systematic organization, in general they have historically been categorized into moral/spiritual, disease, and learning models. At the heart of the controversies about addiction lies the issue of *control*, and the (possibly oversimplistic) question of whether *choice* or *compulsion* drives the initiation and perpetuation of these behaviors; the complexities of human behavior and the very definition of "choice" (or compulsion) itself render it unlikely that a clear-cut answer will ever be arrived at. There is a growing sense that both may be true, just as light is both particle and wave.

In this chapter we will follow the general outline of models based on choice vs. compulsion and attempt to frame major theories within the context of these two opposing viewpoints as applicable. Integrated into the section on condition/learning is a brief discussion of the observation that addiction generally follows a biphasic course of positive reinforcement/reward followed by negative reinforcement (withdrawal phenomena) which to many forms a bridge or transition between the bipolar constructs of choice vs. compulsion. More recently, social and system models have been proposed and are briefly introduced as well, as they are certainly germane to public health if not individual prevention efforts. The chapter concludes with consideration of the complex phenomenon of motivation as a critical consideration in the analysis and prevention/treatment of OUD.

Cardinal Phenomena of Addiction and Related Questions

To date, there has never been a reported case of congenital addiction. Whether or not the condition is heritable or latent may be debated until the end of time, but it is clear that an initial exposure initiates the process. While outliers of truly forcible exposure (not mere "peer pressure") undoubtedly exist, for the most part this introduction to the substance follows a conscious decision, often facilitated by some perceived well-being deficit, whether pain, emotional distress, or simply boredom. Not everyone exposed, however, whether once or repetitively, goes on to develop dependence and addiction. Despite multiple substances with addictive potential, people furthermore generally seek out and develop a dependence upon a "drug of choice" or a limited combination thereof (e.g., alcohol and tobacco, or opioids and benzodiazepines).

In those in whom addiction develops, a well-documented progression from a "positive" reward-chasing cycle to one of "negative" pursuit of the habituated substance to avoid withdrawal phenomena exists. During the initial reward-mediated phase, powerful cravings for the substance generally develop that are inversely proportional to an inevitable experience of diminishing returns. This satisfaction-resistant drive supersedes/subjugates all others, and the pursuit of the substance becomes singular at the expense of all other goals and priorities. Ultimately (sometimes within a very short period) the switch to negative reinforcement occurs, mediated by powerful withdrawal symptoms both psychological and physical, and avoidance of this discomfort becomes the primary motivating factor. More often than not, the individual struggles with this increasing captivity and makes efforts to resist and desist to some degree. Relapse after varying periods of sobriety is common.

Questions to consider include:

- What makes some people more prone than others to develop addiction?
- Why do youth appear to be disproportionately vulnerable?
- What are the psychological processes (and risk factors) involved in the development and maintenance of addiction?
- What are the neurobiological processes (and risk factors) involved in the development and maintenance of addiction?
- What are the social processes (and risk factors) involved in the development and maintenance of addiction?
- How much overlap is there between choice and compulsion in the development and maintenance of addiction?
- How much common ground do the many apparent distinct "pathways to addiction" including different initial motivations, different substances, different biochemical/genetic profiles, etc. share?
- Are we doing enough to educate individual patients or the populace as a whole about the manifold dangers of addiction?
- What motivates people to succumb to addictive behavior?
- How do we help confer resistance/immunity to addiction?
- How do we best intervene when addiction has developed? Is there a single best approach or multiple options best tailored to individual situations?

Addiction Theories and Models: Choice

The viewpoint of addiction in the West was dominated by choice models up until the latter part of the twentieth century. Until modern era tobacco-related mortality (coupled with its ubiquity—there are 33 million daily American tobacco users in 2014 vs. 16 million "heavy" alcohol users [11]) commandeered public health attention and monies, alcoholism has historically served as the prototypical and most studied addiction. Excessive use of alcohol has been viewed as aberrant since antiquity, with recognition of adverse physical health consequences as well as relational and societal damage documented for millennia in the Hebrew Scriptures and other sacred texts. The prevalent spiritual/religious influence on human behavior in most pre-industrial societies was generally associated with a viewpoint on behavioral excesses in general as immoral and deliberately defiant of a Divinely prescribed order. Inherent in that transgression is the concept of choice.

Choice in common parlance involves an independent decision free of predetermination or constraint. It exemplifies the concept of free will and an internal locus of control. Choice is not necessarily at odds with habituation nor indeed with vulnerability nor predisposition to certain behavioral patterns. It does not imply rational/logical thought nor self-interest.

The determination of whether decisions or behaviors are rational or irrational depends of course upon the definition of those terms and concepts. Closely linked with this evaluation is whether the party rendering such judgment appeals to an external comparison standard of good/best/right and whether that comparison standard is absolute or relative. Relevant questions include:

- Does rational choice require full comprehension of risks, benefits, and alternatives?
- How can such comprehension be determined/does simple verbal assent really signify understanding?
- Is the standard the highest good of the individual or that of their local or larger society?
- Does highest good mean absolute absence of negative/harmful actions or the "best we can do/lesser of two evils" in terms of balancing competing benefits and harms?
- Does highest good entail conformity/compliance with an external code of behavior?

Some thought leaders (and certainly a multitude of individual users) take the position that substance abuse and dependence/addiction may in certain situations be adaptive rather than maladaptive. Addiction models mirroring this stance propose that underlying the behavior lies a rational choice to escape from/self-medicate physical or emotional pain, stress and anxiety, concentration/resolve difficulties, angst, or simple boredom. Again, such calculated decisions do not necessarily reflect a fully informed position nor one accurately weighing the relative cost of future consequences against current perceived needs. The etymologic origin of the word rational however stems from the Latin *ratio*, involving a reckoning/calculating, and thus to be true to the language, any decision weighing pros and cons is technically rational, regardless of the scope of information considered or the degree of foresight involved.

The traditional (and general current consensus) viewpoint however is that the unregulated behavior of addiction in general, and in the context of this book, opioid use disorder specifically is irrational. Individual adverse effects abound as discussed in Chap. 3, and addiction almost universally results in harm to the addict's wider psychosocial context as well, including strained family and societal relationships, loss of productivity, and criminal issues. Most consensus definitions of addiction have invariably included compromise of these arenas; the current DSM-5 substance use disorder social impairment category [5] includes:

- Repeatedly unable to carry out major obligations at work, school, or home due to substance use
- Continued use despite persistent or recurring social or interpersonal problems caused or made worse by substance use
- Stopping or reducing important social, occupational, or recreational activities due to substance use

Among its criteria, all are generally deemed irrational by both professional and lay communities. In Dr. Jim Orford's words, addiction "spoils many lives, and often shortens them" [12].

Choice models recognize a continuum of impaired decision-making generally beginning with initial experimentation and frequent underestimation of the addictive potential of the substance in question. At this stage, prior to the development of habit or compulsion, regardless of the latitude of behavioral and biologic philosophy, it is patently difficult to attribute use to anything but choice.

During the reward-seeking phase of addiction, in which ongoing and generally increasing use is reinforced by "positive" but diminishing effect, it is similarly difficult to refute the element of choice without essentially denying the human capacity/function of the will, despite the presence of potentially overwhelming desire and craving. Craving may be simply a matter of unregulated, "excessive appetite" [12] although it is, as alluded to above, an "acquired taste" reinforced by psychological conditioning and neural adaptation [13]. During this period there is a transition from "unstable preferences" [14] in competition with each other to solidification of purpose with ascension of the addictive pursuit to supremacy. The degree to which conflicting desires and ideology exert opposition is as unique as each individual and is based on varying levels of information, worldview and conviction, relevance and potency of competing motives (in many cases "I've got too much to lose" is sufficient disincentive), etc. Numerous neurobiological processes and adaptations are at work during this period as well, as discussed in greater detail later. Regardless of the relative inputs and interface between the biologic/physical and the psychologic/metaphysical, decision-making and choice play a paramount role in indulgence vs. abstinence and in the progression vs. abatement of addiction.

Addiction as Learned Behavior

There is no doubt that conditioning forms an essential part of the addictive process. There is much disagreement (as with most aspects of addiction) as to whether such learning/behavioral habituation represents compulsion or choice. While many regard conditioning as an ever-increasing state of helplessness, it clearly involves reinforcement of volitional behaviors and as such these models are considered under the rubric of addiction as choice in this survey.

Reinforcement of behavior is generally considered to occur as a result of direct pairing of a stimulus with a positive or negative response in the memory of the learner. This instrumental or operant conditioning is at the heart of habit formation and transcends the conscious/unconscious barrier, as evidenced by people lighting up a cigarette without even realizing it. Classical (Pavlovian) conditioning, whereby a secondary stimulus (e.g., Pavlov's bell or a particular setting) becomes associated with the primary stimulus (e.g., meat or drug use), is well known to scientists, clinicians, and lay counselors alike to play a powerful role in addiction development and maintenance. These cues (e.g., "people, places, things" in the Alcoholics Anonymous lingo) often generally operate at the level of the subconscious and may well develop greater motivational power than the substance itself, especially as tolerance to the substance builds. The *incentive sensitization* theory formulated by Robinson and Berridge [15, 16] recognizes a distinction between wanting the substance vs. liking it, especially as time progresses and the reward diminishes, yet desire increases. This increasing "incentive salience" is postulated as underlying the overpowering cravings for the substance that develop despite waning positive reinforcement.

The well-known and consistent phenomenon of progression from a positive reinforcement-/reward-driven state to one of negative reinforcement avoidance involves "macro-level" psychobiological adaptations that presumably occur in concert with "micro-level" conditioning. Neurobiological correlates (and their ever-evolving nature) thought to be associated with this transition are discussed below; from a broader theoretical perspective, the opponent process theory of Solomon and Corbit [17] has been widely adapted to the field of addictionology. In general this theory proposes that highly pleasurable (or unpleasant) experiences generate an antagonistic or opponent response to restore emotional homeostasis; over time, desensitization to the initial stimulus occurs while the strength and duration of the opposing force appears to increase. In the context of addiction, tolerance and/or other mechanisms reduce the positive reinforcement; however, both physical and psychological withdrawal (opponent processes) gain increasing motivational power. Koob and Le Moal added to this general framework with their allostatic theory, postulating that a "chronic deviation of reward threshold" [18] occurs as a result of both decrease in reward sensitivity with repeated exposure and an augmented reactionary hormonal stress response. This altered hedonic threshold drives further drug-seeking not so much to achieve pleasure any longer but rather in an attempt to return to baseline.

Addiction as a Spiritual/Religious Problem

Spiritual/religious models for the most part fall under the (irrational) choice rubric as well. Inherently irrational deviation from an absolute (or even relative) standard of good/right behavior defines this perspective. It is an overly simplistic and ill-informed criticism of spiritual/religious models however to characterize them across the board as pure choice models prescribing improved willpower as the solution to overcoming addictive or other maladaptive behaviors. The widely acclaimed 12-step model introduced by Alcoholics Anonymous in the 1930s begins with the famous "I have a problem" confession (We admitted we were powerless over alcohol—that our lives had become unmanageable [19]) and is much more congruent (as is the quote from St. Paul gracing the Part heading) with an understanding of solidified behavior patterns that have escaped the control of the individual. "Voluntary slavery" as described by Welch [20] describes a potency of compulsion at least equal to that of any biologic model and furthermore carries a more broad theoretical construct invoking the possibility of external control hearkening back to Martin Luther [21], St. Augustine [22], and holy writings centuries older than that.

The defining characteristic of spiritual/religious models is a deviation from right, not just choice. Many of these models recognize (and have helped draw attention to) the progressive loss of control. Key foci also include values and motivation (increasing in popularity both within addiction theory as well as therapeutic approaches). Addiction is often conceptualized in terms of a suboptimal attempt to meet valid needs/fill a void and in some paradigms even an aberrant form of worship [20, 23].

Addiction Theories and Models: Compulsion

As with choice, what comprises compulsion is hazy and fluid. Collins Dictionary of Law [24] defines compulsion as "the forcible inducement to act." In the legal arena, this generally indicates that significant threat to the individual's life or well-being is under exercise by an external source. Such extremis, of course, rarely applies to the realm of psychology and behavioral disorders, and Oxford's "softer" definition [25]—"an irresistible urge to behave in a certain way, especially against one's conscious wishes"—encompasses reasonable pressures exerted upon the psyche by internal forces (not exclusive of external influence).

The underlying thesis of compulsion models is that powerful psychobiological forces drive the addicted (and in some models, even the naïve but genetically predisposed) individual to engage in repetitive and uncontrolled behaviors over which they have lost control, if ever they possessed it.

Introduction to Biologic/Disease Models

The current addictionology landscape is dominated by the viewpoint that addiction is a medical illness caused (or at least explainable) by perturbations of normal cerebral function. While not equivalent concepts, these terms "disease model" and "biologic model" are used jointly/interchangeably throughout this book to refer to the evolving concept that addiction is the result of functional or even structural abnormalities within the brain. Observations regarding the similarity of alcoholism to other known disease states began to find expression in the nineteenth century [26–28], but it was not until the American Medical Association's House of Delegates in 1956 first declared alcoholism an "illness" [29] (subsequently labeling it a "disease" in 1966) that the door opened to a gradual and widespread reconceptualization of addiction among the medical and scientific communities. Supporters of this viewpoint drew attention to the fact that alcoholism exhibits a well-defined pattern of symptoms (and sequelae), with a generally chronic and progressive course, and may be treatable although shows significant vulnerability to relapse. The most notorious proponent of the alcoholism-as-disease theory was E.M. Jellinek, whose landmark treatise "The Disease Concept of Alcoholism" [30] in 1960 is still widely credited with bringing this theory into its current place of prominence. Jellinek's work and even credentials however have fallen into disrepute lately as it appears that much of both were fabricated, and there are allegations that much of his published data were heavily biased and influenced by third party agendas [31–34].

Regardless of the veracity or reliability of Jellinek's work and construct, the disease model's ascension to prominence has facilitated considerable scientific and medical research, shedding light on neurobiologic substrates and genetic expressions that appear to be associated with increased addictive behaviors.

Genetic Models

Some of the earliest evidence suggesting a biologic basis for addiction arose from observations that predisposition (and in extreme cases predetermination) to addiction is heritable. Clustering of behavior patterns within families and apparent preservation of the association despite early overhaul of the environment, e.g., adoption of the offspring by non-addicted parents, led to the hypothesis of a genetic vulnerability to addiction.

The explosive advances in DNA sequencing technology over the past three decades have facilitated the identification of numerous genes associated with substance use disorders and dependence/addiction including the well-studied *DAT1* gene (encoding the dopamine transporter), polymorphisms of which have been linked to numerous pathologic states involving dopaminergism including conditions as diverse as alcoholism, Parkinson's disease, and schizophrenia [35]. Several

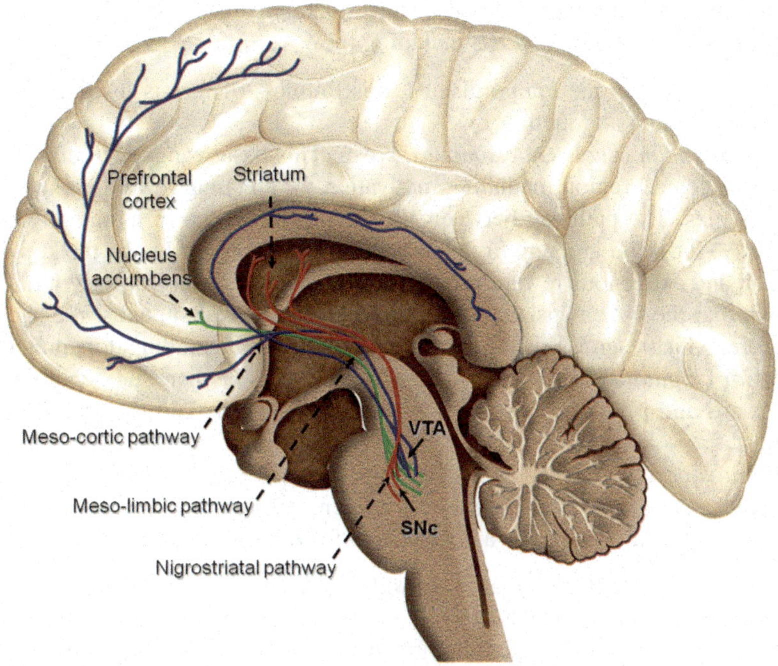

Fig. 9.3 Reward and addiction pathways in the brain. SNc, substantia nigra; VTA, ventral tegmental area. Reprinted from Arias-Carrión O, Stamelou M, Murillo-Rodríguez E, Menéndez-González M, Pöppel E. Dopaminergic reward system: a short integrative review. International Archives of Medicine 2010, 3:24. © Arias-Carrión et al. 2010. http://www.biomedcentral.com/1755-7682/3/24/, CC BY 3.0, https://commons.wikimedia.org/w/index.php?curid=44695433

other allelic variants encoding various dopamine receptor and metabolic function including the *ANKK1* gene *Taq*IA1 variant [LAWF1, MOY1], the *DRD2* gene *rs6277* variant [36], and the *DBH* gene *rs1611115* variant [37] have all been associated with opioid and other substance use disorders.

Numerous covariates exist of course, and given the complexities of the subject, it is entirely conceivable that currently identified (or as of yet undiscovered) candidate biomarkers/genes themselves are confounders. Recent discoveries of exposure-related differential transcription factor activity (e.g., ΔFosB) and epigenetic influences are discussed below (Fig. 9.3).

The Dopamine Theory

As introduced in Chap. 5, the past two decades of addiction neurobiology research suggested a central role for *dopamine (DA)* and dopaminergic neurons within the ventral tegmental area (VTA) of the midbrain. VTA dopaminergic neurons project superiorly along the medial forebrain bundle (nicknamed the "hedonic highway") to various limbic and executive areas including the:

- *Amygdala:* Within the temporal lobe, this limbic structure is involved in emotional processing and memory.
- *Ventral striatum* (*nucleus accumbens*, NAc): This basal ganglia structure is held to be the central region mediating motivation for pursuing rewarding substances or activities. The pathway between VTA and NAc is known as the *mesolimbic pathway* (shown in green in Fig. 9.3) and has long been held to be the key link in natural and exogenous reward/reinforcement and addiction. Recently it has been shown that the NAc consists of two anatomic/functional subunits, the shell and the core, which exercise differing responses to stimuli including dopaminergism.
- *Anterior cingulate cortex:* This paralimbic region is involved in the anticipation of reward and plays a key role in integrating emotions with painful stimuli as well.
- *Prefrontal cortex (PFC):* This "executive center" of the brain is involved in decision-making based on integration of sensory and limbic inputs as well as memory and is thought to be a critical area for reinforcing drug effects.

Until recently, the theory that mesolimbic DA activity is responsible for both hedonic conditioning and also the development of dependence to virtually all addictive substances/pleasurable activities [38–40] has reigned unchallenged within the neuropsychiatric arena, and highlights of its development are presented herein. This common dopaminergic pathway has been implicated in the development of addiction to substances with activities as divergent as the profound stimulants cocaine and methamphetamines as well as sedative/depressant drugs such as alcohol, benzodiazepines and barbiturates, and opioids. The former have been thought to induce reward primarily by direct increases (induced release or reuptake inhibition) within the NAc, with the latter exerting an indirect effect via depression of VTA gamma amino butyric acid (GABA)-mediated inhibition of NAc dopaminergism [41, 42].

Intracerebral administration of DA agonists in rodent models results in reward-seeking behavior including self-administration and conditioned place preference [43–46]. Conversely, cerebral (or systemic) DA antagonism in multiple species including humans results in aversive behaviors [47–49]. As discussed in Chap. 5, evidence for the centrality of the VTA in opioid dependence specifically is also both positive (intra-VTA opioid administration induces reward-seeking behaviors in rodents [50–53]) and negative (intra-VTA opioid antagonists or genetic MOR knockout results in loss of these behaviors [54, 55]).

Beyond simply mediating reward, dopaminergic activity has been postulated to underlie incentive salience and the development of cravings, conditioning, motivational changes, impaired control/inhibition, and tolerance [56]. The phenomenon of classic conditioning has been linked to increased activity of DA in the striatum (as well as cortical circuits associated with motivation and executive function) in response to the conditioned stimulus (cue) also. Interestingly, in addicted (human) subjects compared to controls, increases in DA as well as subjective reward are significantly reduced with exposure to the drug but significantly increased with exposure to cues, beyond the original response to the unconditioned stimulus [56]. This apparent decreasing reward to the original addictive substance in the face of increased incentive salience attributed to the cue may underlie an increasingly unsatisfying yet frantic pursuit of the drug. This amplification of salience attribution to anticipation may in effect reflect "addiction to the addiction." A central role in motivational phenomena has also been attributed to DA, with evidence of complex dopaminergic interactions between several target regions, including NAc and the anterior cingulate, orbitofrontal and dorsolateral prefrontal cortices, as well as the amygdala, dorsal striatum, and ventral pallidum [56, 57].

The NAc itself has recently been shown to consist of two distinct anatomic regions (shell and core) which appear to be differentially and complementarily engaged in the reward circuit and motivational input. As of yet the complex individual and joint functions of the structure are not well understood, but it appears that the shell mediates value assignment/reward quantification to pleasurable stimuli, whereas the core is more involved with goal-directed memory and learning/conditioning and also "computational" motivation and decision-making with regard to the pursuit of those stimuli [58, 59].

Chronic exposure to drugs of abuse appears to confer decreased DA receptor density (especially the D2 receptor, DRD2) within the striatum [56, 60, 61] which in turn appears to be associated with decreased DA activity within the cortical regions [62–66]. It has been proposed that these widespread alterations collectively result in compromise of inhibitory control/emotion regulation and decision-making and loss of control. In addition, this reduced dopaminergism in the tolerant/dependent state appears to confer diminishing substance-related reward as well as decreased sensitivity to pleasurable stimuli overall [67–69] (congruent with the concept of altered hedonic threshold) and may explain in part the general lassitude to normal motivations/goals observed in addicts. Besides these perturbations in "positive"/reward mechanisms, "negative" adaptations involving apparent sensitization to stress, at least that associated with withdrawal may be mediated in part by attenuated DA responsiveness throughout the system [70, 71]. Analogous to (and conceivably even linked with) the distinct phenomena of tolerance and opioid-induced hyperalgesia, these dual adaptations parallel and may underlie the shift from pleasure-seeking to withdrawal avoidance.

Rethinking Dopamine

However, several recent lines of evidence indicate that there is far more to the neurobiologic picture than dopamine simply burning the imprint of pleasure/salience onto the psyche/neural network. To quote Wanat [72], "the dopamine system is associated with a diverse array of natural and appetitive behaviors… [and] likely subserves various functions depending upon the anatomical location, context, and duration of its release." While almost certainly serving as "oil in the machine" of addiction (to quote Koob quoting Fibiger [73]), dopamine's role in learning and behavioral reinforcement is exceedingly complex, and the literature bears witness to the ever-changing understanding of the interactions between (and even functions of) different brain regions.

Not all NAc dopaminergism is rewarding; several agents (delta-opioid receptor agonists, cholecystokinin, glial-derived neurotrophic factor) increase DA in the NAc but do not result in reward-seeking behavior [74], and furthermore even the administration of MOR antagonists sufficient to cause aversive behaviors also results in NAc DA increases [75, 76]. There is also indication that opioid reinforcement can occur in the absence of mesolimbic dopaminergism [77–80]. Interestingly, dopaminergic neuronal activity in response to MOR agonism has been shown to increase in anesthetized animals but decrease in awake animals [74]. Similarly, MOR-mediated inhibition of reward-seeking by DA antagonism has been shown in opioid-dependent rodents, whereas opioid-naïve animals do not lose these behaviors [81]. In addition, stimulation of VTA dopaminergic neurons has been shown to also result in release of other neurotransmitters including glutamate and GABA [82–84].

Recent research has focused on differences between phasic versus tonic dopamine release, with fair evidence linking the former to incentive salience and reinforcement learning, and alterations of the latter somehow involved in modulating response [72, 85].

The counterintuitive recent discoveries of decreased striatal dopamine receptor density and release in addicts [56, 60, 61, 86] have led to speculation (in the absence of longitudinal data) that perhaps these perturbations were present a priori and represent a predisposing vulnerability rather than a cumulative drug effect [86].

Epigenetic activity likely plays a critical role as well, and while numerous molecules have been shown to alter relevant gene expression, the *ΔFosB* variant transcription factor has received the most attention as a potential key player in the development of addiction. This truncated moiety accumulates in various brain regions including the NAc and frontal cortical regions in the context of chronic drug use (and other repetitive pleasurable pursuits) and persists for weeks to months [87, 88]. Numerous drugs including amphetamines and methamphetamine, cocaine, ethanol, nicotine, opioids, and D9-tetrahydrocannabinol have all been shown to result in an increase in ΔFosB [88]. Animal subjects that express higher levels of this variant show increased substance pursuit and drug effects, and it has been proposed that ΔFosB acts as a "molecular switch" in the development and maintenance of addiction [89, 90].

It bears mention that virtually all of the data associating ΔFosB have been provided by murine models, and thus extrapolation to human neurobiology is just that. Furthermore, as discussed previously, whether these "biomarker" alterations represent etiologic mechanisms or merely indicators of other, yet undiscovered, processes remains unclear. Nonetheless, our rapidly increasing understanding of how environmental factors affect and even regulate genetic expression should serve to remind all parties to the discussion of addiction that the old adage "nature and nurture" likely holds true at every level of human experience.

Limitations of Biology

The biologic/disease model is perhaps in the best position to explain some if not all of the neuropsychiatric phenomena associated with addiction, such as euphoria, withdrawal, and the shift from a positive reinforcement/reward pursuit to the avoidance of negative reinforcement/withdrawal once dependence is established. It has provided indisputable objective insights into the physical components of the pathophysiology of addiction. It also provides the best reproducible/demonstrable explanation to date for clustering of addiction within families.

Association does not equal causality, however; while invaluable, the conceptual provenience of the model remains unproven. The presence of statistically significant increases in neurotransmitter activity or functional imaging signal changes among addicted individuals does not substantiate mechanism.

The main limitation of the biologic/disease model (or perhaps more accurately the current wholesale capitulation of the medical community to it) is its effective monism. *Homo sapiens* is certainly on the one hand a physical creature subject to physiologic processes and whose perceptions and cognition/emotion are certainly intertwined with the material. Compartmentalization of human thought, emotion, behavior, etc. to the realm of the corporeal however is absurdly reductionist and in contrast/conflict with the greater wisdom and thought process of intellectual and scholarly disciplines throughout all cultures and time periods. The discipline of psychiatry has come under internal criticism lately [91–97] for gravitating toward an exclusively neurobiologic paradigm, i.e., one that proposes that cognitive and emotional processes are nothing more than neurotransmitter activity and psychopathology comprises "brain disorders" (without acknowledging existential mind, heart, soul, and spirit). This physicalist retreat from a dualistic mind-body philosophy is likely due in part to numerous pressures upon the discipline including perceived need for comparative objective validation and a sense of legitimacy within the increasingly technologically driven medical world, economic/reimbursement trends which favor "medical" diagnoses, and pharmaceutical industry influence [98–102].

This trend toward reductive physicalism ironically has occurred during a period of renaissance of awareness of the immaterial within medicine and the biologic sciences. Just as the gate theory and subsequent development of biopsychosocial-spiritual pain models have superseded the simple Cartesian stimulus-perception pain construct (as discussed in Chap. 6), it is clear that a more comprehensive framework acknowledging the nonquantifiable complexities of human behavior is required.

The most obvious criticism leveled against the addiction-as-disease paradigm is that it minimizes or even eliminates the role of the will and characterizes the addicted individual as merely a victim of DNA or neurotransmitters. It has in essence supplanted the concept of addiction as something that people do with the notion of addiction as something that happens to people [103]. To be fair, many of the thought leaders propounding the model acknowledge uncertainty as to the primacy of illness characteristics and observations and biomarkers. Edwards and Gross, who contributed a foundational medical overview of the disease model in 1976, did admit in their now classic paper, "It is unclear… whether the experience is truly one of losing control rather than one of deciding not to exercise control" [104].

The disease model has also been impugned from a sociologic standpoint. Besides absolution of responsibility for the addicted individual, its determinism may also mislead other involved parties such as family members who can blame their loved ones' problem on a physiologic illness rather than psychopathology or potential relational dysfunction, etc. It has also been criticized for providing a "politically safe" paradigm for policymakers to direct attention and efforts while avoiding passing moral judgments, and an unassailable harbor for the medical addictionology community to justify its research, therapeutic approaches, and even existence.

Addiction Theories and Models: Social Systems

Numerous sociologic theories addressing addiction exist, and as might be expected, many display a scope of theory and analysis far beyond the limitations of this work; the reader is referred to the excellent review by Adrian [105] for a sweeping survey. The discipline provides both individual and population-level insights into the process of addiction, and as such holds significant clinical and epidemiologic relevance, with a proven track record of utility in the arena of rehabilitation, and an even greater potential for preventive benefit.

Relationships and Substance Abuse

Substance abuse and addiction are behaviors that develop and persist for the most part in the context of personal interaction of some form or another. Modeling of use is almost invariably present and contributory to the initiation and maintenance of use; while genetic predisposition appears to be gaining credibility and certainly enjoys widespread support, the influence of parental, sibling, and peer example is not to be dismissed. Bandura's seminal work on social learning [106, 107] has provided foundational understanding of how behaviors, especially deviant ones, are "transmitted."

The individual's social context is also invariably involved to some extent to motivation for use. While plasticity of the young brain is proposed by proponents of the biologic model to account for the apparent greater vulnerability of this demographic [108, 109], the profound social acceptance pressures of the peri-adolescent period are incontrovertible to anyone who has survived secondary education and college. The increasing stressors of normal adult life form an assumed rationale for various "self-medication" strategies taken for granted by most patients and need to be assessed by the prescriber as part of every evaluation as discussed in Chaps. 6 and 8. Strained, dysfunctional and all too often abusive relationships may confer tremendous impetus to seek relief from psychological, emotional, and in some cases physical suffering.

The addict's world changes in many ways, with a replacement of former relationships and circles by a new society of drug suppliers and users. Besides reinforcement, these "people, places, things" comprise potent triggers for relapse as every Alcoholics Anonymous or Narcotic Anonymous member will attest to.

The advent of the internet and instant wireless communication has opened up new sociologic dimensions pertinent to substance misuse and abuse, including universally available information, and increased availability of substances (particularly prescription drugs [110, 111]). Multiple surveys suggest that approximately 3% of prescription drug abusers purchased their medications online, and a recent interesting study showed that for every 10% increase in high-speed internet use at the state level, associated treatment facility admissions for prescription drug abuse rose by 1% [111]. The development of online communities and "social networking" has been criticized for both creating and filling voids of traditional interpersonal relationships and communities which may encourage substance misuse and abuse; specific drug-related forums and sites abound and undoubtedly present a source of reinforcement and identity.

The Subculture of Substance Abuse

While substance use and abuse have existed to varying degrees among different population elements in societies around the world for millennia, the twentieth and twenty-first centuries have seen what is likely the historically unique development of a drug subculture within the West primarily. One of the more intriguing perspectives on this twentieth and twenty-first century phenomenon came from the Chicago School of Sociology in the 1960s; among many of the unorthodox theories arising from there was the thesis that deviancy from social norms arises directly as a reactionary result of the label applied [112] not unlike a self-fulfilling prophecy or a curse (although such value judgments were not proposed). More recent work from Britain primarily has focused on the "normalization" of substance abuse within youth culture [113, 114] and the observation that postindustrial leisure and consumerism have fostered a "new economy" of hedonistic experimentation and pursuits [115–118]. By way of contrast, societies that place high value upon productivity (as well as greater adherence to social norms) such as Japan demonstrate a markedly reduced prevalence of drug abuse [119].

Motivational Theory and Addiction

No consideration of substance abuse and addiction would be complete without the acknowledgment that regardless of the relative contributions of biology, choice, learning/conditioning, and other societal factors, understanding of underlying motivation is essential to understanding addiction and to preventive and rehabilitative efforts. Motivation is defined as the process that initiates, guides, and maintains goal-oriented behaviors [120].

Philosophers and psychologists will likely always debate the nature of and overlap between motivation and will; one analogy is that will is the machine that moves the individual and motivation is the fuel that fires the machine. Suffice it to say they are distinct but intertwined and generally subject to competing desires and goals within the addict or any human being. West's PRIME theory of motivation [10], represented graphically and in summary table below, provides an excellent framework within which to consider the complex interactions between the "unstable preferences" and conflicting motives that form the dynamic world of the individual struggling with addiction (Fig. 9.4).

As Dr. West laments, "When giving a psychological account of motivation, it is impossible to avoid making statements that sound just like common sense" [10]. Similarly, discussion of the central role of the will—not neurobiologic impulses and drives—in addiction is generally regarded as passe at best (and often met with a reactionary disdain) by those who champion pure biologic compulsion.

While having largely fallen out of favor over the past half century, basic psychoanalytic constructs provide a useful and familiar platform from which to consider some of the basic "commonsense" issues involved. Freud's id vs. superego tension accurately describes the conflicting elements of self-gratification vs. alignment with external mores. The will's exercise of self-control, while not equivalent in depth psychology to the ego, may be considered in a similar governance role over primal urges. It seems a fascinating commonsense observation that abstinence, advocated by proponents of the disease and biologic models, is a choice executed by the will.

Summary

The prevalence of opioid use disorder (OUD) continues to increase, and at the heart of this epidemic lies the hosts' loss of control. Success in reversing the crisis will require cultivation of "resistance" to misuse and abuse vulnerability analogous to immunity within a host population. The grim statistics on relapse bear witness to the power of both initial hedonic motivation and the subsequent inevitable withdrawal avoidance drive. Whether choice or compulsion mediates the development and maintenance of OUD comprises the main philosophical watershed whereby most addiction theories may be categorized, with the currently popular biologic/disease model leaning strongly toward the latter pole. Moral and spiritual, biologic/disease, learned behavior, and social models have all yielded valuable contributions into our understanding of the complex behavioral disorder, that is, substance abuse; social models provide population-level insights that are highly relevant to a public health perspective.

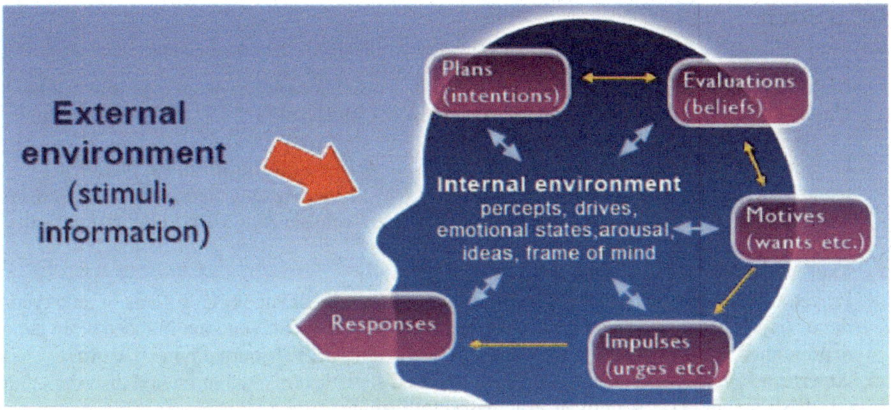

Key Propositions from PRIME Theory (Summarized)

1. At every moment we act in pursuit of what we most desire.
2. Wants and needs involved imagined futures and associated feelings of anticipated pleasure/satisfaction or relief from mental or physical discomfort.
3. Beliefs only influence actions if they generate desires that are strong enough to overwhelm those arising from other sources (e.g., drives and emotions) or impulses and inhibitions rising automatically out of learned or unlearned associations.
4. Plans provide overarching structure to our actions but in order to direct our behavior, they need to be recalled and generate desires at relevant moments that are sufficiently powerful to overcome desires and impulses arising from other sources.
5. The motivational system can be characterized in terms of dispositions for its components to respond in particular ways to internal and external inputs. Processes that lead to changes in dispositions include associative learning, habituation, sensitization, direct imitation, analysis and inference.
6. Identity is an important source of desires and provides a degree of stability to our behavior.
7. Identity change is a starting point for deliberate behavior change.
8. Deliberate behavior change is sustained when desires arising from the new identity are stronger at each relevant moment than the desires arising from other sources to revert to the previous behavior pattern, or are able to overwhelm habitual or instinctive impulses.
9. When identity change results from self-conscious beliefs about what is good and bad, maintaining behavior change requires 'self-control': the effortful generation of desire to adhere to a rule that is sufficiently powerful to overcome desires arising from other sources.
10. Personal rules that have clear boundaries and a strong connection with components of identity that involve strong emotional attachments will generate more powerful desires when required and better suppress countervailing desires and so have a stronger lasting impact on behavior.

Fig. 9.4 Dr. Robert West's PRIME theory of motivation. Reprinted from http://www.primetheory.com/summary-prime-motivation.php, with permission from Dr. West

References

1. Rudd RA, Seth P, David F, Scholl L. Increases in drug and opioid-involved overdose deaths—United States, 2010–2015. MMWR. 2016;65(50-51):1445–52. doi:10.15585/mmwr.mm655051e1.
2. Executive Office of the President, Office of National Drug Control Policy. National Drug Control Budget: FY 2017 Funding Highlights. Washington, DC, February 2016. https://www.whitehouse.gov/sites/default/files/ondcp/press-releases/fy_2017_budget_highlights.pdf. Accessed 26 Dec 2016.
3. Thomas Sydenham, Observationes medicae, 1676.
4. Pravetoni M, Pentel PR, Potter DN, Chartoff EH, Tally L, LeSage MG. Effects of an oxycodone conjugate vaccine on oxycodone self-administration and oxycodone-induced brain gene expression in rats. PLoS One. 2014;9(7):e101807. doi:10.1371/journal.pone.0101807.
5. American Psychiatric Association. Diagnostic and statistical manual of mental disorders. 5th ed. Washington, D.C.: American Psychiatric Publishing; 2013.
6. Weissman DE, Haddox JD. Opioid pseudoaddiction-an iatrogenic syndrome. Pain. 1989;36:363–6.
7. Greene MS, Chambers RA. Pseudoaddiction: fact or fiction? An investigation of the medical literature. Curr Addict Rep. 2015;2:310–7.
8. Passik SD, Kirsh KL, Webster L. Pseudoaddiction revisited: a commentary on clinical and historical considerations. Pain Manag. 2011;1:239–48.
9. Bell K, Salmon A. Pain, physical dependence and pseudoaddiction: redefining addiction for 'nice' people? Int J Drug Policy. 2009;20:170–8.
10. West RJ, Brown J. Theory of addiction. 2nd ed. West Sussex, UK: Wiley Blackwell Addiction Press; 2013.
11. Center for Behavioral Health Statistics and Quality. (2015). Behavioral health trends in the United States: results from the 2014 National survey on drug use and health (HHS Publication No. SMA 15-4927, 11 Series H-50). Retrieved from http://www.samhsa.gov/data/
12. Orford J. Addiction as excessive appetite. Addiction. 2001;96:15–31.
13. Drummond DC. Theories of drug craving, ancient and modern. Addiction. 2001;96:33–46.
14. Skog OJ. Addicts' choice. Addiction. 2000;95:1309–14.
15. Robinson TE, Berridge KC. The neural basis of drug craving: an incentive-sensitization theory of addiction. Brain Res Brain Res Rev. 1993;18:247–91.
16. Berridge KC, Robinson TE. Liking, wanting, and the incentive-sensitization theory of addiction. Am Psychol. 2016;71:670–9.
17. Solomon RL, Corbit JD. An opponent-process theory of motivation. Am Econ Rev. 1978;68:12–24.
18. Koob GF, Le Moal M. Drug addiction, dysregulation of reward, and allostasis. Neuropsychopharmacology. 2001;24:97–129.
19. Alcoholics Anonymous. Alcoholics anonymous. 1st ed. New York: Works Publishing Company; 1939.
20. Welch ET. Addictions: a banquet in the grave. Phillipsburg, NJ: P&R Publishing Company; 2001.
21. Luther M. The bondage of the will, translated by Packer JI, Johnston OR. Revell: Westwood, NJ; 1957.
22. Saint Augustine. The confessions, vol. 8., translated by Burton P. New York: Everyman's Library; 2001.
23. Shaw M. The heart of addiction: a biblical perspective. Bemidji, MN: Focus Publishing; 2008.
24. Stewart WJ. Compulsion. In: Collins dictionary of law. 3rd ed. Glasgow: Collins; n.d. p. 2006. Retrieved 30 Dec 2016 from: http://legal-dictionary.thefreedictionary.com/compulsion.
25. Oxford Dictionaries Online. Compulsion. Oxford: Oxford University Press; 2016. Retrieved 30 Dec 2016 from: https://en.oxforddictionaries.com

26. Trotter T. An essay, medical, philosophical, and chemical, on drunkenness and its effects on the human body. London: Printed for T.N. Longman, and O. Rees; 1804.
27. Rush B. An inquiry into the effects of ardent spirits upon the human body and mind: with an account of the means of preventing, and of the remedies for curing them. Philadelphia: Thomas Dobson; 1808.
28. Huss M. Alcoholismus chronicus. Stockholm: 1852.
29. Niven RG. Alcoholism—a problem in perspective. JAMA. 1984;252:1912–4.
30. Jellinek EM. The disease concept of alcoholism. New Haven: Hillhouse; 1960.
31. Peele S. Jellinek was a cheat! The stanton peele addiction website. http://www.peele.net/lib/jellinek.html. Accessed 31 Dec 2016.
32. Roizen REM. Jellinek and all that! A brief look back at the origins of post-repeal alcohol science in the United States. Nordisk alkohol narkotikatidskrift. 2000;17:355–66.
33. Baldwin Research Institute. Alcoholism is not a disease. http://www.baldwinresearch.com/alcoholism.cfm. Accessed 31 Dec 2016..
34. Greenberg G. The creation of disease. The New Yorker, 30 Apr 2013.
35. Patriquin MA, Bauer IE, Soares JC, Graham DP, Nielsen DA. Addiction pharmacogenetics: a systematic review of the genetic variation of the dopaminergic system. Psychiatr Genet. 2015;25:181–93.
36. Doehring A, Hentig N, Graff J, Salamat S, Schmidt M, Geisslinger G, Harder S, Lotsch J. Genetic variants altering dopamine D2 receptor expression or function modulate the risk of opiate addiction and the dosage requirements of methadone substitution. Pharmacogenet Genomics. 2009;19:407–14.
37. Xie X, Xu L, Liu H, Chen W, Zhuang D, Zhang J, Duan S, Zhou W. Positive association between--1021TT genotype of dopamine beta hydroxylase gene and progressive behavior of injection heroin users. Neurosci Lett. 2013;541:258–62.
38. Wise RA, Bozarth MA. Brain mechanisms of drug reward and euphoria. Psychiatr Med. 1985;3:445–60.
39. Koob GF, Bloom FE. Cellular and molecular mechanisms of drug dependence. Science. 1988;242:715–23.
40. Volkow ND, Fowler JS, Wang GJ, Swanson JM, Telang F. Dopamine in drug abuse and addiction: results of imaging studies and treatment implications. Arch Neurol. 2007;64:1575–9.
41. Johnson SW, North RA. Opioids excite dopamine neurons by hyperpolarization of local interneurons. J Neurosci. 1992;12:483–8.
42. Bourdy R, Barrot M. A new control center for dopaminergic systems: pulling the VTA by the tail. Trends Neurosci. 2012;35:681–90.
43. Wise RA, Gardner EL. Functional anatomy of substance-related disorders. In: D'haenen H, den Boer JA, Willner P, editors. Biological psychiatry. New York: Wiley; 2002. p. 509–22.
44. Corbett D, Wise RA. Intracranial self-stimulation in relation to the ascending dopaminergic systems of the midbrain: a moveable electrode mapping study. Brain Res. 1980;185:1–15.
45. Wise RA, Bozarth MA. Action of drugs of abuse on brain reward systems: an update with specific attention to opiates. Pharmacol Biochem Behav. 1982;17:239–43.
46. Bozarth MA, Wise RA. Neural substrates of opiate reinforcement. Prog Neuro-Psychopharmacol Biol Psychiatry. 1983;7(4-6):569–75.
47. Gardner EL. Introduction: addiction and brain reward and anti-reward pathways. Adv Psychosom Med. 2011;30:22–60.
48. Schechter MD, Meechan SM. Conditioned place aversion produced by dopamine release inhibition. Eur J Pharmacol. 1994;260:133–7.
49. Shippenberg TS, Bals-Kubik R, Huber A, Herz A. Neuroanatomical substrates mediating the aversive effects of D-1dopamine receptor antagonists. Psychopharmacology. 1991;103:209–14.
50. Wise RA. Opiate reward: sites and substrates. Neurosci Biobehav Rev. 1989;13:129–33.
51. McBride WJ, Murphy JM, Ikemoto S. Localization of brain reinforcement mechanisms: intracranial self-administration and intracranial place-conditioning studies. Behav Brain Res. 1999;101:129–52.

52. Bozarth MA, Wise RA. Intracranial self-administration of morphine into the ventral tegmental area in rats. Life Sci. 1981;28:551–5.
53. Zangen A, Ikemoto S, Zadina JE, Wise RA. Rewarding and psychomotor stimulant effects of endomorphin-1: anteroposterior differences within the ventral tegmental area and lack of effect in nucleus accumbens. J Neurosci. 2002;22:7225–33.
54. Olmstead MC, Franklin KB. The development of a conditioned place preference to morphine: effects of microinjections into various CNS sites. Behav Neurosci. 1997;111:1324–34.
55. Zhang Y, Landthaler M, Schlussman SD, Yuferov V, Ho A, Tuschl T, et al. Mu opioid receptor knockdown in the substantia nigra/ventral tegmental area by synthetic small interfering RNA blocks the rewarding and locomotor effects of heroin. Neuroscience. 2009;158:474–83.
56. Volkow ND, Wang G-J, Fowler JS, Tomasi D, Telang F. Addiction: beyond dopamine reward circuitry. PNAS. 2011;108:15037–42.
57. Salamone JD, Correa M, Farrar A, Mingote SM. Effort-related functions of nucleus accumbens dopamine and associated forebrain circuits. Psychopharmacology. 2007;191:461–82.
58. Espana RA, Jones SR. Presynaptic dopamine modulation by stimulant self-administration. Front Biosci. 2013;5:261–76.
59. Saddoris MP, Sugam JA, Cacciapaglia F, Carelli RM. Rapid dopamine dynamics in the accumbens core and shell: learning and action. Front Biosci. 2013;5:273–88.
60. Volkow ND, Wang GJ, Fowler JS, Logan J, Hitzemann R, Ding YS, et al. Decreases in dopamine receptors but not in dopamine transporters in alcoholics. Alcohol Clin Exp Res. 1996;20:1594–8.
61. Wang GJ, Volkow ND, Fowler JS, Logan J, Abumrad NN, Hitzemann RJ, et al. Dopamine D2 receptor availability in opiate-dependent subjects before and after naloxone-precipitated withdrawal. Neuropsychopharmacology. 1997;16:174–82.
62. Volkow ND, Fowler JS, Wang GJ, Hitzemann R, Logan J, Schlyer DJ, et al. Decreased dopamine D2 receptor availability is associated with reduced frontal metabolism in cocaine abusers. Synapse. 1993;14:169–77.
63. Volkow ND, Chang L, Wang GJ, Fowler JS, Ding YS, Sedler M, et al. Low level of brain dopamine D2 receptors in methamphetamine abusers: association with metabolism in the orbitofrontal cortex. Am J Psychiatry. 2001;158:2015–21.
64. Volkow ND, Wang GJ, Telang F, Fowler JS, Logan J, Jayne M, et al. Profound decreases in dopamine release in striatum in detoxified alcoholics: possible orbitofrontal involvement. J Neurosci. 2007;27:12700–6.
65. Volkow ND, Fowler JS. Addiction, a disease of compulsion and drive: involvement of the orbitofrontal cortex. Cereb Cortex. 2000;10:318–25.
66. Goldstein RZ, Volkow ND. Drug addiction and its underlying neurobiological basis: neuroimaging evidence for the involvement of the frontal cortex. Am J Psychiatry. 2000;159:1642–52.
67. Hägele C, Schlagenhauf F, Rapp M, Sterzer P, Beck A, Bermpohl F, et al. Dimensional psychiatry: reward dysfunction and depressive mood across psychiatric disorders. Psychopharmacology. 2015;232:331–41.
68. Hyatt CJ, Assaf M, Muska CE, Rosen RI, Thomas AD, Johnson MR, et al. Reward-related dorsal striatal activity differences between former and current cocaine dependent individuals during an interactive competitive game. PLoS One. 2012;7(5):e34917.
69. Konova AB, Moeller SJ, Tomasi D, Parvaz MA, Alia-Klein N, Volkow ND, et al. Structural and behavioral correlates of abnormal encoding of money value in the sensorimotor striatum in cocaine addiction. Eur J Neurosci. 2012;36:2979–88.
70. Koob GF, Le Moal M. Plasticity of reward neurocircuitry and the 'dark side' of drug addiction. Nat Neurosci. 2005;8:1442–4.
71. Kaufling J, Aston-Jones G. Persistent adaptations in afferents to ventral tegmental dopamine neurons after opiate withdrawal. J Neurosci. 2015;35:10290–303.
72. Wanat MJ, Willuhn I, Clark JJ, Phillips PEM. Phasic dopamine release in appetitive behaviors and drug abuse. Curr Drug Abuse Rev. 2009;2:195–213.
73. Wise RA, Koob GF. The development and maintenance of drug addiction. Neuropsychopharmacology. 2014;39:254–62.

74. Fields HL, Margolis EB. Understanding opioid reward. Trends Neurosci. 2015;38:217–25.
75. Devine DP, Leone P, Wise RA. Mesolimbic dopamine neurotransmission is increased by administration of mu-opioid receptor antagonists. Eur J Pharmacol. 1993;243:55–64.
76. Shippenberg TS, Bals-Kubik R. Involvement of the mesolimbic dopamine system in mediating the aversive effects of opioid antagonists in the rat. Behav Pharmacol. 1995;6:99–106.
77. Bechara A, van der Kooy D. A single brain stem substrate mediates the motivational effects of both opiates and food in nondeprived rats but not in deprived rats. Behav Neurosci. 1992;106:351–63.
78. Olmstead MC, Munn EM, Franklin KB, Wise RA. Effects of pedunculopontine tegmental nucleus lesions on responding for intravenous heroin under different schedules of reinforcement. J Neurosci. 1998;18:5035–44.
79. Laviolette SR, Gallegos RA, Henriksen SJ, van der Kooy D. Opiate state controls bi-directional reward signaling via $GABA_A$ receptors in the ventral tegmental area. Nat Neurosci. 2004;7:160–9.
80. Hnasko TS, Sotak BN, Palmiter RD. Morphine reward in dopamine-deficient mice. Nature. 2005;438:854–7.
81. Nader K, van der Kooy D. Deprivation state switches the neurobiological substrates mediating opiate reward in the ventral tegmental area. J Neurosci. 1997;17:383–90.
82. Tecuapetla F, Patel JC, Xenias H, English D, Tadros I, Shah F, et al. Glutamatergic signaling by mesolimbic dopamine neurons in the nucleus accumbens. J Neurosci. 2010;30:7105–10.
83. Gorelova N, Mulholland PJ, Chandler LJ, Seamans JK. The glutamatergic component of the mesocortical pathway emanating from different subregions of the ventral midbrain. Cereb Cortex. 2012;22:327–36.
84. Root DH, Mejias-Aponte CA, Zhang S, Wang HL, Hoffman AF, Lupica CR, et al. Single rodent mesohabenular axons release glutamate and GABA. Nat Neurosci. 2014;17:1543–51.
85. Grace AA. The tonic/phasic model of dopamine system regulation and its implications for understanding alcohol and psychostimulant craving. Addiction. 2000;95(Suppl 2):S119–28.
86. Nutt DJ, Lingford-Hughes A, Erritzoe D, Stokes PR. The dopamine theory of addiction: 40 years of highs and lows. Nat Rev Neurosci. 2015;16:305–12.
87. Jorissen HJ, Ulery PG, Henry L, Gourneni S, Nestler EJ, Rudenko G. Dimerization and DNA-binding properties of the transcription factor DeltaFosB. Biochemistry. 2007;46:8360–72.
88. Ruffle JK. Molecular neurobiology of addiction: what's all the (Δ)FosB about? Am J Drug Alc Abuse. 2014;40:428–37.
89. Nestler EJ, Barrot M, Self DW. DeltaFosB: a sustained molecular switch for addiction. PNAS. 2001;98:11042–6.
90. Robison AJ, Nestler EJ. Transcriptional and epigenetic mechanisms of addiction. Nat Rev Neurosci. 2011;12:623–37.
91. Pam A. Biological psychiatry: science or pseudoscience?. In Ross C, Pam A. Pseudoscience in biological psychiatry: blaming the body. New York: Wiley & Sons; 1995.
92. Brendel DH. Philosophy of mind in the clinic: the relation between causal and meaningful explanation in psychiatry. Harv Rev Psychiat. 2000;8:184–91.
93. Bracken P, Thomas P. Postpsychiatry: a new direction for mental health. BMJ. 2001;322:724–7.
94. Kendler KS. A psychiatric dialogue on the mind-body problem. Am J Psychiatry. 2001;158:989–1000.
95. Kendler KS. Toward a philosophical structure for psychiatry. Am J Psychiatry. 2005;162:433–40.
96. Walter H. The third wave of biological psychiatry. Front Psychol. 2013;4:582.
97. Stier M. Normative preconditions for the assessment of mental disorder. Front Psychol. 2013;4:611.
98. Sharfstein SS. Big pharma and American psychiatry: the good, the bad, and the ugly. Psychiatr News. 2005;40:3.
99. Zipkin DA, Steinman MA. Interactions between pharmaceutical representatives and doctors in training: a thematic review. J Gen Intern Med. 2005;20:777–86.

100. Lacasse JR, Leo J. Serotonin and depression: a disconnect between the advertisements and the scientific literature. PLoS Med. 2005;2(12):e392. doi:10.1371/journal.pmed.0020392.
101. Nys TR, Nys MG. Psychiatry under pressure: reflections on psychiatry's drift towards a reductionist biomedical conception of mental illness. Med Health Care Philos. 2006;9:107–15.
102. Whitaker R, Cosgrove L. Psychiatry under the influence. New York: Palgrave Macmillan; 2015.
103. Davies J. The myth of addiction. Amsterdam: Harwood Academic Publishers; 1997.
104. Edwards G, Gross MM. Alcohol dependence: provisional description of a clinical syndrome. Br Med J. 1976;1:1058–61.
105. Adrian M. How can sociological theory help our understanding of addictions? Subst Use Misuse. 2003;38(10):1385–423.
106. Bandura A. Social learning and personality development. New York: Holt, Rinehart, and Winston; 1963.
107. Bandura A. Social learning theory. Oxford, England: Prentice-Hall; 1977.
108. Spear LP. The adolescent brain and age-related behavioral manifestations. Neurosci Biobehav Rev. 2000;24:417–63.
109. Volkow ND, Li TK. Drugs and alcohol: treating and preventing abuse, addiction and their medical consequences. Pharmacol Ther. 2005;108:3–17.
110. Forman RF, Marlowe DB, McLellan AT. The internet as a source of drugs of abuse. Curr Psychiatr Rep. 2006;8:377–82.
111. Jena AB, Goldman DP. The United States growing internet use may help explain the rise in prescription drug abuse. Health Aff. 2011;30:1192–9.
112. Becker HS. Outsiders: studies in the sociology of deviance. New York: Macmillan; 1963.
113. Parker H, Williams L, Aldridge J. The normalization of sensible recreational drug use: further evidence from the north West England longitudinal study. Sociology. 2002;36:941–64.
114. Measham F, Shiner M. The legacy of 'normalisation': the role of classical and contemporary criminological theory in understanding young people's drug use. Int J Drug Policy. 2009;20:502–8.
115. Parker H, Aldridge J, Measham F. Illicit leisure: the normalization of adolescent recreational drug use. London: Routledge; 1998.
116. Young J. The exclusive society: social exclusion, crime and difference in late modernity. London: Sage; 1999.
117. Rojek C. Leisure and culture. Basingstoke: Macmillan; 2000.
118. Gershuny J. Changing times: work and leisure in post-industrial society. Oxford: Oxford University Press; 2000.
119. Greberman SB, Wada K. Social and legal factors related to drug abuse in the United States and Japan. Public Health Rep. 1994;109:731–7.
120. Nevid J. Psychology: concepts and applications. Wadworth: Belmont, CA; 2013.

Chapter 10
Opioid Dependence Risk Factors and Risk Assessment

While staffing a local urgent care clinic on a Friday evening, you encounter a 46-year-old female who presents mild apparent distress, reporting that she has just moved to town following a "really bad divorce." She states that she is "really glad to see you" as she has "heard such great things about this clinic" and "can already tell you are a really great doctor."

She is a somewhat difficult historian but lists complaints of diffuse dorsalgia with bilateral sciatica, polymyalgias, and arthralgias and a history of a "broken neck and back" which she states was sustained in a previous abusive relationship. She has undergone ACDF and also lumbar fusion remotely. She otherwise reports a history of migraine, asthma, and interstitial cystitis. She has also status post hysterectomy and reports a history of endometriosis. Medication list includes oxycodone, alprazolam, carisoprodol, cyclobenzaprine, and albuterol. Allergies include NSAIDs, tramadol, codeine and morphine, bupropion, sertraline, escitalopram, topiramax, lamotrigine, levetiracetam, risperidone, and "steroids." She admits to tobacco and marijuana use and reports no employment secondary to disability. Family history is notable for paternal alcoholism and hypertension and maternal "rheumatic arthritis" and bipolar disorder. ROS is positive for insomnia, numbness and tingling, cough, abdominal pain, nausea, diarrhea, polyuria and dysuria, and multiple musculoskeletal complaints.

She presents with an out-of-state driver's license, and the PDMP is negative for any controlled prescriptions.

H.B. McAnally, *Opioid Dependence*, DOI 10.1007/978-3-319-47497-7_10

On exam, you note a thin female appearing older than her stated age, well-groomed and dressed, with a strong odor of tobacco and a frequent dry cough. Her gait is brisk and without compromise. Pupils are 7 mm, and although there is no tremulousness nor evident agitation, she appears fairly anxious. There is a well-healed ACDF scar and a right carpal tunnel release scar. There is yellowish discoloration/clubbing of the fingernails bilaterally, with faint ecchymoses in various stages of resolution over the left humerus, and numerous well-healed linear scars over the left dorsal forearm. There are no track marks nor fresh punctate marks. Her visible joints do not display edema, erythema, and no significant tenderness. She does exhibit fairly pronounced global myofascial tenderness. There is a well-healed midline linear lumbosacral scar. Cervical and lumbar range of motion are both rather limited in flexion and extension by pain. Straight leg raise is positive at 30° bilaterally for sciatica to the ankle. Neurologic exam is otherwise grossly unremarkable with the exception of a positive Hoffman sign on the left.

Introduction

Opioid-related deaths reached an all-time high in 2015, surpassing 33,000 [1]. We have previously suggested that while not without merit and some degree of benefit, modification of the agent (rendering prescription opioids less addictive) and the vector (improving prescribing practice) does not comprise the most effective means of reducing either individual- or population-level opioid dependence. Adaptation of the host(s) is required if this crisis is to be contained and reversed. Reductions in both vulnerability and exposure behavior must occur.

As also discussed previously, it is only within recent human history that we have been able to engineer immunity with vaccinations, etc.; historically, innate or acquired immunity and natural selection have been the sole mediators of vulnerability reduction. There are always individuals within a population blessed with resistance to specific agents' pathogenicity, either congenitally or from passive (acquired maternal antibodies) immunity or overcoming the disease themselves. Identifying these individuals a priori is currently impossible however, and as such most population-critical vaccines (e.g., polio, DPT, MMR) are administered to the entire populace indiscriminately. Other vaccines (e.g., Pneumovax, shingles) are currently reserved for high-risk demographics. (Opioid vaccines have been conjectured and even developed, as discussed briefly in Chap. 9; it is unlikely in the author's opinion that this tactic will yield significant public health benefit.) While general opioid risk reduction strategies should be applied across the board, more intensive preventive measures should be considered for those known to be more vulnerable, which of course assumes such knowledge. The first section of this chapter addresses the known epidemiology of opioid vulnerability.

The vast majority of patients seeking opioid prescriptions from providers do so ostensibly for pain complaints, and as such a solid understanding of proper assessment of all major common pain complaints (e.g., lumbago with or without lower extremity symptoms, cervicalgia with or without extremity features, headaches, joint pain, abdominopelvic pain, neuropathic pain, etc.) should be within the scope of any provider planning to prescribe opioids. However, given the complexity of chronic pain, with its broad cognitive and emotional substrate, and tremendously prevalent psychiatric comorbidities, some facility in assessing psychosocial pathology is equally if not more important in keeping with the dictum of primum non nocere. A brief literature survey of risk factors for opioid misuse and dependence shows that the vast majority of identifiable vulnerability has its basis in distress affecting the whole person, rarely confined to (or even generated by) the biological/physical component; presentation of these data forms the first section of this chapter.

The second section examines current risk assessment or stratification tools, the use of which are indicated at every level of the prevention continuum. As discussed in Chap. 8 and as recommended by various advisory bodies (e.g., the recent CDC guidelines [2] and other professional society guidelines [3, 4]), the use of these instruments (standardized questionnaires, prescription drug monitoring programs, and urine drug testing) forms an essential part of the comprehensive biopsychosocial assessment required for adequate risk assessment when considering opioid prescription.

Risk Factors for Opioid Misuse and Dependence

It had been proposed [5–7] during the late twentieth and first few years of the twenty-first century that the vast majority of patients exposed to short-term prescription opioids for acute pain (postoperative, injury/trauma-related) and even chronic opioid prescription did not go on to develop opioid dependence. One of the more well-known proponents of more aggressive opioid prescription was widely quoted as citing an addiction rate of "less than one percent" [8].

Descriptive statistics are limited and crude, but current estimates place the number of individuals with an opioid use disorder (OUD) somewhere near 5 million [9, 10], whereas the amount of opioid prescriptions written exceeds that by two to three orders of magnitude over the past two decades [11, 12]. However, high-consumption individuals are receiving not only recurrent (e.g., monthly) but also multiple (e.g., an extended-release/long-acting opioid in conjunction with an immediate-release opioid) thus likely reducing the number of individuals prescribed opioids to something on the order of 20–30 million, assuming high-consumption individuals comprise half of recipients and are issued 20 prescriptions per year. In that case, there are roughly 5 million individuals with OUD in the face of some 20–30 million individuals who have been prescribed opioids in the past couple years, which suggests a much more significant risk of iatrogenic addiction than previously believed. One of the more influential studies referenced above [7] has been criticized from a methodologic standpoint (including the exclusion of chronic pain patients), and component data show a wide range of addiction and other aberrant behavior from 0 to 45% [13]. Other recent reviews similarly suggest a rate of abuse between 9 and 41% [14, 15].

Nonetheless, not everyone prescribed opioids becomes dependent. Vulnerability to OUD is multifactorial, and as introduced in the previous chapter, risk factors include far more than just genetic predispositions; psychosocial contributors as well as amount and chronicity of exposure play enormous roles as well.

Genetic Risk Factors

While discussed in greater detail in the previous chapter, there are some genetic factors that appear to confer greater vulnerability toward opioid use disorder. Polymorphisms of dopamine receptor and opioid receptor genes, including *DRD2*, *DRD3*, *DRD4*, *OPRM1*, *OPRK1*, and *OPRD1*, have all been implicated in some studies with predisposition to various behavioral disorders and in some cases outright opioid dependence, although evidence is inconsistent [16]. "Poor metabolizers" at the CYP2D6 locus (within the cytochrome P450 family; see Chap. 2) seem to be less vulnerable to opioid dependence than those with more robust activity of this enzyme [17]. This is intuitively logical given that such individuals are exposed to less dynamic and lower plasma levels of active metabolites of tramadol, codeine, hydrocodone, oxycodone, and methadone. However, as discussed below, the only strictly genetic predictor variable shown with any consistency within population-level studies is male gender.

Biological Risk Factors

Most clinicians with any degree of experience in caring for people suffering with chronic pain carry an unspoken list of conditions they associate with increased opioid seeking/OUD. It is well-established, however, that disease and injury confer a highly variable spectrum of pain perception and suffering among different individuals, and to date, there exists no proof of specific physical pathophysiology as an independent risk factor for OUD. Chronic pain is considered independently below.

An ambitious attempt to examine biological risk factors for opioid dependence was carried out recently [18] using data from the National Epidemiologic Survey on Alcohol and Related Conditions (NESARC) Waves 1 (2001–2002) and 2 (2004–2005), a longitudinal survey of adults (18 years or older) conducted by the National Institute on Alcohol Abuse and Alcoholism. Over 43,000 civilian, noninstitutionalized adult individuals were interviewed in Wave 1, with almost 35,000 participants in the follow-up Wave 2. Fifty-three hundred of the original respondents were either non-locatable or refused follow-up interview, and 3100 were excluded due to being "institutionalized, mentally/physically impaired, on active duty in the armed forces throughout the Wave 2 interview period, deceased, or deported" [19].

By far, the strongest predictor variables in this dataset included sociodemographic and psychiatric ones, namely, male gender, younger age, non-Hispanic white ethnicity, comorbid substance use disorders, and Axis I and II psychiatric disorders [18, 20].

Katz et al. report that after adjusting for sociodemographic variables and both Axis I and II disorders, "cardiovascular disease" was predictive of incident non-medical prescription opioid use (NMPOU), whereas "all chronic physical conditions except gastrointestinal disease [18]" significantly predicted incident OUD, with greater number of conditions correlating with increasing odds. These conditions included atherosclerosis, hypertension, cirrhosis or other hepatic disease, angina pectoris or non-cardiac chest pain, tachycardia, myocardial infarction, "any other form of heart disease," gastritis or peptic ulcer disease, arthritis, and schizophrenia or other psychotic illness or episode. They report that hepatic disease could not be examined due to limited statistical power.

The authors do note several limitations of the study, including both potential false positives/low specificity due to lay interviewers, rather than clinicians gathering the data; conversely there may be false negatives/low sensitivity due to exclusion of "subclinical manifestations" of psychiatric disease. It is unclear from the report whether tachycardia was included in the "cardiovascular disease" category variable, which would of course invalidate any conclusions drawn regarding the association of cardiovascular disease with NMPOU, as this state may be associated with a host of other conditions both organic and psychiatric. Self-report comprises a very significant weakness of most studies investigating substance use issues; studies relying on NESARC data suffer the additional weakness of self report of physical conditions as well, with suspect sensitivity/specificity as mentioned previously. The authors also note that NESARC does not include chronic pain data; self-reported pain interference was captured with a single question asking the respondent to identify how much physical pain interferes with normal work and other activities over the previous month.

A recent Australian study [21] using similar population-based longitudinal (3 months) survey methodology and employing quite complex data analysis strategies sheds a little more light onto the question of whether biological issues confer independent risk for OUD. Specific diagnoses were not captured in this study; however predictor variables included physical condition categories including back and neck problems, arthritis/rheumatism, headaches, and visceral pain conditions. Patients (n = 1514) prescribed opioids for longer than 6 weeks were stratified into four groups:

1. Those reporting poor physical functioning alone (poor physical functioning only group, 27%)
2. Those reporting poor physical functioning in combination with poor coping strategies and social support (poor coping and physical functioning group, 35%)
3. Those reporting a substance use disorder (SUD group, 14%)
4. Those reporting multiple comorbid problems (multiple comorbid problems group, 25%)

The former (poor physical functioning only) group was chosen to serve as a reference and was statistically significantly more likely to be older and employed. Likelihood of musculoskeletal complaints did not differ significantly among all four groups; the reference group did have statistically significantly lower incidence of headaches than the other three groups. The reference group (poor physical functioning only) showed the lowest incidence of medication noncompliance/aberrant behavior, with rates doubling in the poor coping and physical functioning and the substance use disorder groups, and highest in the multiple comorbid problems group [21]. These data may be interpreted as indicative of relatively less importance of physical pathology compared to psychosocial dysfunction in terms of OUD risk.

In brief, it is highly unlikely that biological factors/disease conditions independently predict OUD; any association thereof must be confounded by pain, which is a nonquantifiable and highly subjective phenomenon with tremendous individual variability and perception of suffering, coping mechanisms, etc. Pain (as well as other psychological variables including emotional suffering/self-medication) is that which drives people to seek opioids in the first place and as discussed below is an independent risk factor for OUD. In conclusion of this section and introduction to the next, Sir William Osler's adage, "it is much more important to know what sort of a patient has a disease than what sort of a disease a patient has," remains as insightful today as when he spoke it two centuries ago.

Psychosocial Risk Factors

The vast majority of literature describing risk factors for OUD has focused on psychological/psychiatric and sociological variables, and as is discussed below, these factors show the greatest degree of predictive value in multivariate logistic regression analysis and other models.

Substance Use Disorders

As discussed later, other *substance use disorders* have been consistently found to confer the highest risk of opioid use disorder [22, 23]. Tobacco and alcohol are the most commonly abused substances in this country with 64 million tobacco users in 2015, 66.7 million "binge," and 17.3 million "heavy" alcohol users [24]. Numerous large studies over the past couple decades have shown fairly consistently that tobacco use is associated with a higher rate of opioid use and abuse [25–27]. A recent large ($n > 24{,}000$) study showed that smokers were greater than three times more likely to report opioid misuse and three to five times more likely to meet OUD criteria relative to non-smokers [27].

While numerous investigations suggest increased risk of OUD among patients with comorbid alcohol use disorder, large-scale epidemiologic data and even smaller individual retrospective or prospective studies are very scarce. This is likely due in part to a number of factors, including ubiquity of alcohol use in the general population, well-documented underreporting of alcohol use, and also lack of consensus for alcohol use disorder definition/cutoffs.

Among 1883 patients using opioids daily in a managed care environment on the West Coast, 12.4% admitted to concurrent use of alcohol, defined as having a drink within 2 h of consuming opioids [28]. Within this study, however, there was no difference between concurrent drinkers vs. nondrinkers in terms of diagnosis or self-report of substance use disorder, other than concurrent drinkers being statistically significantly more likely to show an AUDIT-C (a self-report tool for quantitation of alcohol consumption) score consistent with alcohol use disorder. Coexisting alcohol use disorder has been reported to be as prevalent as one-third among patients undergoing opioid maintenance therapy [29]. Daily alcohol use has been associated with increased risk of prescription drug misuse in general [30], and an early investigation using NESARC data reported a 5% and 15% prevalence of prescription opioid misuse among alcohol-abusing and alcohol-dependent individuals, respectively, compared to 0.6% for those who had abstained from alcohol in the previous year [31]. A recent study using data from NESARC Waves 1 and 2 shows an association between early-onset alcohol abuse and later development of prescription drug, including opioid misuse, [32] and makes a strong case for the frequently cited "gateway" phenomenon of drugs such as alcohol and marijuana leading to OUD and other substance use disorders.

Cannabis is the most commonly illicit substance of abuse in this country, and its use has been shown in several recent investigations to be strongly predictive of opioid use [33–35].

Benzodiazepines are frequently co-prescribed with opioids; the ever-growing body of evidence [36–38] from emergency department visit and postmortem analyses of overdose victims demonstrates the tremendous and generally unacceptable risk of this combination. Nonetheless, the practice often continues, not infrequently due to ignorance of (hopefully not apathy concerning) other providers' treatment plans that may include benzodiazepines. The use of benzodiazepines has been shown in multiple investigations to confer increased risk of opioid use disorder [39, 40], and a large (n = 17,074) Norwegian study published at the beginning of this decade showed an unadjusted odds ratio of 7:7 for chronic opioid use from previous benzodiazepine prescription [41]. After adjusting for alcohol and tobacco use, chronic pain, and socioeconomic variables, the effect was reduced by a little over 50% (odds ratio 3.1); nonetheless this sample suggested that benzodiazepine use exceeds even chronic pain as a risk factor for opioid use.

Anxiety

Benzodiazepine use of course probably bears significant association with opioid use in that it is a surrogate for anxiety and a predilection for "chemical coping" with distress. The association between anxiety disorders and opioid use disorders has been reported for decades [42–45]. Whether pre-existing anxiety (or other psychiatric disorder) precedes and predicts the development of OUD or vice versa has been debated in the literature, and support for both pathways exists, as discussed below. "Self-medication" of emotional distress including anxiety by opioids has long been recognized as a significant issue driving OUD; conversely, anxiety almost universally accompanies the development of dependence and withdrawal states. A common underlying vulnerability to both issues has also been postulated but awaits proof. The recent availability of large-scale population databases (e.g., NESARC) has allowed for some attempt to investigate the temporal directions/progression of these associations. One investigation examining the question of whether psychiatric disorders including anxiety preceded the development of OUD or vice versa showed support for both directional hypotheses [46]. In this study using NESARC Wave 1 data, nonmedical use of opioids was associated with a threefold higher rate of development of anxiety, and on the other hand, the odds of developing OUD was 6-fold higher in patients with anxiety disorders in general and nearly 11-fold higher in patients with generalized anxiety disorder. A follow-up study using NESARC Waves 1 and 2 showed similar results [47].

A cognitive distortion common to anxiety disorders (and also PTSD, discussed below, which was previously categorized within the anxiety disorders in the DSM-IV) is *pain catastrophization*, defined as a negative perceptual filter applied to actual or anticipated pain. Components include feelings and thoughts of inevitability of and helplessness about pain, rumination on pain, and magnification of pain. Pain catastrophization has been associated in numerous studies with increased incidence and severity of chronic pain [48–50] and also independently with increased risk of opioid misuse and OUD [51–53]. In the study by Martel et al., catastrophizing conferred statistically significant risk for opioid misuse even after controlling for pain severity, anxiety, and depressive symptoms [52].

Post-Traumatic Stress Disorder

Post-traumatic stress disorder (PTSD) as defined in the DSM-5 is a syndrome of persistent reexperiencing of distress (including nightmares, intrusive thoughts, flashbacks, etc.) and other symptom clusters of avoidance, negative alterations in cognition and mood, and alterations in arousal and reactivity following exposure to actual or threatened death, serious injury, or sexual violence [54].

PTSD has strong independent associations with chronic pain [55–57] and has been shown for decades to be associated with higher rates of substance abuse. PTSD confers a higher risk of heroin use [58], and those with this dual diagnosis are more prone to overdose and otherwise show worse treatment outcomes [59]. More recently, specific association of PTSD with general opioid misuse and OUD has been shown in both military and civilian populations [60–63], although the latter two studies, both using NESARC data, showed that full-blown OUD (again, subject to that database's limitations of self-report and lay interviewers) occurred in the PTSD population only among females.

Depression/Bipolar Disorder

Moderate to severe depression has long been understood to both contribute to and also stem from chronic pain [64–66], and, similarly, earlier literature on the association between depression and opioid misuse could not clearly identify/support directionality of risk [67, 68]. As discussed in Chap. 4, more recent data support a causal association between chronic opioid use and resultant depression [69, 70], whereas the converse (depression increasing risk for opioid misuse/OUD) has also been shown [46, 47]. Given the depressant effects of opioids, it seems intuitively less likely that patients suffering with depressive disorders would self-medicate with this drug class compared to those with anxiety and PTSD, and the odds ratios bear that out. Complex comorbidities abound however, with depression often intertwined with chronic pain, substance use disorders in general, anxiety, and other risk factors. Fink et al. used data from the 2011–2012 National Survey of Drug Use and Health (n = 113,665) to show that patients suffering from comorbid depression and OUD were more likely to be female, of low annual income, not currently married, and to report an alcohol use disorder or other drug use [71]; numerous confounders between these variable exist of course, rendering conclusions difficult.

Associations between bipolar disorder and chronic pain are far less frequently reported, although some reports exist [72]. Substance use disorders on the other hand are extremely comorbid with bipolar disorder; their coexistence is regarded by many as "the norm" [73]. While opioids do not appear to be the drug of choice among this population, with international literature showing a preference for alcohol, cannabis, and cocaine all greater than opioids [74], the condition does remain a significant risk factor for the development of OUD [46, 47].

Personality Disorders

Personality disorders have been associated with OUD; borderline personality disorder (BPD) in particular has shown some consistency as a predictive variable within the literature [75–77]. Heightened sensitivity to physical pain sensation in addition to lowered emotional distress threshold and heightened impulsivity have both been suggested as contributors to this association. A recent population-based review using NESARC data identified borderline, schizotypal, and antisocial personality disorders as all being predictive of opioid misuse and OUD [78].

Various personality factors have also been reported to confer both increased and decreased risk for opioid misuse and OUD. As indicated above, impulsivity appears to be associated with OUD irrespective of DSM diagnosis [79–81]. A study of 312 opioid addicts in Serbia (compared to 346 controls) linked high novelty seeking and low reward dependence, as well as self-transcendence to OUD [82]. A Dutch study comparing 161 opioid misusers without a diagnosis of OUD to 402 methadone- or heroin-maintained addicts (and a third group of 135 non-heroin users) found that the misusers were more likely to report increased novelty seeking, self-transcendence, harm avoidance, and less self-directedness than healthy non-using controls. Conversely, they reported greater social reward dependence and self-directedness than diagnosed addicts [83].

Other Sociodemographic Risk Factors

Domestic Developmental Factors

Disruption of normal childhood development by various aberrancies has long been held to confer later-life psychological/psychiatric dysfunction. Plentiful evidence of childhood sexual and physical abuse leading to various disturbances including substance abuse and dependence exist and are considered in a later section. Harm needs not occur solely in the context of these gross violations; however, verbal and emotional abuse and neglect may also predict opioid misuse and OUD. An Australian study of nearly 1000 opioid-dependent individuals showed an odds ratio of 1.9 for frequent emotional abuse in male OUD subjects (no difference for female OUD subjects vs. controls) [84]. Outright child neglect, as well as detached/disengaged parenting styles, has been shown to increase the risk of substance abuse in general [85, 86] as has a less encouraging/more rejecting parental role [87]. (Significant overlap between nonphysical forms of abuse with physical and sexual abuse exists of course, which confounds the associations.) Parental loss through death or divorce and even family discord seem to increase the risk as well [85, 88], and adoptee status is associated with nearly a twofold increase in substance use disorder risk, with an adjusted odds ratio of 2.2 for opioids specifically [89]. A fascinating link between childhood parental loss (and separation anxiety disorder in general) with disruption of the endogenous opioid system has been elucidated by the panic disorder research community [90, 91]. This deficiency in endogenous opioid activity, with its complex ramifications upon the neuroimmunoendocrine system, may explain in part the vulnerability of these individuals to exogenous opioids in later life.

Gender Issues

Data show that women receive more opioid prescriptions than men [92, 93] perhaps associated with a higher incidence of severe pain complaints [94, 95]. Numerous studies over the past decade have investigated whether gender is associated with opioid misuse and dependence [24, 25, 96–101]. Despite variability in settings, most show a consistent pattern of increased prescription opioid misuse and dependence in men compared to women. A recent large investigation using NESARC data [62] revealed greater prevalence of opioid misuse among men than women but no difference in the prevalence of OUD between the sexes.

Jamison et al. reported similar degrees of aberrant opioid use between men and women, but a greater association among women to misuse opioids is "due to emotional issues and affective distress while men tend to misuse opioids due to legal and problematic behavioral issues [98]."

Human Rights Violations

Among numerous tragic consequences of childhood physical and sexual abuse, a substantial body of literature bears witness to markedly increased rates of substance abuse in victims [102–105]. More recently childhood physical and sexual abuse has been linked with increased risk of opioid abuse and dependence, specifically [84, 106]. So well known is this association that screening for preadolescent sexual abuse is a component of opioid misuse risk stratification instruments, such as the Opioid Risk Tool (ORT) discussed below. While self-medication of physical pain symptoms (not uncommon in abusive relationships, which tend to correlate with substance abuse) is certainly present in many situations, the literature on the subject draws considerable attention/lends support to the very plausible theory that a tremendous amount of opioid misuse stems from an attempt to long-standing emotional wounds and distress.

While not as well represented in the literature, there is growing awareness that post-childhood sexual abuse [107–109] and other interpersonal violence particularly toward women [110] are associated with an increased incidence of opioid misuse and dependence. Unidirectional association of abuse preceding opioid misuse/OUD clearly seen in children (who do not use opioids for the most part) is not as clear with adults, in whom there is likely a circular pattern of abuse preceding opioid misuse and that misuse likely facilitating further abuse, etc.

Chronic Pain and Opioid Use Disorder

Not surprisingly, chronic pain is associated with opioid misuse and the development of OUD, as borne out in multiple studies [15, 111, 112]. Greater severity of pain rating, number of complaints, and reported impairments also correlate with increased risk of misuse [113, 114]. The potential bidirectionality of the association however must be considered; it has been shown for some time that opioid-dependent patients display reduced pain tolerance [115, 116], possibly owing to opioid-induced hyperalgesia. Furthermore, given the complexities of chronic pain as discussed in Chap. 6, and the disproportionately high degree of comorbid psychiatric conditions among chronic pain patients [117, 118], significant confounding almost certainly exists within these associations. As such, any conclusions regarding chronic pain and opioid misuse/OUD risk must be interpreted cautiously and with a full biopsychosocial "filter."

Prescription Factors and Opioid Use Disorder Risk

Numerous studies consistently cite high-dose [119–122], higher abuse liability as predicted by controlled substance schedule [119] escalation of dose [123, 124] and duration of therapy [119, 121, 125] as risk factors for the development of OUD. There is less agreement in the literature regarding the association of immediate-release/short-acting opioids vs. extended-release/long-acting opioids as risk factors, although there is some evidence implicating the former [120, 125] and the Food and Drug Administration recently released an "enhanced" warning indicating higher risk of misuse, abuse, and dependence with immediate-release opioids [122].

Population-Level Analyses

There exist within the literature a handful of large, primarily retrospective case-control studies comparing individuals with known OUD to those for whom that diagnosis has not been established. One of the earlier investigations of OUD risk factors was the TROUP (Trends and Risks of Opioid Use for Pain) study, which analyzed patients receiving chronic opioid therapy (COT) excluding buprenorphine for chronic non-cancer pain (CNPC) between 2000 and 2005. The base population comprised over 46,000 nationwide privately insured and Arkansas Medicaid populations, and roughly 3% of this population had documented OUD diagnostic codes. Predictor variables assessed included both physical and mental health/substance abuse diagnoses, sociodemographic factors, and prescription factors. Statistically significant risk factors included age younger than 65 and especially younger than age 50, pre-existing substance abuse diagnoses, other pre-existing mental health disorders, chronic back pain and headaches, and increasing dose and duration of COT [119].

White et al. [123] examined 875 patients with an OUD diagnosis in Maine between 2005 and 2006 and compared them to over 15,000 patients without that diagnosis who also received opioid prescriptions that year. Younger age, male gender, multiple prescriptions, multiple pharmacies, escalating doses, and other evidences of aberrancy including early refills were all associated with OUD. Substance abuse and other psychiatric diagnoses and history of viral hepatitis were also associated.

Boscarino et al. [126] evaluated 705 of 2139 patients receiving COT within the Geisinger Health System in Pennsylvania and found similar results, with age less than 65, history of opioid abuse, "pain impairment," major depression, and psychotropic medication use all conferring statistically significant risk for OUD.

Rice et al. [127] compared 6380 patients with a diagnosis of OUD within a large compilation of privately insured patients to over 800,000 patients without this diagnosis, between the years of 2007 and 2009. Statistically significant risk factors included prior opioid prescriptions, at least one prior prescription of buprenorphine or methadone, non-opioid drug abuse, or other psychiatric diagnosis, hepatitis, and family history of opioid abuse. Of note, patients with OUD were also far more likely than those without that diagnosis to have received a prescription for oxycodone (40.8% vs 13.4%).

Dufour et al. [128] evaluated 3500 cases of OUD identified within the Humana database from 2010–2011 and determined that both younger age and male gender were independent risk factors for OUD, as were substance abuse and other psychological disorders and a history of viral hepatitis.

Cochran et al. [125] examined nearly 3000 commercially and Medicare-insured patients (geographic locations not disclosed) with OUD for individual predictor variables and subsequently applied multivariate risk models based on these factors to both cases and controls ($n = 2.8$ million). Individual risk factors included younger age and male gender, economic dependent status, increased healthcare utilization variables, substance abuse and other mental health diagnoses, and psychotropic medication use. Predictive multivariate models were constructed based on diagnostic codes, medical utilization, pharmacy data, and mental health variables; the latter provided nearly an 80% positive predictive value for OUD diagnostic codes. Within this category, substance dependence (especially benzodiazepines/barbiturate dependence) conferred by far the highest risk of opioid misuse, followed by mood disorders, anxiety disorders, and chronic pain diagnoses.

A recent study [129] of 2067 OUD patients drawn from a sample of nearly 700,000 patients receiving at least one opioid prescription via a nationwide pharmacy benefit manager (excluding those with a prior diagnosis of OUD or cancer) found both chronic and high-dose usage, non-opioid substance (including alcohol) use, mental illness, younger age, and male gender to all confer increased risk.

Turk et al. [22] reviewed 15 well-conducted English language studies for risk factors for OUD. They reported that a personal history of substance abuse has been the most consistent predictor found in the literature and also noted strong correlations with other psychiatric diagnoses and history of legal troubles in multiple studies. Family history of drug abuse, personal history of childhood sexual abuse, and other aberrant prescription-related behaviors showed strongly positive association but were not widely investigated.

A recent large study by Quinn et al. examining over 10 million patients receiving chronic opioid therapy without a diagnosis of cancer showed statistically significant increased risk of chronic opioid use (not necessarily OUD) with common psychiatric diagnoses including anxiety, depression, and substance use disorders [130]. Despite the lack of specific OUD outcome data, the known association between chronic opioid use and OUD along with the immense statistical power of this study further highlights the need for comprehensive assessment and careful therapeutic planning among patients suffering with psychological and emotional distress issues and disorders.

All of these studies suffer from the common limitation of reliance upon reported diagnostic codes, with insensitivity of diagnosis certainly diluting the strength of statistical associations.

Primary Preventive Risk Assessment Approaches

Beyond thorough history (including psychosocial assessment), examination, and corroborating diagnostic imaging and laboratory tests, numerous clinical screening approaches have been developed and published. Atlari and Sudarshan [131] published a set of six criteria (in non-standardized instrument format) that were developed for pain management settings in particular and shown to be highly predictive of opioid misuse in the chronic pain patient population [131–133]. They include focus on opioids, opioid overuse, other substance use, nonfunctional status, unclear etiology of pain, and exaggeration of pain. These criteria should be considered by anyone prescribing opioids for pain but are not easily defined in many cases and are open to highly subjective interpretation.

Standardized instruments designed for stratification of patients' risk for opioid misuse, abuse, and dependence have proliferated within the literature recently as awareness of the problem expands. Three of these tools are reviewed below.

Instruments for Initial Risk Assessment

Opioid Risk Tool

The *Opioid Risk Tool (ORT)*, published in 2005 by Dr. Lynn Webster, was designed specifically "to predict the probability of a patient displaying aberrant behaviors when prescribed opioids for chronic pain" [134]. The ORT is a self-report questionnaire designed specifically for new (not at all synonymous with opioid-naïve) patient screening and assesses both personal and family history of substance abuse including alcohol, prescription and illicit drugs, age, history of preadolescent sexual abuse, and specific psychiatric diagnoses. Positive answers are assigned a weighted point value for overall risk contribution, and the sum is tabulated and categorized into low-risk (score 0–3), moderate-risk (score 4–7), and high-risk (score >7) groups. This original publication reported results from a sample of 185 patients new to the authors' pain clinic. Subsequent aberrant drug-related behaviors (including soliciting prescriptions from other providers, using unauthorized/illicit opioids, abnormal drug screening, unsanctioned dose escalation, missing visits) were identified after a 12-month period in 6% of patients categorized as low risk, 28% of patients categorized as moderate risk, and 91% of those categorized as high risk. Increasing number of aberrant behaviors also correlated with increasing score.

Moore et al. [135] conducted a small but important study of 48 patients new to their pain clinic who were initially prescribed opioids but subsequently had opioid therapy terminated for aberrant behaviors. Besides an initial interview by one of the psychologists, the sample was subjected to the ORT, and two other risk assessment tools described below in a head-to-head comparison of the instruments' sensitivity for predicting aberrancy. In this analysis, when evaluating patients assigned an initial ORT risk category of moderate or high risk, the instrument showed a sensitivity value of 0.45 (21 of the 48 patients accurately identified a priori.) The sensitivity was reduced to 0.10 when evaluating only patients categorized as high risk by the instrument.

Two follow-up studies comparing the same instruments in larger samples ($n = 132$ and 263) and using the same methodology [136] showed similar low sensitivity for the ORT (0.10 and 0.18, respectively) but superior specificity (0.88) among the screening tools. Thus, while more likely to miss patients at risk for opioid misuse and abuse, the ORT has the lowest likelihood of false positives among commonly used tools.

A German study evaluating a cancer population (n = 114) compared the predictive value of the ORT for urine drug testing (UDT) abnormalities [137]. This study found a higher proportion of aberrant UDT (positive primarily for cannabis) in patients categorized as moderate risk (69%) and high risk (59%) compared to those categorized as low risk (7%). Significant limitations of this analysis however included the fact that some patients did not fill out the ORT themselves, with questionnaire completed retrospectively by staff. Furthermore, not all patients underwent urine drug screening, with the test biased toward those patients assigned a higher-risk categorization (79% of high-risk patients undergoing UDT compared to 52% in the moderate-risk group and 21% in the low-risk group).

Screener and Opioid Assessment for Patients with Pain

The *Screener and Opioid Assessment for Patients with Pain (SOAPP)* is a self-report questionnaire designed to predict opioid misuse and abuse among chronic pain patients considered for long-term opioid therapy. The original instrument (SOAPP) was designed using eight concept clusters listed here in descending order of predictive importance: antisocial behaviors/history, substance abuse history, medication-related behaviors, doctor-patient relationship factors, psychiatric history, emotional attachment to pain medicine, personal care and lifestyle issues, and finally psychosocial problems [138].

An initial validation study by the developers [138] reported good sensitivity (0.91) and specificity (0.69) at a cutoff score of 7 or greater in predicting aberrant drug-related behaviors after 6 months. A second validation study by the same group [139] showed markedly lower performance, with sensitivity of 0.68 and specificity of 0.39 for a cutoff score of 8 or greater; the authors reported however that 10% of the sample did not complete the form and were excluded, and the comparison standard (UDT) was not applied to all patients in this sample.

In the analysis of Moore et al. [135], the SOAPP achieved a relatively high sensitivity value (0.73), with 35 of 48 of the aberrancy-displaying/discharged patients having received a high-risk rating (score greater than 6) at baseline.

The initial version, however, was perceived to be excessively vulnerable to deceptive answers and furthermore was conceptually flawed in that predictive validity which was tested primarily against self-reported aberrant behaviors at follow-up [140]. As such, SOAPP subsequently underwent revision *(SOAPP-R)* which included a focus on eliminating "admission of socially unacceptable behaviors" and incorporating more "subtle" predictors (deemed less transparent to respondents) from the literature such as impulsivity, anger, resentment, and boredom to complement or update the initial instrument (Fig. 10.1). Scoring categories based upon subsequent analysis introduced below include low-risk (score <10), moderate-risk (score 10–21), and high-risk (score >21).

In the initial validation study [140], an outcome measure ("aberrant drug behavior index" or ADBI) was created with score based upon self-report, physician assessment, and UDT. In the final analysis, 223 patients' SOAPP-R data were compared to their ADBI score, and at the recommended cutoff score (18) for positivity, sensitivity was shown to be 0.81 with a specificity of 0.68. Subsequent cross-validation analysis in a different sample showed comparable predictive value and reliability [141].

SOAPP®-R

The following are some questions given to patients who are on or being considered for medication for their pain. Please answer each question as honestly as possible. There are no right or wrong answers.

	Never	Seldom	Sometimes	Often	Very Often
	0	1	2	3	4
1. How often do you have mood swings?	○	○	○	○	○
2. How often have you felt a need for higher doses of medication to treat your pain?	○	○	○	○	○
3. How often have you felt impatient with your doctors?	○	○	○	○	○
4. How often have you felt that things are just too overwhelming that you can't handle them?	○	○	○	○	○
5. How often is there tension in the home?	○	○	○	○	○
6. How often have you counted pain pills to see how many are remaining?	○	○	○	○	○
7. How often have you been concerned that people will judge you for taking pain medication?	○	○	○	○	○
8. How often do you feel bored?	○	○	○	○	○
9. How often have you taken more pain medication than you were supposed to?	○	○	○	○	○
10. How often have you worried about being left alone?	○	○	○	○	○
11. How often have you felt a craving for medication?	○	○	○	○	○
12. How often have others expressed concern over your use of medication?	○	○	○	○	○

	Never	Seldom	Sometimes	Often	Very Often
	0	1	2	3	4
13. How often have any of your close friends had a problem with alcohol or drugs?	○	○	○	○	○
14. How often have others told you that you had a bad temper?	○	○	○	○	○
15. How often have you felt consumed by the need to get pain medication?	○	○	○	○	○
16. How often have you run out of pain medication early?	○	○	○	○	○
17. How often have others kept you from getting what you deserve?	○	○	○	○	○
18. How often, in your lifetime, have you had legal problems or been arrested?	○	○	○	○	○
19. How often have you attended an AA or NA meeting?	○	○	○	○	○
20. How often have you been in an argument that was so out of control that someone got hurt?	○	○	○	○	○
21. How often have you been sexually abused?	○	○	○	○	○
22. How often have others suggested that you have a drug or alcohol problem?	○	○	○	○	○
23. How often have you had to borrow pain medications from your family or friends?	○	○	○	○	○
24. How often have you been treated for an alcohol or drug problem?	○	○	○	○	○

Fig. 10.1 Screener and Opioid Assessment for Patients in Pain (SOAPP). Copyright 2015 Inflexxion, Inc. Used with permission

In the analysis of Jones et al. [136], their first study showed that 32% of patients discharged for aberrant drug-related behavior were assigned a high-risk category by cutoff score of 18 on the SOAPP-R a priori; despite this poor performance, it remained the most sensitive of the standardized instruments in the analysis, outperforming the Pain Medication Questionnaire (not discussed in this chapter) and the ORT in terms of sensitivity. In the second study, the SOAPP-R remained the most sensitive standardized instrument (0.39) but showed the lowest specificity at 0.69.

The SOAPP-R was recently evaluated in an emergency department patient population (n = 82) in comparison to PDMP data (with aberrancy definition chosen as four or more prescriptions from four or more providers) [142]. Thirty-three percent were determined to be "at risk" (score ≥18) by SOAPP-R, and 16% met the study's PDMP criteria for aberrant behavior. Of the latter, 54% had SOAPP-R scores ≥18. Weaknesses of the study included small numbers, and while the point was not to validate the instrument, the comparison standard chosen was arbitrary and arguably one of very low sensitivity.

SOAPP has more recently undergone further reduction to a five-question short form (*SOAPP Version 1.0-SF*). The advantage lies of course in its brevity which in practical terms should translate into greater potential of widespread adoption/utilization. A cutoff score of 4 on this instrument showed a sensitivity of 0.86 and specificity of 0.67 [143], which is comparable to the SOAPP-R (0.91 and 0.69, respectively.)

To date no study validating the short form has been published. This version however was evaluated for overall agreement with other predictor variables in a sample of 522 patients at MD Anderson Cancer Center in Houston [144]. Twenty-nine percent of patients in this sample were identified as high risk, with a score at or greater than 4, and this subgroup were statistically significantly more likely to be younger (with 55 years being the cutoff), endorse more pain, receive higher opioid doses, and report more symptoms of depression and anxiety.

Diagnosis, Intractability, Risk, and Efficacy

The *Diagnosis, Intractability, Risk, and Efficacy (DIRE) Score* was created in 2007 by Dr. Miles Belgrade to "predict efficacy of analgesia and patient compliance with long-term opioid analgesic treatment" (Fig. 10.2) [145]. It is a provider-scored instrument that may be completed without direct input from the patient and evaluates issues related to objective severity of diagnosis; patient's history of multimodal therapy, engagement, and self-efficacy; "risk" profile based on psychological stability, substance use tendency, reliability, and social support; and efficacy of both analgesia

D.I.R.E. Score: Patient Selection for Chronic Opioid Analgesia

For each factor, rate the patient's score from 1-3 based on the explanations in the right hand column.

Score	Factor	Explanation
	Diagnosis	1 = Benign chronic condition with minimal objective findings or no definite medical diagnosis. Examples: fibromyalgia, migraine headaches, nonspecific back pain. 2 = Slowly progressive condition concordant with moderate pain, or fixed condition with moderate objective findings. Examples: failed back surgery syndrome, back pain with moderate degenerative changes, neuropathic pain. 3 = Advanced condition concordant with severe pain with objective findings. Examples: severe ischemic vascular disease, advanced neuropathy, severe spinal stenosis.
	Intractability	1 = Few therapies have been tried and the patient takes a passive role in his/her pain management process. 2 = Most customary treatments have been tried but the patient is not fully engaged in the pain management process, or barriers prevent (insurance, transportation, medical illness). 3 = Patient fully engaged in a spectrum of appropriate treatments but with inadequate response.
	Risk	(R = Total of P + C + R + S below)
	Psychological:	1 = Serious personality dysfunction or mental illness interfering with care. Example: personality disorder, severe affective disorder, significant personality issues. 2 = Personality or mental health interferes moderately. Example: depression or anxiety disorder. 3 = Good communication with clinic. No significant personality dysfunction or mental illness.
	Chemical Health:	1 = Active or very recent use of illicit drugs, excessive alcohol, or prescription drug abuse. 2 = Chemical coper (uses medications to cope with stress) or history of CD in remission. 3 = No CD history. Not drug-focused or chemically reliant.
	Reliability:	1 = History of numerous problems: medication misuse, missed appointments, rarely follows through. 2 = Occasional difficulties with compliance, but generally reliable. 3 = Highly reliable patient with meds, appointments & treatment.
	Social Support:	1 = Life in chaos. Little family support and few close relationships. Loss of most normal life roles. 2 = Reduction in some relationships and life roles. 3 = Supportive family/close relationships. Involved in work or school and no social isolation.
	Efficacy score	1 = Poor function or minimal pain relief despite moderate to high doses. 2 = Moderate benefit with function improved in a number of ways (or insufficient info – hasn't tried opioid yet or very low doses or too short of a trial). 3 = Good improvement in pain and function and quality of life with stable doses over time.

___ Total score = D + I + R + E

Score 7-13: Not a suitable candidate for long-term opioid analgesia
Score 14-21: May be a candidate for long-term opioid analgesia

Fig. 10.2 Diagnosis, Intractability, Risk, and Efficacy (DIRE) Score. Copyright 2005 Dr. Miles Belgrade. Used with permission

and functional improvement. Higher scores are expected to predict a more successful prescribing process with respect to patient compliance and efficacy of treatment. The initial validation study ($n = 61$) compared DIRE scores to three different outcome measures including clinicians' global impression of compliance/aberrancy with the prescribing process, global impression of efficacy of opioid analgesia, and disposition with respect to continuation of opioids at the time of the last clinical contact [145]. Spearman correlation coefficient between DIRE score and compliance assessment was high at 0.76 and moderate (0.58) for efficacy assessment. The Wilcoxon rank sum test was used to compare DIRE score to the two disposition categories of continued vs. discontinued opioid prescribing and showed significant correlation as well. The authors reported that a score of 13 was determined as the cutoff point at or below which chronic opioid therapy would not be recommended. At this cutoff point, sensitivities for compliance, efficacy, and disposition were 94%, 81%, and 86%, respectively. Specificities were 87%, 76%, and 73%, respectively.

In Moore et al.'s analysis DIRE score yielded a low sensitivity of 0.17; it should be remembered however that the instrument was created not only to predict aberrancy vs. compliance but also treatment efficacy, and in the words of the authors, "The DIRE score is more than simply an addiction risk tool, and some of its items may not be germane to predicting early dismissal for medication misuse [137]."

Nonetheless, it bears mention that despite concerns for the reliability of self-report, the literature would seem to indicate that at least some self-report instruments (e.g., SOAPP-R) show at least as good if not better predictive value than some clinician-scored instruments based on currently available data.

A systematic review [146] of these instruments (as well as the ongoing compliance/aberrancy monitoring instruments discussed below) by the American Pain Society (APS) and American Academy of Pain Medicine (AAPM) published in 2009 evaluated the quality of data from these studies using the United States Preventive Services Task Force (USPSTF) criteria [147]. They found "higher-quality" evidence for validity of SOAPP and SOAPP-R in predicting increased likelihood for future aberrant drug-related behaviors, with lower-quality evidence supporting the validity of the ORT. Studies evaluating other instruments did not meet USPSTF criteria for data quality.

Prescription Drug Monitoring Programs and Urine Drug Testing

While comprising obvious and essential requirements for ongoing compliance/aberrancy monitoring as discussed below, the use of *Prescription Drug Monitoring Programs (PDMP)* and *urine drug testing (UDT)* in initial risk assessment is increasingly recommended (and legislated in the case of PDMP) by numerous authorities. While their purpose is primarily to identify those with an existing problem, and contributing therefore to secondary (and tertiary) prevention efforts, there remains a substantial role for these tools in primary prevention as well, as they may identify patients who have not yet developed an opioid misuse/abuse problem but who are displaying problematic behaviors related to other drugs with abuse potential (e.g., benzodiazepines, stimulants, etc.).

While not recommended as part of routine assessment, it should be mentioned that the use of widely available internet-based technology such as the CourtView Justice Solutions database may provide invaluable insight into a patient's risk of either abuse or diversion.

Stratification of patients into low-, medium-, and high-risk categories for opioid abuse has been suggested for over a decade [4, 148, 149] to improve characterization of risk-benefit ratios for individuals being considered for opioid prescription and also to help inform more appropriate monitoring strategies. Table 10.1 presents a suggested stratification paradigm that, interestingly, came from the initial article [148] urging "universal precautions" in the context of pain management (the two concepts are of course not mutually exclusive.)

Secondary Preventive/Aberrancy Assessment Approaches

The risk factor analyses and instruments reviewed above serve the purpose of initial screening/risk stratification—i.e., to predict misuse. While they have relevance to both primary and secondary prevention (discussed in Chap. 11), they are intended to help identify patients at risk of opioid misuse and abuse prior to initiation of therapy and thus comprise an important part of primary prevention efforts.

Ongoing risk assessment to identify active misuse/abuse and dependence in patients being treated with opioids is essential for secondary prevention efforts at an individual level, as well as population-level reduction of opioid misuse and dependence. While

Table 10.1 Suggested compliance and aberrancy monitoring when prescribing opioids, by risk category[a]

Risk category	Risk factors	Care team	Suggested management parameters
Low	No personal history of substance abuse	PCP	q1–3-month visits
	No or minimal comorbid psychiatric conditions		PDMP check per state law
			Baseline and q6–12-month random UDT
Moderate	Past (not current) personal history of substance abuse	PCP and/or pain specialist, +behavioral health, ± addictionologist	q1 month visits
	Moderate comorbid psychiatric conditions		PDMP check per state law, or at least quarterly
			Baseline and q1–6-month random UDT
			Random pill counts
High	Current substance abuse	Interdisciplinary pain center and/or addictionologist	q1 week to 1 month visits
	Unstable comorbid psychiatric conditions		PDMP check with each prescription
			Baseline and q1–3-month random UDT
			Random pill counts

[a]Adapted from [148]

diverters of prescription opioids technically fall under the category of vector rather than host in the epidemiologic model used throughout this book, it is clear that a great number of diverters are also dependent upon (or at least misusing) opioids and from a more pragmatic standpoint, it is generally impossible in the absence of thorough and ongoing risk assessment to differentiate between those seeking opioids primarily for personal use vs. entrepreneurial activity or other illicit currency/purpose.

Problematic behaviors predictive of opioid misuse and abuse have been identified and discussed in the literature for the past two decades [150, 151]. Behaviors with lower predictive value (greater sensitivity but lower specificity) include unwillingness to trial multimodal approaches, aggressive complaining about the need for more opioids, drug hoarding, unsanctioned dose escalation with frequent early refill requests, and problems with personal and social responsibilities including work. Stealing or borrowing opioids, forging prescriptions, frequently alleging lost prescriptions, and resisting changes to therapy despite adverse side effects are more worrisome indicators [150]. As with primary screening tools, several instruments have been developed and tested for clinical use in monitoring compliance/aberrancy.

Instruments to Monitor Compliance/Identify Current Aberrancy

Pain Medication Questionnaire

The *Pain Medication Questionnaire (PMQ)* is a 26-question self-report instrument developed and analyzed extensively at Southwestern Medical Center, focusing on "potentially dysfunctional attitudes and aberrant behaviors surrounding the use of pain medication" including non-opioid analgesics, and was first published in 2004 [152]. The initial report of the index testing group ($n = 184$) compared questionnaire scores to outcome measures of physician ratings of risk for opioid misuse obtained at initial medical evaluation and self-admitted misuse or diagnosis reported by referring physician. Objective measures such as urinalysis were not reported. Participants were categorized by tertile PMQ score into low-, middle-, and high-scoring groups, with the high-scoring group correlating with substantially higher likelihood of both being treated with opioids and also known history of substance abuse. Comparing data captured by standardized psychological assessments including the Beck Depression Inventory and the Minnesota Multiphasic Personality Inventory, patients falling in the high-scoring group were significantly more likely to have interpersonally distressed or dysfunctional coping styles, depression, anxiety, physical preoccupation, and a sense of social alienation. Comparing data captured by standardized functional assessments including the Oswestry Pain Disability Questionnaire and the SF-36 form, patients falling in the high-scoring group were significantly more likely to be collecting disability income. This observation led the authors to hypothesize that "the same diminished coping strategies that undermine a patient's motivation to return to work also place that person at greater risk for opioid misuse" [152].

A follow-up validity study examining 271 patients selected for interdisciplinary pain management (i.e., behavioral and physiotherapy in addition to medical care) at the same institution compared PMQ scores to physician assessment of risk, patients' requests for early refill of pain medications, and compliance with interdisciplinary treatment [153]. Higher PMQ scores were associated with both a known substance abuse history and also more frequent requests for early refills of pain medication. Of interest, in longitudinal analysis PMQ scores were seen to significantly decrease over time with the completion of the interdisciplinary pain management program.

The original PMQ was criticized for being overly cumbersome, and more recently a revised version consisting of 23 questions (three less than the original) was tested by the authors on a sample of 1200 patients, showing essentially identical results in terms of correlation with known substance abuse history and early refill requests [154]. Again, completion of the multidisciplinary program resulted in reduced PMQ score over time.

Current Opioid Misuse Measure

The *Current Opioid Misuse Measure (COMM)* is another instrument for ongoing aberrancy monitoring, developed by Inflexxion (who created the SOAPP for initial risk assessment) using similar concept mapping methodology (Fig. 10.3). Preliminary analysis identified the three most important concept areas as medication misuse/noncompliance (evasiveness related to UDT, reports of stolen or lost prescriptions, pharmacy aberrancies) followed by evidence of lying and illicit drug use and finally emotional problems/psychiatric issues (reports of anger or impulse control issues, emotional instability, suicidality, emerging family or marital problems, etc.) [155]. The COMM comprises a 17-item, self-administered questionnaire analyzing six key areas derived from the concept mapping (signs and symptoms of intoxication, emotional volatility, evidence of poor response to medications, addiction, healthcare use patterns, and problematic medication behavior. COMM scores were compared in the original validation study to the same aberrant drug behavior

Current Opioid Misuse Measure (COMM)®

Please answer each question as honestly as possible. Keep in mind that we are only asking about the **past 30 days**. There are no right or wrong answers. If you are unsure about how to answer the question, please give the best answer you can.

Please answer the questions using the following scale:	Never	Seldom	Sometimes	Often	Very Often
	0	1	2	3	4
1. In the past 30 days, how often have you had trouble with thinking clearly or had memory problems?	o	o	o	o	o
2. In the past 30 days, how often do people complain that you are not completing necessary tasks? (i.e., doing things that need to be done, such as going to class, work or appointments)	o	o	o	o	o
3. In the past 30 days, how often have you had to go to someone other than your prescribing physician to get sufficient pain relief from medications? (i.e., another doctor, the Emergency Room, friends, street sources)	o	o	o	o	o
4. In the past 30 days, how often have you taken your medications differently from how they are prescribed?	o	o	o	o	o
5. In the past 30 days, how often have you seriously thought about hurting yourself?	o	o	o	o	o
6. In the past 30 days, how much of your time was spent thinking about opioid medications (having enough, taking them, dosing schedule, etc.)?	o	o	o	o	o

Please answer the questions using the following scale:	Never	Seldom	Sometimes	Often	Very Often
	0	1	2	3	4
7. In the past 30 days, how often have you been in an argument?	o	o	o	o	o
8. In the past 30 days, how often have you had trouble controlling your anger (e.g., road rage, screaming, etc.)?	o	o	o	o	o
9. In the past 30 days, how often have you needed to take pain medications belonging to someone else?	o	o	o	o	o
10. In the past 30 days, how often have you been worried about how you're handling your medications?	o	o	o	o	o
11. In the past 30 days, how often have others been worried about how you're handling your medications?	o	o	o	o	o
12. In the past 30 days, how often have you had to make an emergency phone call or show up at the clinic without an appointment?	o	o	o	o	o
13. In the past 30 days, how often have you gotten angry with people?	o	o	o	o	o
14. In the past 30 days, how often have you had to take more of your medication than prescribed?	o	o	o	o	o
15. In the past 30 days, how often have you borrowed pain medication from someone else?	o	o	o	o	o
16. In the past 30 days, how often have you used your pain medicine for symptoms other than for pain (e.g., to help you sleep, improve your mood, or relieve stress)?	o	o	o	o	o
17. In the past 30 days, how often have you had to visit the Emergency Room?	o	o	o	o	o

Fig. 10.3 Current Opioid Misuse Measure (COMM). Copyright 2015 Inflexxion, Inc. Used with permission

index (based upon self-report, physician assessment, and UDT) used to validate SOAPP, and a score equal to or greater than 9 was shown to have a sensitivity of 0.77 and specificity of 0.68 [155]; the negative predictive value at this score is 0.95 indicating very low likelihood of false negatives. Cross-validation in another population showed essentially the same results [156].

Patient Drug Use Questionnaire

The *Patient Drug Use Questionnaire (PDUQ)* is a 42-item clinician-administered instrument created specifically to try to help clinicians determine whether patients treated with chronic opioids, the majority of whom are physically and/or psychologically dependent, are in fact addicted [157, 158]. First published in 1996, it remains the most commonly used benchmark device in research for comparison measurement of aberrancy reporting and is furthermore unique in that it has been validated against clinical expert diagnosis of substance use disorders [159]. It assesses pain complaints/factors, opioid use patterns, social and family factors, family history of pain and substance abuse syndromes, patient history of substance abuse, and psychiatric history. The PDUQ has been shown to distinguish addicted and nonaddicted patients using modified DSM-4 criteria such that subjects scoring below 11 "did not meet criteria for a substance disorder" and those scoring 15 or greater "had a substance use disorder." The original PDUQ is a 20 min interview, and this has limited its use in clinical settings. More recently, a 31-question, self-administered version has been developed to circumvent these issues [159].

A large study of chronic pain patients on opioids in a general medical population [160] showed poor internal reliability of the PDUQ, and these investigators opined that there may be significant differences between chronic pain patient populations (in which the PDUQ was developed and tested initially) and general practice patients that explain the differences in results. In this study, three overall factor groups appeared to best predict aberrancy and included addiction-related behaviors (illicit procurement, illicit use, history of other substance problems), addiction-related concerns (whether on the part of patients, family, or physician), and "pain treatment problems" which included believing that pain was inadequately treated, self-increasing dose, and being angry with one's doctor.

In the APS/AAPM systematic review referenced above [146], "higher-quality" evidence by USPSTF criteria supported the validity of COMM in accurately identifying current aberrant drug-related behaviors. Studies evaluating other instruments did not meet USPSTF criteria for data quality.

Prescription Monitoring Programs and Urine Drug Testing

Behavioral assessment tools, the use of PDMPs, and UDT form the primary means of ongoing risk assessment at present, and this multifaceted approach has been recommended for some time now by professional societies [161, 162] and more recently in the proliferation of clinical practice guidelines introduced in Chap. 8.

The regular use of PDMPs in ongoing risk monitoring is being increasingly advised and in many states now legislated. PDMPs are uniquely able to demonstrate the aberrant behavior of "doctor shopping" and may aid in identifying lying behaviors as well. While these do not in and of themselves constitute misuse and abuse (they may well signify diversion, medication losses, memory losses, etc.), it is fairly universal practice to accept PDMP aberrancies as indicative of abuse, and they furthermore comprise violations of most opioid treatment agreements mandating single prescriber, no early prescription reissuing, etc.

UDT remains the "gold standard" for assessing aberrancy but is not foolproof; patients have found numerous means of defeating this surveillance with common means including the addition of medication directly into the sample, provision of "clean" urine from another source, and in extreme cases going so far as to instill urine from other people into their own urinary bladders for witnessed specimen provision [163]. Nonetheless, it is held to be the most reliable and accurate noninvasive means of assessing compliance and aberrancy. "Point-of-care" immunoassay tests can determine the presence or absence of particular substances according to a predetermined threshold and are available at low cost (generally in multiple assay systems such as 5-, 10-, 13-panel collection cups) and provide data within a matter of minutes. Problems with immunoassay methods however include variable and imperfect sensitivity and specificity and lack of availability of many immunoreagents for specific drugs. Cross-reactivity with other substances may yield false positives, and discrimination of specific drugs within a class is essentially impossible when drugs share similar structure and hence are bound by the same antibody. Furthermore, immunoassays do not provide information on the presence or absence of metabolites, which may be essential information in assessing compliance, e.g., samples positive for the parent drug without metabolites are indicative of tampering/adulteration. Most of these potential problems with point-of-care/immunoassay testing are solved by submitting the urine sample for "confirmatory testing" which usually uses gas or liquid chromatography in conjunction with mass spectroscopy for significantly greater sensitivity and specificity as well as the ability to detect metabolites and also provide quantitative levels. Confirmatory testing is more expensive and does not provide immediate results; thus it is inappropriate to rely on as a sole means of monitoring.

Recommended frequency of UDT has been the subject of much debate lately, partially due to the increased prevalence/awareness of substance abuse in our nation and also due to financial abuses of over-testing for profit's sake. Most of the advisory guidelines discussed in the previous chapter recommend at least initial baseline screening with subsequent random testing depending on the assessed level of risk. A recent expert panel consensus report recommends testing at a minimum of every 6 months in low-risk patients and at least every 3 months in medium- to high- risk patients [164].

Summary

Reduction of individual- and population-level opioid dependence will require adaptation of the host(s) if the opioid epidemic is to be contained and reversed. Attempts to alter abuse liability of opioids (agent virulence) and prescription patterns (vector transmission) are reasonable but ultimately insufficient interventions. Attenuation of both host vulnerability and exposure behavior must occur. This is a joint effort between patient and provider, and from the provider's standpoint, it must begin with a thorough understanding of risk factors for opioid misuse and dependence. Most of the risk factors identified in the literature are psychosocial in nature and have been incorporated into various standardized screening instruments. The use of prescription drug monitoring programs and urine drug testing comprise other essential risk assessment and monitoring tools. Risk stratification—with ongoing assessment for both compliance and aberrancy—must become standard practice for every provider that prescribes opioids.

References

1. Rudd RA, Seth P, David F, Scholl L. Increases in drug and opioid-involved overdose deaths — United States, 2010–2015. MMWR. 2016;65(50–51):1445–52. doi:10.15585/mmwr.mm655051e1.
2. Dowell D, Haegerich TM, Chou R. CDC guideline for prescribing opioids for chronic pain – United States, 2016. MMWR. 2016;65:1–49.
3. Washington Agency Medical Directors Group. Interagency guideline on opioid dosing for chronic non-cancer pain. 2010. Available from: http://www.agencymedicaldirectors.wa.gov/Files/OpioidGdline.pdf
4. Manchikanti L, Kaye AM, Knezevic NN, McAnally H, Slavin K, Trescot AM, et al. Responsible, safe, and effective prescription of opioids for chronic non-cancer pain: American Society of Interventional Pain Physicians (ASIPP) guidelines. Pain Physician. 2017;20(2S):S3–S92.
5. Porter J, Jick H. Addiction rare in patients treated with narcotics. N Engl J Med. 1980;302:12.
6. Portenoy RK, Foley KM. Chronic use of opioid analgesics in non-malignant pain: report of 38 cases. Pain. 1986;25:171–86.
7. Fishbain DA, Cole B, Lewis J, Rosomoff HL, Rosomoff RS. What percentage of chronic nonmalignant pain patients exposed to chronic opioid analgesic therapy develop abuse/addiction and/or aberrant drug-related behaviors? A structured evidence-based review. Pain Med. 2008;9:444–59.
8. Quinones S. Dreamland: the true tale of America's opiate epidemic. New York: Bloomsbury Press; 2015.
9. Kolodny A, Courtwright DT, Hwang CS, Kreiner P, Eadie JL, Clark TW, et al. The prescription opioid and heroin crisis: a public health approach to an epidemic of addiction. Annu Rev. Public Health. 2015;36:559–74.
10. Alexander GC, Frattaroli S, Gielen AC, editors. The prescription opioid epidemic: an evidence-based approach. Baltimore, MD: Johns Hopkins Bloomberg School of Public Health; 2015.
11. https://www.drugabuse.gov/about-nida/legislative-activities/testimony-to-congress/2016/prescription-opioid-heroin-abuse. Accessed 4 Feb 2017.
12. https://www.hhs.gov/sites/default/files/Factsheet-opioids-061516.pdf. Accessed 4 Feb 2017.
13. Database of Abstracts of Reviews of Effects (DARE): Quality-assessed Reviews [Internet]. York (UK): Centre for Reviews and Dissemination (UK); 1995. https://www.ncbi.nlm.nih.gov/pubmedhealth/PMH0025656/. Accessed 24 Jan 2017.
14. Manchikanti L, Cash KA, Damron KS, Manchukonda R, Pampati V, McManus CD. Controlled substance abuse and illicit drug use in chronic pain patients: an evaluation of multiple variables. Pain Physician. 2006;9:215–25.

15. Boscarino JA, Rukstalis MR, Hoffman SN, Han JJ, Erlich PM, Ross S, et al. Prevalence of prescription opioid-use disorder among chronic pain patients: comparison of the DSM-5 vs. DSM-4 diagnostic criteria. J Addict Dis. 2011;30:185–94.
16. Mistry CJ, Bawor M, Desai D, Marsh DC, Samaan Z. Genetics of opioid dependence: a review of the genetic contribution to opioid dependence. Curr Psychiatr Rev. 2014;10:156–67.
17. Khokhar JY, Ferguson CS, Zhu AZ, Tyndale RF. Pharmacogenetics of drug dependence: role of gene variations in susceptibility and treatment. Annu Rev. Pharmacol Toxicol. 2010;50:39–61.
18. Katz C, El-Gabalawy R, Keyes KM, Martins SS, Sareen J. Risk factors for incident nonmedical prescription opioid use and abuse and dependence: results from a longitudinal nationally representative sample. Drug Alcohol Depend. 2013;132:107–13.
19. National Institute on Alcohol Abuse and Alcoholism. Alcohol use and alcohol use disorders in the United States, a 3-year follow-up: main findings from the 2004–2005 wave 2 national epidemiologic survey on alcohol and related conditions (NESARC). 2010. https://pubs.niaaa.nih.gov/publications/nesarc_drm2/nesarc2drm.pdf. Accessed 12 Feb 2017.
20. Blanco C, Rafful C, Wall MM, Jin CJ, Kerridge B, Schwartz RP. The latent structure and predictors of non-medical prescription drug use and prescription drug use disorders: a national study. Drug Alcohol Depend. 2013;133:473–9.
21. Peacock A, Degenhardt L, Campbell G, Larance B, Nielsen S, Hall W, et al. A typology of predictive risk factors for non-adherent medication-related behaviors among chronic non-cancer pain patients prescribed opioids: a cohort study. Pain Physician. 2016;19(3):E421–34.
22. Turk DC, Swanson KS, Gatchel RJ. Predicting opioid misuse by chronic pain patients: a systematic review and literature synthesis. Clin J Pain. 2008;24:497–508.
23. Boscarino JA, Hoffman SN, Han JJ. Opioid-use disorder among patients on long-term opioid therapy: impact of final DSM-5 diagnostic criteria on prevalence and correlates. Subst Abuse Rehabil. 2015;6:83–91.
24. Center for Behavioral Health Statistics and Quality. Key substance use and mental health indicators in the United States: Results from the 2015 National Survey on Drug Use and Health (HHS Publication No. SMA 16–4984, NSDUH Series H-51); 2016. Available from: http://www.samhsa.gov/data/
25. Huang B, Dawson DA, Stinson FS, Hasin DS, Ruan WJ, Saha TD, et al. Prevalence, correlates, and comorbidity of nonmedical prescription drug use and drug use disorders in the United States: results of the national epidemiologic survey on alcohol and related conditions. J Clin Psychiatry. 2006;67:1062–73.
26. Skurtveit S, Furu K, Selmer R, Handal M, Tverdal A. Nicotine dependence predicts repeated use of prescribed opioids. Prospective population-based cohort study. Ann Epidemiol. 2010;20:890–7.
27. Zale EL, Dorfman ML, Hooten WM, Warner DO, Zvolensky MJ, Ditre JW. Tobacco smoking, nicotine dependence, and patterns of prescription opioid misuse: results from a nationally representative sample. Nicotine Tob Res. 2015;17:1096–103.
28. Saunders K, Von Korff M, Campbell CI, Banta-Green CJ, Sullivan MD, Merrill JO, et al. Concurrent use of alcohol and sedatives among persons prescribed chronic opioid therapy: prevalence and risk factors. J Pain. 2012;13:266–75.
29. Soyka M. Alcohol use disorders in opioid maintenance therapy: prevalence, clinical correlates and treatment. Eur Addict Res. 2015;21:78–87.
30. Simoni-Wastila L, Strickler G. Risk factors associated with problem use of prescription drugs. Am J Public Health. 2004;94:266–8.
31. McCabe SE, Cranford JA, Boyd CJ. The relationship between past-year drinking behaviors and nonmedical use of prescription drugs: prevalence of co-occurrence in a national sample. Drug Alcohol Depend. 2006;84:281–8.
32. Arterberry BJ, Horbal SR, Buu A, Lin HC. The effects of alcohol, cannabis, and cigarette use on the initiation, reinitiation and persistence of non-medical use of opioids, sedatives, and tranquilizers in adults. Drug Alcohol Depend. 2016;159:86–92.

33. Reisfield GM, Wasan AD, Jamison RN. The prevalence and significance of cannabis use in patients prescribed chronic opioid therapy: a review of the extant literature. Pain Med. 2009;10:1434–41.
34. Fiellin LE, Tetrault JM, Becker WC, Fiellin DA, Desai RA. Prior use of alcohol, cigarettes, and marijuana and subsequent abuse of prescription opioids in young adults. J Adolesc Health. 2013;52(2):158–63. doi:10.1016/j.jadohealth.2012.06.010.
35. Moss HB, Chen CM, Yi H. Early adolescent patterns of alcohol, cigarettes, and marijuana polysubstance use and young adult substance use outcomes in a nationally representative sample. Drug Alcohol Depend. 2014;136:51–62.
36. Day C. Benzodiazepines in combination with opioid pain relievers or alcohol: greater risk of more serious ed visit outcomes. 2014 Dec 18. In: The CBHSQ report. Rockville (MD): Substance Abuse and Mental Health Services Administration (US); 2013. Available from: https://www.ncbi.nlm.nih.gov/books/NBK384672/?report=classic.
37. Hwang CS, Kang EM, Kornegay CJ, Staffa JA, Jones CM, McAninch JK. Trends in the concomitant prescribing of opioids and benzodiazepines, 2002-2014. Am J Prev Med. 2016;51:151–60.
38. Yarborough BJ, Stumbo SP, Janoff SL, Yarborough MT, McCarty D, Chilcoat HD, et al. Understanding opioid overdose characteristics involving prescription and illicit opioids: a mixed methods analysis. Drug Alcohol Depend. 2016;167:49–56.
39. Nielsen S, Lintzeris N, Bruno R, Campbell G, Larance B, Hall W, et al. Benzodiazepine use among chronic pain patients prescribed opioids: associations with pain, physical and mental health, and health service utilization. Pain Med. 2015;16:356–66.
40. Park TW, Saitz R, Nelson KP, Xuan Z, Liebschutz JM, Lasser KE. The association between benzodiazepine prescription and aberrant drug-related behaviors in primary care patients receiving opioids for chronic pain. Subst Abus. 2016;37:516–20.
41. Skurtveit S, Furu K, Bramness J, Selmer R, Tverdal A. Benzodiazepines predict use of opioids--a follow-up study of 17,074 men and women. Pain Med. 2010;11:805–14.
42. Regier DA, Rae DS, Narrow WE, Kaelber CT, Schatzberg AF. Prevalence of anxiety disorders and their comorbidity with mood and addictive disorders. Br J Psychiatry Suppl. 1998;34:24–8.
43. Castle DJ. Anxiety and substance use: layers of complexity. Expert Rev. Neurother. 2008;8:493–501.
44. Fatséas M, Denis C, Lavie E, Auriacombe M. Relationship between anxiety disorders and opiate dependence--a systematic review of the literature: implications for diagnosis and treatment. J Subst Abus Treat. 2010;38:220–30.
45. Wolitzky-Taylor K, Operskalski JT, Ries R, Craske MG, Roy-Byrne P. Understanding and treating comorbid anxiety disorders in substance users: review and future directions. J Addict Med. 2011;5:233–47.
46. Martins SS, Keyes KM, Storr CL, Zhu H, Chilcoat HD. Pathways between nonmedical opioid use/dependence and psychiatric disorders: results from the national epidemiologic survey on alcohol and related conditions. Drug Alcohol Depend. 2009;103:16–24.
47. Martins SS, Fenton MC, Keyes KM, Blanco C, Zhu H, Storr CL. Mood/anxiety disorders and their association with non-medical prescription opioid use and prescription opioid use disorder: longitudinal evidence from the national epidemiologic study on alcohol and related conditions. Psychol Med. 2012;42:1261–72.
48. Quartana PJ, Campbell CM, Edwards RR. Pain catastrophizing: a critical review. Expert Rev. Neurother. 2009;9:745–58.
49. Theunissen M, Peters ML, Bruce J, Gramke HF, Marcus MA. Preoperative anxiety and catastrophizing: a systematic review and meta-analysis of the association with chronic postsurgical pain. Clin J Pain. 2012;28:819–41.
50. Wertli MM, Eugster R, Held U, Steurer J, Kofmehl R, Weiser S. Catastrophizing-a prognostic factor for outcome in patients with low back pain: a systematic review. Spine J. 2014;14:2639–57.

51. Morasco BJ, Turk DC, Donovan DM, Dobscha SK. Risk for prescription opioid misuse among patients with a history of substance use disorder. Drug Alcohol Depend. 2013;127:193–9.
52. Martel M, Wasan A, Jamison R, Edwards R. Catastrophic thinking and increased risk for prescription opioid misuse in patients with chronic pain. Drug Alcohol Depend. 2013;132:335–41.
53. Darnall BD. Pain psychology and pain catastrophizing in the perioperative setting: a review of impacts, interventions and unmet needs. Hand Clin. 2016;32:33–9.
54. American Psychiatric Association. Diagnostic and statistical manual of mental disorders. 5th ed. Arlington: American Psychiatric Association; 2013.
55. Moeller-Bertram T, Keltner J, Strigo IA. Pain and post traumatic stress disorder - review of clinical and experimental evidence. Neuropharmacology. 2012;62:586–97.
56. Brennstuhl MJ, Tarquinio C, Montel S. Chronic pain and PTSD: evolving views on their comorbidity. Perspect Psychiatr Care. 2015;51:295–304.
57. Fishbain DA, Pulikal A, Lewis JE, Gao J. Chronic pain types differ in their reported prevalence of post-traumatic stress disorder (PTSD) and there is consistent evidence that chronic pain is associated with PTSD: an evidence-based structured systematic review. Pain Med. 2016;18(4):711–35.
58. Cottler LB, Compton WM, Mager D, Spitznagel EL, Janca A. Posttraumatic stress disorder among substance users from the general population. Am J Psychiatry. 1992;149:664–70.
59. Mills KL, Mills M, Lynskey M, Teesson J, Ross S, Darke S. Post-traumatic stress disorder among people with heroin dependence in the Australian treatment outcome study (ATOS): prevalence and correlates. Drug Alcohol Depend. 2005;77:243–9.
60. Seal KH, Shi Y, Cohen G, Cohen BE, Maguen S, Krebs EE, Neylan TC. Association of mental health disorders with prescription opioids and high-risk opioid use in US veterans of Iraq and Afghanistan. JAMA. 2012;307:940–7.
61. Meier A, Lambert-Harris C, McGovern MP, Xie H, An M, McLeman B. Co-occurring prescription opioid use problems and posttraumatic stress disorder symptom severity. Am J Drug Alcohol Abuse. 2014;40:304–11.
62. Kerridge BT, Saha TD, Chou SP, Zhang H, Jung J, Ruan WJ, et al. Gender and nonmedical prescription opioid use and DSM-5 nonmedical prescription opioid use disorder: results from the National Epidemiologic Survey on alcohol and related conditions–III. Drug Alcohol Depend. 2015;156:47–56.
63. Smith KZ, Smith PH, Cercone SA, McKee SA, Homish GG. Past year non-medical opioid use and abuse and PTSD diagnosis: interactions with sex and associations with symptom clusters. Addict Behav. 2016;58:167–74.
64. Bair MJ, Robinson RL, Katon W, Kroenke K. Depression and pain comorbidity: a literature review. Arch Intern Med. 2003;163:2433–45.
65. Gureje O, Von Korff M, Kola L, Demyttenaere K, He Y, Posada-Villa J, et al. The relation between multiple pains and mental disorders: results from the world mental health surveys. Pain. 2008;135:82–91.
66. Demyttenaere K, Reed C, Quail D, Bauer M, Dantchev N, Montejo AL, et al. Presence and predictors of pain in depression: results from the FINDER study. J Affect Disord. 2010;125:53–60.
67. Becker WC, Sullivan LE, Tetrault JM, Desai RA, Fiellin DA. Non-medical use, abuse and dependence on prescription opioids among U.S. adults: psychiatric, medical and substance use correlates. Drug Alcohol Depend. 2008;94:38–47.
68. Goldner EM, Lusted A, Roerecke M, Rehm J, Fischer B. Prevalence of Axis-1 psychiatric (with focus on depression and anxiety) disorder and symptomatology among non-medical prescription opioid users in substance use treatment: systematic review and meta-analyses. Addict Behav. 2014;39:520–31.
69. Scherrer JF, Salas J, Copeland LA, Stock EM, Ahmedani BK, Sullivan MD, et al. Prescription opioid duration, dose, and increased risk of depression in 3 large patient populations. Ann Fam Med. 2016;14:54–62.

70. Scherrer JF, Salas J, Schneider FD, Bucholz KK, Sullivan MD, Copeland LA, et al. Characteristics of new depression diagnoses in patients with and without prior chronic opioid use. J Affect Disord. 2017;210:125–9.
71. Fink DS, Hu R, Cerdá M, Keyes KM, Marshall BDL, Galea S, et al. Patterns of major depression and nonmedical use of prescription opioids in the United States. Drug Alcohol Depend. 2015;153:258–64.
72. Stubbs B, Eggermont L, Mitchell AJ, De Hert M, Correll CU, Soundy A, et al. The prevalence of pain in bipolar disorder: a systematic review and large-scale meta-analysis. Acta Psychiatr Scand. 2015;131:75–88.
73. Hunt GE, Malhi GS, Cleary M, Lai HM, Sitharthan T. Prevalence of comorbid bipolar and substance use disorders in clinical settings, 1990-2015: systematic review and meta-analysis. J Affect Disord. 2016;206:331–49.
74. Hunt GE, Malhig GS, Cleary M, Lai HM, Sitharthan T. Comorbidity of bipolar and substance use disorders in national surveys of general populations, 1990–2015: systematic review and meta-analysis. J Affect Disord. 2016;206:321–30.
75. Tragesser SL, Jones RE, Robinson RJ, Stutler A, Stewart A. Borderline personality disorder features and risk for prescription opioid use disorders. J Personal Disord. 2013;27:427–41.
76. Frankenburg FR, Fitzmaurice GM, Zanarini MC. The use of prescription opioid medication by patients with borderline personality disorder and axis II comparison subjects: a 10-years follow-up study. J Clin Psychiatry. 2014;75:357–61.
77. Campbell G, Bruno R, Darke S, Degenhardt L. Associations of borderline personality with pain, problems with medications and suicidality in a community sample of chronic non-cancer pain patients prescribed opioids for pain. Gen Hosp Psychiatry. 2015;37:434–40.
78. Saha TD, Kerridge BT, Goldstein RB, Chou SP, Zhang H, Jung J, et al. Nonmedical prescription opioid use and DSM-5 nonmedical prescription opioid use disorder in the United States. J Clin Psychiatry. 2016;77:772–80.
79. Robles E, Huang BE, Simpson PM, McMillan DE. Delay discounting, impulsiveness, and addiction severity in opioid-dependent patients. J Subst Abus Treat. 2011;41:354–62.
80. Nielsen DA, Ho A, Bahl A, Varma P, Kellogg S, Borg L, et al. Former heroin addicts with or without a history of cocaine dependence are more impulsive than controls. Drug Alcohol Depend. 2012;124:113–20.
81. Marino EN, Rosen KD, Gutierrez A, Eckmann M, Ramamurthy S, Potter JS. Impulsivity but not sensation seeking is associated with opioid analgesic misuse risk in patients with chronic pain. Addict Behav. 2013;38:2154–7.
82. Milivojevic D, Milovanovic SD, Jovanovic M, Svrakic DM, Svrakic NM, Svrakic SM, et al. Temperament and character modify risk of drug addiction and influence choice of drugs. Am J Addict. 2012;21:462–7.
83. Zaaijer ER, Bruijel J, Blanken P, Hendriks V, Koeter MW, Kreek MJ, et al. Personality as a risk factor for illicit opioid use and a protective factor for illicit opioid dependence. Drug Alcohol Depend. 2014;145:101–5.
84. Conroy E, Degenhardt L, Mattick RP, Nelson EC. Child maltreatment as a risk factor for opioid dependence: comparison of family characteristics and type and severity of child maltreatment with a matched control group. Child Abuse Negl. 2009;33:343–52.
85. Nurco DN, Kinlock TW, O'Grady KE, Hanlon TE. Differential contributions of family and peer factors to the etiology of narcotic addiction. Drug Alcohol Depend. 1998;51:229–37.
86. Becoa E, Martinez U, Calafat A, Juan M, Fernandez-Hermida JR, Secades-Villa R. Parental styles and drug use: a review. Drugs Educ Prev Polic. 2012;19(1):1–10.
87. Barnow S, Schuckit MA, Lucht M, John U, Freyberger HJ. The importance of a positive family history of alcoholism, parental rejection and emotional warmth, behavioral problems and peer substance use for alcohol problems in teenagers: a path analysis. J Stud Alcohol. 2002;63:305–15.
88. Denton WH, Adinoff BH, Lewis D, Walker R, Winhusen T. Family discord is associated with increased substance use for pregnant substance users. Subst Use Misuse. 2014;49:326–32.

89. Yoon G, Westermeyer J, Warwick M, Kuskowski MA. Substance use disorders and adoption: findings from a national sample. PLoS One. 2012;7(11):e49655. doi:10.1371/journal.pone.0049655.
90. Preter M, Klein DF. Panic, suffocation false alarms, separation anxiety and endogenous opioids. Prog Neuro-Psychopharmacol Biol Psychiatry. 2008;32(3):603–12.
91. Preter M, Klein DF. Lifelong opioidergic vulnerability through early life separation: a recent extension of the false suffocation alarm theory of panic disorder. Neurosci Biobehav Rev. 2014;46:345–51.
92. Sullivan MD, Edlund MJ, Steffick D, Unutzer J. Regular use of prescribed opioids: association with common psychiatric disorders. Pain. 2005;119:95–103.
93. Kelly JP, Cook SF, Kaufman DW, Anderson T, Rosenberg L, Mitchell AA. Prevalence and characteristics of opioid use in the US adult population. Pain. 2008;138:507–13.
94. Greenspan J, Craft R, LeResche L, Arendt-Nielsen L, Berkley K, Fillingim R, et al. Studying sex and gender differences in pain and analgesia: a consensus report. Pain. 2007;132:S26–45.
95. Tsang A, Von Korff M, Lee S, Alonso J, Karam E, Angermeyer MC, et al. Common chronic pain conditions in developed and developing countries: gender and age differences and comorbidity with depression-anxiety disorders. J Pain. 2008;9:883–91.
96. Tetrault JM, Desai RA, Becker WC, Fiellin DA, Concato J, Sullivan LE. Gender and non-medical use of prescription opioids: results from a national US survey. Addiction. 2007;103:258–68.
97. Back SE, Payne RL, Simpson AN, Brady KT. Gender and prescription opioids: findings from the national survey on drug use and health. Addict Behav. 2010;235:1001–7.
98. Jamison RN, Butler SF, Budman SH, Edwards RR, Wasan AD. Gender differences in risk factors for aberrant prescription opioid use. J Pain. 2010;11:312–20.
99. Campbell CI, Weisner C, LeResche L, Ray GT, Saunders K, Sullivan MD, et al. Age and gender trends in long-term opioid analgesic use for noncancer pain. Am J Public Health. 2010;100:2541–7.
100. Substance Abuse and Mental Health Services Administration. Results from the 2013 national survey on drug use and health – detailed tables. Rockville, MD: Substance Abuse and Mental Health Services Administration; 2014.
101. Manubay J, Davidson J, Vosburg S, Jones J, Comer S, Sullivan M. Sex differences among opioid-abusing patients with chronic pain in a clinical trial. J Addict Med. 2015;9:46–52.
102. Dembo R, Dertke M, LaVoie L, Borders S, Washburn M, Schmeidler J. Physical abuse, sexual victimization and illicit drug use: a structural analysis among high risk adolescents. J Adolesc. 1987;10:13–33.
103. Brown GR, Anderson B. Psychiatric comorbidity in adult inpatients with childhood histories of sexual and physical abuse. Am J Psychiatry. 1991;148:55–61.
104. Paone D, Chavkin W, Willets I, Friedman P, DesJarlais D. The impact of sexual abuse: implications for drug treatment. J Women's Health. 1992;1:149–53.
105. Bennett EM, Kemper KJ. Is abuse during childhood a risk factor for developing substance abuse problems as an adult? Develop Behav Pediatr. 1994;15:426–9.
106. Heffernan K, Cloitre M, Tardiff K, Marzuk PM, Portera L, Leon AC. Childhood trauma as a correlate of lifetime opiate use in psychiatric patients. Addict Behav. 2000;25:797–803.
107. Balousek S, Plane MB, Fleming M. Prevalence of interpersonal abuse in primary care patients prescribed opioids for chronic pain. J Gen Intern Med. 2007;22:1268–73.
108. Young A, Grey M, Boyd CJ, McCabe SE. Adolescent sexual assault and the medical and nonmedical use of prescription medication. J Addict Nurs. 2011;11:25–31.
109. Lawson KM, Back SE, Hartwell KJ, Maria MM-S, Brady KT. A comparison of trauma profiles among individuals with prescription opioid, nicotine or cocaine dependence. Am J Addict. 2013;22:127–31.
110. Smith PH, Homish GG, Leonard KE, Cornelius JR. Intimate partner violence and specific substance use disorders: findings from the national epidemiologic survey on alcohol and related conditions. Psychol Addict Behav. 2012;26:236–45.

111. Blanco C, Wall MM, Okuda M, Wang S, Iza M, Olfson M. Pain as a predictor of opioid use disorder in a nationally representative sample. Am J Psychiatry. 2016;173:1189–95.
112. Sehgal N, Manchikanti L, Smith HS. Prescription opioid abuse in chronic pain: a review of opioid abuse predictors and strategies to curb opioid abuse. Pain Physician. 2012;15(3 Suppl):ES67–92.
113. Jamison RN, Link CL, Marceau LD. Do pain patients at high risk for substance misuse experience more pain? A longitudinal outcomes study. Pain Med. 2009;10:1084–94.
114. Liebschutz JM, Saitz R, Weiss RD, Averbuch T, Schwartz S, Meltzer EC, et al. Clinical factors associated with prescription drug use disorder in urban primary care patients with chronic pain. J Pain. 2010;11:1047–55.
115. Liebman PM, Lehofer M, Schönauer-Cejpek M, Legl T, Pernhaupt G, Moser M, et al. Pain sensitivity in former opioid addicts. Lancet. 1994;344:1031–2.
116. Compton P, Charuvastra VC, Kintaudi K, Ling W. Pain responses in methadone-maintained opioid abusers. J Pain Symptom Manag. 2000;20:237–345.
117. Wasan AD, Butler SF, Budman SH, Benoit C, Fernandez K, Jamison RN. Psychiatric history and psychologic adjustment as risk factors for aberrant drug-related behavior among patients with chronic pain. Clin J Pain. 2007;23:307–15.
118. Manchikanti L, Giordano J, Boswell MV, Fellows B, Manchukonda R, Pampati V. Psychological factors as predictors of opioid abuse and illicit drug use in chronic pain patients. J Opioid Manag. 2007;3:89–100.
119. Edlund MJ, Martin BC, Fan M-Y, Devries A, Braden JB, Sullivan MD. Risks for opioid abuse and dependence among recipients of chronic opioid therapy: results from the TROUP study. Drug Alcohol Depend. 2010;112:90–8.
120. Sullivan MD, Edlund MJ, Fan M-Y, DeVries A, Braden JB, Martin BC. Risks for possible and probable opioid misuse among recipients of chronic opioid therapy in commercial and Medicaid insurance plans: the TROUP study. Pain. 2010;150:332–9.
121. Edlund MJ, Martin BC, Russo JE, Devries A, Braden JB, Sullivan MD. The role of opioid prescription in incident opioid abuse and dependence among individuals with chronic noncancer pain: the role of opioid prescription. Clin J Pain. 2014;30:557–64.
122. Food and Drug Administration, Public Health Service, U.S. Department of Health and Human Services. FDA boxed warning for immediate-release opioids. J Pain Pall Care Pharmacother. 2016;30:141–5.
123. White AG, Birnbaum HG, Schiller M, Tang J, Katz NP. Analytic models to identify patients at risk for prescription opioid abuse. Am J Manag Care. 2009;15:897–906.
124. Henry SG, Wilsey BL, Melnikow JA, Iosif A-M. Dose escalation during the first year of long-term opioid therapy for chronic pain. Pain Med. 2015;16:733–44.
125. Cochran BN, Flentje A, Heck NC, Van Den Bos J, Perlman D, Torres J, et al. Factors predicting development of opioid use disorders among individuals who receive an initial opioid prescription: mathematical modeling using a database of commercially-insured individuals. Drug Alcohol Depend. 2014;138:202–8.
126. Boscarino JA, Rukstalis M, Hoffman SN, Han JJ, Erlich PM, Gerhard GS, et al. Risk factors for drug dependence among out-patients on opioid therapy in a large US health-care system. Addiction. 2010;105:1776–82.
127. Rice JB, White AG, Birnbaum HG, Schiller M, Brown DA, Roland CL. A model to identify patients at risk for prescription opioid abuse, dependence, and misuse. Pain Med. 2012;13:1162–73.
128. Dufour R, Mardekian J, Pasquale MK, Schaaf D, Andrews GA, Patel NC. Understanding predictors of opioid abuse: predictive model development and validation. Am J Pharmacy Benefits. 2014;6:208–16.
129. Ciesielski T, Iyengar R, Bothra A, Tomala D, Cislo G, Gage BF. A tool to assess risk of de novo opioid abuse or dependence. Am J Med. 2016;129:699–705.
130. Quinn PD, Hur K, Chang Z, Krebs EE, Bair MJ, Scott EL, et al. Incident and long-term opioid therapy among patients with psychiatric conditions and medications: a national study of commercial health care claims. Pain. 2017;158:140–8.

131. Atluri SL, Sudarshan G. Development of a screening tool to detect the risk of inappropriate prescription opioid use in patients with chronic pain. Pain Physician. 2004;7:333–8.
132. Manchikanti L, Singh V, Damron KS, Beyer CD, Pampati V. Screening for controlled substance abuse in interventional pain management settings: evaluation of an assessment tool. Pain Physician. 2003;6:425–33.
133. Manchikanti L, Pampati V, Damron KS, McManus CD. Evaluation of variables in illicit drug use: does a controlled substance abuse screening tool identify illicit drug use? Pain Physician. 2004;7:71–5.
134. Webster LR, Webster RM. Predicting aberrant behaviors in opioid-treated patients: preliminary validation of the opioid risk tool. Pain Med. 2005;6:432–42.
135. Moore TM, Jones T, Browder JH, Daffron S, Passik SD. A comparison of common screening methods for predicting aberrant drug-related behavior among patients receiving opioids for chronic pain management. Pain Med. 2009;10:1426–33.
136. Jones T, Moore T, Levy JL, Daffron S, Browder JH, Allen L, et al. A comparison of various risk screening methods in predicting discharge from opioid treatment. Clin J Pain. 2012;28:93–100.
137. Barclay JS, Owens JE, Blackhall LJ. Screening for substance abuse risk in cancer patients using the opioid risk tool and urine drug screen. Support Care Cancer. 2014;22:1883–8.
138. Butler SF, Budman SH, Fernandez K, Jamison RN. Validation of a screener and opioid assessment measure for patients with chronic pain. Pain. 2004;112:65–75.
139. Akbik H, Butler SF, Budman SH, Fernandez K, Katz NP, Jamison RN. Validation and clinical application of the screener and opioid assessment for patients with pain (SOAPP). J Pain Symptom Manag. 2006;32:287–93.
140. Butler SF, Fernandez K, Benoit C, Budman SH, Jamison RN. Validation of the revised screener and opioid assessment for patients with pain (SOAPP-R). J Pain. 2008;9:360–72.
141. Butler SF, Budman SH, Fernandez KC, Fanciullo GJ, Jamison RN. Cross-validation of a screener to predict opioid misuse in chronic pain patients (SOAPP-R). J Addict Med. 2009;3:66–73.
142. Weiner SG, Horton LC, Green TC, Butler SF. A comparison of an opioid abuse screening tool and prescription drug monitoring data in the emergency department. Drug Alcohol Depend. 2016;159:152–7.
143. Screener and Opioid Assessment for Patients with Pain (SOAPP)® Version 1.0-SF https://www.nhms.org/sites/default/files/Pdfs/SOAPP-5.pd
144. Koyyalagunta D, Bruera E, Aigner C, Nusrat H, Driver L, Novy D. Risk stratification of opioid misuse among patients with cancer pain using the SOAPP-SF. Pain Med. 2013;14:667–75.
145. Belgrade MJ, Schamber CD, Lindgren BR. The DIRE score: predicting outcomes of opioid prescribing for chronic pain. J Pain. 2006;7:671–81.
146. Chou R, Fanciullo GJ, Fine PG, Miaskowski C, Passik SD, Portenoy RK. Opioids for chronic noncancer pain: prediction and identification of aberrant drug-related behaviors: a review of the evidence for an American pain society and American academy of pain medicine clinical practice guideline. J Pain. 2009;10:131–46.
147. Harris RP, Helfand M, Woolf SH, Lohr KN, Mulrow CD, Teutsch SM, et al. Current methods of the third US preventive services task force. Am J Prev Med. 2001;20:21–35.
148. Gourlay DL, Heit HA, Almahrezi A. Universal precautions in pain medicine: a rational approach to the treatment of chronic pain. Pain Med. 2005;6:107–12.
149. Brown J, Setnik B, Lee K, Wase L, Roland CL, Cleveland JM, et al. Assessment, stratification, and monitoring of the risk for prescription opioid misuse and abuse in the primary care setting. J Opioid Manag. 2011;7:467–83.
150. Portenoy RK. Opioid therapy for chronic non-malignant pain: a review of the critical issues. J Pain Symptom Manag. 1996;11:203–17.
151. Savage SR. Long-term opioid therapy: assessment of consequences and risks. J Pain Symptom Manag. 1996;1:274–86.
152. Adams LL, Gatchel RJ, Robinson RC, Polatin P, Gajraj N, Deschner M, et al. Development of a self-report screening instrument for assessing potential opioid medication misuse in chronic pain patients. J Pain Symptom Manag. 2004;27:440–59.

153. Holmes CP, Gatchel RJ, Adams LL, Stowell AW, Hatten A, Noe C, et al. An opioid screening instrument: long-term evaluation of the utility of the pain medication questionnaire. Pain Pract. 2006;6:74–88.
154. Buelow AK, Haggard R, Gatchel RJ. Additional validation of the pain medication questionnaire in a heterogeneous sample of chronic pain patients. Pain Pract. 2009;9:428–34.
155. Butler SF, Budman SH, Fernandez KC, Houle B, Benoit C, Katz N, et al. Development and validation of the current opioid misuse measure. Pain. 2007;130:144–56.
156. Butler SF, Budman SH, Fanciullo GJ, Jamison RN. Cross validation of the current opioid misuse measure (COMM) to monitor chronic pain patients on opioid therapy. Clin J Pain. 2010;26:770–6.
157. Miotto K, Compton P, Ling W, Conolly M. Diagnosing addictive disease in chronic pain patients. Psychosomatics. 1996;37:223–35.
158. Compton P, Darakjian MA, Miotto K. Screening for addiction in patients with chronic pain and "problematic" substance use: evaluation of a pilot assessment tool. J Pain Symptom Manag. 1998;16:355–63.
159. Compton PA, Wu SM, Schieffer B, Pham Q, Naliboff BD. Introduction of a self-report version of the prescription drug use questionnaire and relationship to medication agreement non-compliance. J Pain Symptom Manag. 2008;36:383–95.
160. Banta-Green CJ, Merrill JO, Doyle SR, Boudreau DM, Calsyn DA. Measurement of opioid problems among chronic pain patients in a general medical population. Drug Alcohol Depend. 2009;104:43–9.
161. Manchikanti L, Alturi S, Trescot AM, Giordano J. Monitoring opioid adherence in chronic pain patients: tools, techniques and utility. Pain Physician. 2008;11:S155–80.
162. Solanki DR, Koyyalagunta D, Shah RV, Silverman SM, Manchikanti L. Monitoring opioid adherence in chronic pain patients: assessment of risk of substance misuse. Pain Physician. 2011;14(2):E119–31.
163. Crumpton SD, Sutheimer CA. Specimen adulteration and substitution in workplace drug testing. Forensic Sci Rev. 2007;19:1–27.
164. Peppin JF, Passik SD, Couto JE, Fine PG, Christo PJ, Argoff C, et al. Recommendations for urine drug monitoring as a component of opioid therapy in the treatment of chronic pain. Pain Med. 2012;13:886–96.

Chapter 11
Addressing Host Factors: Primary, Secondary, and Tertiary Prevention of Opioid Dependence

Your practice administrator brings you a notecard mailed from a former heroin-addicted patient whom you had provided medication-assisted treatment (buprenorphine) to in the context of intensive one-on-one counseling in the office, as well as required professional substance abuse rehabilitation counseling, and also participation in community-based mutual support group.

You have not heard from this patient in over a year, and despite successful wean off of substitution therapy (with abstinence from heroin) she did not follow through with extended-release naltrexone injections as advised. For months you feared she had relapsed, and over time you forgot about her.

The notecard is brief but poignant, expressing gratitude for the firm and directive therapy and counseling you delivered in a caring and nonjudgmental manner. She recounts that despite her trepidation and fears, she "came clean" with her family and fiancé and to her relief found not only forgiveness and healing of old relational wounds but also accountability and structure. She has managed to keep her job, and she writes the notecard on her 1-year work anniversary there. She has continued in an active participation role within a "Celebrate Recovery" group in her city and expresses interest in assuming a position of leadership therein.

H.B. McAnally, *Opioid Dependence*, DOI 10.1007/978-3-319-47497-7_11

She has been heroin-free now for over 2 years and states in the closing sentences of the card that she has found resolution of her shame and that the "track marks" on her arms that she previously went to great efforts to conceal now serve as both reminder to her of choices and a lifestyle she cannot see ever returning to. She states that the acceptance and care from her fiancé, family, and new faith community (and its sponsored Celebrate Recovery group) provide her with a sense of fulfillment and purpose that she desires to share with others who struggle with opioid addiction.

Introduction

While pertinent to infectious diseases, the concept of prevention strata (primary, secondary, tertiary) has been widely adopted for many noncommunicable diseases of significance (e.g., diabetes, hypertension, coronary disease, cancer, etc.) and more recently has been proposed as a reasonable schema to organize efforts targeted at reductions in opioid (and other substance) dependence [1, 2].

Primary prevention is that which seeks to avert the onset of disease or injury in individuals who have not yet experienced it; this is prevention as most people know it. Modification of risk factors when possible (e.g., vaccination, quarantine of infected individuals, lifestyle modifications) comprises the essence of primary prevention. Opioid exposure reduction, while ultimately the responsibility of the individual host, is obviously also a function of vector (prescriber) modification in this paradigm and comprises the bulk of the subject matter of Part III of this book. Nonetheless, it is considered again in this chapter in the context of the host, as the actual physical exposure to the agent is a function of the host using the medication either in compliance with or in deviation from the prescription. As discussed in Chap. 1, a critical and assumed ingredient in a population's effort to end an epidemic is the inherent desire of the vulnerable population to avoid the agent. Unfortunately in the case of addiction, rational self-preservation instincts are surrendered or are conquered by the overwhelming compulsion to seek the addictive substance (or activity) regardless of the results, as discussed in some detail in Chap. 9.

Screening for those at risk of developing, or those who have already developed mild to moderate, or at least clandestine opioid dependence was discussed in the previous chapter. *Secondary prevention* aims to identify (generally by screening programs) and reverse if possible the early effects of the disease or injury state or at least retard its progression. Examples from the noncommunicable disease world include diet and exercise changes as well as antiplatelet pharmacotherapy in cases of known coronary disease and similar lifestyle modifications and hypoglycemic pharmacotherapies in cases of known diabetes.

Without clear-cut objective biomarkers for opioid dependence (such as are available for most infectious and noncommunicable diseases) determining the absence vs. presence of disease is difficult at best, often rendering the line between primary and secondary prevention blurry. Furthermore, interventions at these levels share considerable overlap. Clinical strategies for both primary prevention and also reversal of early/mild opioid dependence are presented again briefly, based on recent national clinical practice guidelines and also the author's experience. More detailed components of these strategies may be found in previous chapters.

Tertiary prevention consists of efforts to attenuate the consequences of established disease ("harm reduction") and comprises the final subject matter of the chapter.

Primary Prevention

Primary prevention can be considered as simply taking steps to ensure that hosts do not develop a disease. It is prevention as most of us think of it. Preventing the development of disease may be a straightforward matter in some situations, such as we have been fortunate enough to have discovered with the development of effective vaccines for several viral and some bacterial infections. In other situations, e.g., Type II diabetes, it may be a very complicated matter without the option of simple immunization, relying instead upon alteration of modifiable risk factors through intensive and sustained lifestyle changes (diet, exercise, and so on.)

As has been discussed previously, elimination of the agent or the vector is neither feasible nor desirable; attenuation of host vulnerability is both. Reducing exposure is one way to reduce host vulnerability, but it is a fragile tactic dependent upon factors (individual and societal/environmental) that are highly unpredictable. Restriction of opioid availability certainly plays a role in the overall effort to reduce dependence, but in addition to the unfeasibility of elimination, the agent may mutate, so to speak. While the analogy breaks down somewhat, just like influenza strains, oxycodone becomes heroin or worse. Similarly, reduction in euphoric/hedonic reward properties of therapeutic opioids is laudable but does not protect against simple shift in drug of choice (or synthesis of new ones).

Reducing vulnerability/risk factors will be required if opioid dependence is to be attenuated. While this has been effectively achieved in the infectious disease world by conferring literal immunity to the agent, in the chronic noninfectious disease world such elegant solutions elude us. Literal vaccination to at least certain "strains" of the agent (e.g., oxycodone) has been explored in animal models [3, 4], and while this author personally finds the notion of elimination of that particular agent a goal worthy of any (Fig. 11.1) [5] and all efforts, it is unlikely to achieve individual- or population-level immunity. Opioid agent classes differ physically enough that immunoassays used for urine drug screening do not recognize molecules with sufficiently diverse chemical structure, and similarly artificial immunity to one class is unlikely to span phenanthrenes, phenylheptylamines, and phenylpiperidines, just as patients' opioid allergies (another immune-mediated phenomenon) tend to be class specific. Furthermore, just as with reduction of availability, simple shift in drug of choice may occur as has been seen with the tremendous surge in heroin use over the past few years as prescription opioids become more difficult to procure.

Where widespread cultivation of actual humoral (antibody-mediated) immunity to exogenous opioids is possible, not only would this be undesirable in that it would

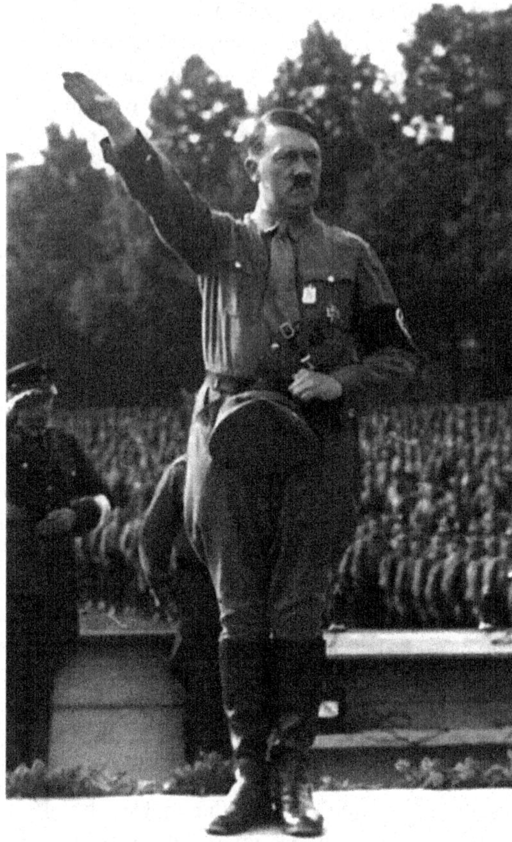

Fig. 11.1 Oxycodone fueled the Führer [5]. By Bundesarchiv, Bild 146–1982-159-22A/ CC-BY-SA 3.0, CC BY-SA 3.0 de, https://commons.wikimedia.org/w/index.php?curid=6699198

render the host now unable to respond to therapeutic opioids, but their own endogenous opioids (β-endorphin, endomorphin) would likely also be rendered nonfunctional. Besides essentially conferring the individual to a life of misery not only from significant pathology but also potentially from inconceivable amplification/sensitization to pain, perturbation of the complex neuroimmunoendocrine system as it interfaces with the endogenous opioid system could result. Development of autoimmune sequelae is not inconceivable either.

Prophylactic mu-receptor antagonism (naltrexone in the water supply) could conceptually fall under the rubric of primary prevention but is neither without risk (hepatotoxicity, inability to respond to necessary therapeutic opioids) nor ethical challenge. This approach is however certainly effective and indicated in addiction recovery, and is discussed below at some length in the section on tertiary prevention.

Primary prevention as applied to opioid misuse and abuse must take the form of risk factor reduction. In a sense, modifiable risk factor reduction as discussed above in the case of chronic noninfectious diseases such as diabetes may be thought of to some degree as the development of *behavioral immunity* [6] to agents (e.g., simple sugars, sedentariness) that elicit or contribute to the pathophysiologic response of insulin resistance and the sequelae of sustained hyperglycemia.

Conferring behavioral immunity to opioid dependence must of course involve reduction or elimination of the desire to seek and use the drug, and this is most effectively achieved via both negative and positive motivators. Negative motivation in terms of the physician-patient relationship is limited essentially to education and includes instillation of respect and even fear of adverse consequences related to opioids (see Chap. 3). Human beings however are not always inclined to make the most logical decisions nor those in their own best interest, as Dostoevsky expresses so unapologetically:

> "...when in all these thousands of years has there been a time when man has acted only from his own interest? What is to be done with the millions of facts that bear witness that men, consciously, that is fully understanding their real interests, have left them in the background and have rushed headlong on another path... another difficult, absurd way, seeking it almost in the darkness..." [7]

Various health behavior models including the health belief model [8] note this universal observation that awareness of adverse consequences is not always enough to ensure healthy choices and behaviors. If the perceived benefits (alleviation of physical or emotional/psychological suffering deemed intolerable otherwise) outweigh perceived negative consequences (physical and psychological health, societal, legal) in the mind of the user, ongoing and progressive use will occur. Perceived susceptibility to and severity of a threat or negative outcome are not the only determinants of health-related (or other) choices; the belief in one's ability to alter an outcome (self-efficacy) and the relative desirability thereof affect the behavior as well [8, 9].

Psychological opinion (and the evidence underlying it) has been divided for decades as to whether punishment or reward is more effective at altering behaviors and choices; regardless it appears that both play an effective role in varying circumstances and presenting patients with all the data is rarely a bad thing.

Positive motivation for opioid avoidance may be instilled by promoting the benefits of a healthy lifestyle and non-opioid means of analgesia and pain management including behavioral strategies, complementary-alternative therapies in some cases, physiotherapy, and other pharmacology and procedural/operative interventions if appropriate. Even more beneficial to the patient is hearing themselves express these things. One of the techniques used in various counseling styles including motivational interviewing (described in greater detail below) is to help the patient/counselee identify and articulate their incentives both for and against instituting or at least pursuing a change of course; having the patient verbalize superseding goals excluding opioid use can be very beneficial to this end. The cultivation of self-efficacy and motivation has been well-documented as a critical component in behavioral change including cessation from substance use and misuse [10–12] and is presumably of positive benefit in prevention as well. While not drawn from the primary prevention literature, a study of 432 individuals from the 1991 to 1993 national Drug Abuse Treatment Outcome Studies (DATOS) sample who completed 5 years follow-up [13] reported that addicts who successfully remained in recovery demonstrated statistically significantly greater perception of self-motivation toward that end; this was in fact the most important discriminating factor in the analysis. Regardless of whether that self-assessment represents a personality "predictor variable" (power of positive thinking) or a "dependent variable" following success, the literature [10, 14, 15] as well as common sense advocates for early and constant attention toward fostering personal initiative and motivation.

Table 11.1 Motivational approaches to opioid dependence prevention in the individual

	Negative motivators aiding avoidance of opioid use	Positive motivators aiding avoidance of opioid use
Incentive theory (operant conditioning) motivators		Positive reinforcement/praise for healthy choices
Expectancy theory motivators	Education on adverse consequences of opioids	Education on benefits of opioid avoidance
Drive theory motivators		Obviation of need through effective pain management and through optimizing psychosocial-spiritual health

An obvious strategy for the prevention of opioid dependence is the efficacious treatment (or better yet, prevention) of pain—physical or otherwise—that might otherwise lead the patient to seek opioids. In psychological terms, this diminution/satisfaction of need is called drive reduction. An overview of prevention and rational/effective pain management addressing all salient pathologic contributors (including overall health deficiencies, organic "pain generator(s)" if applicable, and psychosocial dysfunction) was presented in Chap. 6. Given the primary role that the latter plays in the establishment of opioid dependence according to the literature and as discussed at some length in Chap. 10, the importance of effective behavioral health management in preventing opioid dependence cannot be overstated. Arguably, based on the strengths of association between other substance use disorders, anxiety, PTSD, various personality disorders, etc. and opioid dependence as discussed previously, the single most important aspect of primary prevention of opioid dependence may be aggressive psychosocial-spiritual screening and referral as indicated.

These strategies along with the motivational theories associated with them are presented in Table 11.1.

Environment is an epidemiologic concept not directly discussed to this point in the framework of this book and one that deserves focused consideration in the context of prevention. Environment in the classic epidemiologic triangle model encompasses any factors distinct from agent and host that influence the interaction between the two. In this book, the chief element of environment considered (given the target audience) has been the prescriber, conceptualized as vector. Other vectors exist of course, and beyond individuals responsible for the transmission of the agent, societal factors that influence both transmission and exposure behavior abound. Some of the more obvious environmental factors include legislation and regulation and public perception and the media. These latter, societal factors may represent the most important arena in which to target preventive efforts by educational campaigns. The impact of "peer pressure" upon behavior is well known to parents and the educational community and is not limited to children and adolescents. Humans are social creatures responding to, and for the most part adhering to norms (hence their existence and persistence) and cultivation of healthy respect/fear of opioids is arguably one of, if not the most important preventive strategies our nation can invest in. Analysis of numerous tobacco cessation campaigns at local and state levels have shown reduction rates as high as 60% in some communities, with most data showing 30–40% reduction [16]. The CDC's 3-month "Tips from Former Smokers" television advertisement campaign resulted in an estimated successful increase in cessation for over 100,000 individuals [17].

Effective environmental intervention however must go beyond simple focus on opioid shunning/negative incentive; viable alternatives for coping with pain and distress (or even boredom) must be presented and instilled into the culture. Beginning with the healthcare environment and extending into the educational system, workplace, and even popular culture, prevention by healthy lifestyle (biopsychosocially and spiritually) is essential and must be championed and demonstrated. Simple education on the profound interactions between poor sleep quality, sedentary state, poor posture and ergonomics, diet, etc. upon pain may be moderately labor-intensive "up front" but pay dividends over the years. In our practice, we have created a systematic (yet tailorable to the individual) program focusing on these basics as well as recognizing and replacing cognitive distortions such as pain catastrophization. Beyond health promotion, interested parties at every level must also be trained to educate (and model) non-opioid means of managing the inevitable and ubiquitous human experiences of physical and psychological/emotional pain. Such an approach should not be restricted to traditional medical/psychological remedies such as pharmacotherapy, physiotherapy, procedures, and cognitive behavioral therapy but should incorporate consideration of and possibly referral for diverse elements including complementary/alternative medicine and "third wave" systems such as the mindfulness method [18]. Education on pain biology/pathophysiology itself (neurophysiology-focused rather than anatomic-based) has been shown in several trials to result in significant improvements in pain perception and functional improvements [19, 20]. Exposing patients to nascent concepts such as adaptive cortical neural plasticity may confer profound benefit in instilling self-efficacy and internal locus of control, which are critical to prevention of opioid-seeking.

While not conducive to a systematic/formulaic approach, in our practice we have found that after establishing rapport with patients, gentle redirection away from the quagmire of external locus of control/passivity and desire for instant gratification to a place of self-efficacy and acceptance—with concomitant improvement in perceived pain—is possible with adequate knowledge, skill, and compassion. "One size does not fit all," and both content and sequence of counsel are highly individual. However, common elements include reassurance and education and gentle challenge/appeal to an ethic of toughness and courage, as well as encouragement toward establishment of community that can provide support and camaraderie.

It must be emphasized again that it is incumbent upon the physician to establish and maintain a good therapeutic relationship. While the merits or fallacies of the paternalistic medical model may be debated (in this author's opinion we have drifted too far from the physician as physician), there is absolutely no justification for valuation of other human beings as inferior and not deserving of respect and compassion.

The old dictum that "people don't care how much you know until they know how much you care" may be nowhere more appropriate than in the realm of chronic pain and suffering, where patients have likely encountered multiple providers in their search for relief, some of whom are more callous and genuinely disinterested than others in the fellow human being seeking their help.

The often-quoted Alcoholics Anonymous phrase "Fake it until you make it" may be worth reminding oneself if compassion does not come naturally or is frequently fatigued. Fuel for such practice may come from the knowledge that not only patient outcome but also physician reputation and even avoidance of litigation are proportional to the degree of empathy and care perceived by the patient [21–25].

While certainly outside the scope of this book, while focusing on environment it would be gross oversight to neglect the observation that at least temporal correlation exists between a global increase in diagnosis of mental health disorders [26] and the rapid rise in psychoactive substance use. Again, while admittedly within the realm of observation and speculation, ignoring the temporal correlation between the unprecedented extensive changes in Western social structures (e.g., family, neighborhoods and community, centrality of organized religion) over the past three decades and the increasing use of drugs both prescription and illicit may be profoundly shortsighted. Indeed, the literature for the past four decades has supported the protective influence of family cohesion and community support [13, 27–30] upon both psychological health and well-being and reduced substance use and abuse, and spirituality/religion has shown consistent positive association toward those ends as well [13, 30–33].

The tremendous success of spirituality-focused and faith-based programs upon substance misuse reduction at least at the tertiary prevention level [13, 30–35] should engender at the very least investigation into the nature of their influence upon environment, as well as exploration of their utility within a comprehensive primary and secondary prevention strategy. In our practice, while respecting the beliefs of each individual, we also advise openness to spiritual issues that may be the missing link, so to speak, in addressing the underlying distress and otherwise unmet needs and drives motivating substance seeking. To neglect the opportunity for prevention of opioid dependence (in human beings who possess far more faculties and dimensions than rats) afforded by philosophic and religious/spiritual growth and development is arguably at least as shortsighted as ignoring the necessity of biological/somatic health maintenance.

Secondary Prevention

The concepts of primary, secondary, and tertiary prevention form a useful paradigm for organizing thought and in many cases implementing intervention. In the "real world," there is considerable overlap in both targeted populations due to a number of difficulties including lack of sensitivity/specificity of measurement as well as inability to categorize what may be a continuous variable. The application of preventive strategy/tactics is accordingly also "blurry." While screening for disease is generally considered part of secondary prevention, in the context of opioid dependence (as with many other infectious and noninfectious conditions), screening for psychosocial diatheses or risk assessment as discussed at some length in the previous chapter is essential for identifying individuals at greater risk for the development of opioid dependence and therefore aiding in risk factor (pain, distress, opioid exposure) reduction. Given that opioid dependence may also in many cases represent a "remitting-relapsing" condition, such risk assessment and risk factor reduction play a role across the continuum.

Nonetheless, adherence to these categorical concepts is useful for organizing thought and at least population-level if not individually focused efforts. If primary prevention is essentially prevention, secondary prevention comprises detection and early treatment. Screening for opioid dependence was discussed at some length in the previous chapter and validated instruments for assessment of an individual's risk of abuse both before initiating an opioid therapy trial and during treatment have been developed and are increasingly utilized in clinical practice. Such ongoing monitoring has been shown to be associated with reduced abuse and misuse [36].

When identified (or suspected), early treatment of opioid dependence must begin with frank and compassionate counseling, reassessment of risk-benefit ratio for ongoing therapy, and in most cases formulation of a plan for weaning and discontinuation ("exit strategy"). A commonly used program is to decrease total daily dose by 10–20% per week. Provision of alternate multimodal means of physical and psychological distress attenuation (including non-opioid analgesics, withdrawal symptom modifying agents such as clonidine, etc.) is generally necessary but should not be limited to the pharmacologic. Direct counseling and encouragement from the provider as well as enlisting the help of behavioral health colleagues to facilitate self-efficacy is of the essence. The physician's responsibility to the opioid-dependent patient does not end with simple opioid weaning and discontinuation; it remains incumbent upon us to offer rational and effective underlying pain issues by multimodal means as discussed in Chap. 6, while recognizing and communicating that often such an end will require a strategic lifestyle overhaul in multiple dimensions including but not limited to the physical and psychological.

While most effective when backed with science, effective opioid dependence counseling is an art that takes quite a bit of time and effort to develop proficiency in. In our experience and that of many clinicians, the "early"-stage opioid-dependent patient poses much more of a management challenge than the floridly "down-and-out" addict discussed in the next section. Such "mildly" dependent individuals who have not "hit rock bottom" (to borrow a phrase from grassroots peer support parlance) are generally much less likely to recognize and admit their dependence (perhaps due to less cumulative burden of adverse effects including work, social, and family consequences) and are often more resistant to discontinuation advice and efforts.

Motivational interviewing, developed by Miller and Rollnick [12], is one of the more widely practiced techniques in substance dependence counseling today and is highly relevant to clinical secondary (and tertiary) prevention of opioid dependence.

Building on humanistic and self-actualization theories from Carl Rogers and others, motivational interviewing (MI) first helps the patient identify discrepancy between ideals and actions, and also ambivalence—the simultaneous presence of desire for and against something. It then seeks to assist the patient strengthen their fully informed and considered position for change and develop motivation and a plan for carrying this out. In our practice, we seek to use many of the principles of MI in helping patients recognize the obstacles to overcoming opioid dependence and the (sometimes subconscious) reasons they wish to remain in that state. These generally ostensibly begin as complaints of physical pain, but with gentle and skillful facilitation issues of emotional distress, restoration of an overall sense of well-being, and both hedonic/positive and withdrawal/negative reinforcements frequently come to light. It is generally easier to recognize and divulge motivations for change, and some of the more common ones expressed by patients include improvements in health, sense of accomplishment and self-esteem, the respect of others, salvaging a relationship or job, and so on. Once patients arrive at a place of honesty and security in articulating both motivations and counter-motivations/saboteurs (hearing oneself verbalize things is generally more powerful than hearing it from others) it is easier to guide them in a course of growing commitment to achieving freedom from opioid dependence.

As with primary prevention, helping patients "stay the course" with opioid weaning and discontinuation is greatly facilitated by effective physical and emotional pain reduction and possibly even more importantly, cultivation of resilience and self-efficacy. While these efforts are obviously best handled by counselors and psychologists, at least basic familiarity with the concepts and techniques are invaluable to the good physician who would help reinforce their patients' healing and wellness.

Tertiary Prevention

Tertiary prevention comprises harm reduction and efforts to reduce consequences of established disease while continuing to attempt reversal. It is in essence synonymous with treatment.

Treatment of Opioid Addiction: General Considerations

The American Society of Addiction Medicine (ASAM) has published recommendations/standards for the treatment of the opioid-addicted patient [37]. ASAM has also published a National Practice Guideline for Medication-Assisted Treatment (MAT) of opioid addiction [38]; there are significant areas of overlap between the two documents; however, the latter communicates significantly greater detail regarding its subject matter and is discussed in greater detail below. Six main components of care are conceptualized within the standards as follows:

- Assessment and diagnosis
- Withdrawal management
- Treatment planning
- Treatment management
- Care transitions and coordination
- Continuing care management

And while consideration of all aspects are certainly warranted in every clinical situation, their applicability and relative importance may vary.

The first component, assessment and diagnosis, should be comprehensive, addressing not only traditional biopsychosocial variables (including substance use history) and addiction history but should also include a "multidimensional assessment" of factors that may facilitate or impede recovery as outlined in the ASAM Treatment Criteria for Addictive, Substance-Related, and Co-occurring Conditions [39]. The six dimensions assessed include:

- Acute intoxication and/or withdrawal potential
- Biomedical conditions/complications
- Emotional/behavioral/cognitive conditions and complications
- Readiness to change
- Relapse/continued use/continued problem potential
- Recovery environment

Physical examination and pertinent laboratory assays should be performed.

The second component, withdrawal management begins with assessment of withdrawal potential or severity if already in process, and must take into account other substances that the patient may be withdrawing from (or intoxicated by) that may complicate treatment decisions and placement recommendations. A decision to palliate withdrawal symptoms and treat potentially harmful consequences and initiate antagonist therapy vs. induction onto full or partial agonist therapy must be made. Typical opioid withdrawal symptoms may be managed with clonidine, antiemetics and antidiarrheals, non-opioid analgesics, and possibly benzodiazepines bearing in mind the increased risks of these drugs both short and long term.

The third and fourth components, treatment planning and management, involve a comprehensive and ongoing determination of benefit-risk ratios from all relevant psychosocial and pharmacological therapies and formulation and implementation of an individualized plan based on multidimensional assessment. Coordination of care among various disciplines and involvement of social support networks including family when available and appropriate are key elements.

The fifth component, care transitions and coordination, involves ensuring appropriate and smooth transitions between levels of care based on comprehensive assessment including history of responses to previous treatment efforts. This may be in response to therapeutic failure or success, with lateral, higher or lower-echelon care depending on treatment response. It is incumbent upon the addictionologist to obtain proper authorization for release of information and to ensure salient information transfer to other providers while complying with all confidentiality requirements.

The sixth element, continuing care management, is oriented toward outlining and ensuring facilitating sustainable recovery self-care upon meeting treatment goals. It is justifiable and in the patient's best interest, given the frequently relapsing nature of addiction to provide ongoing monitoring and periodic "wellness checks."

Treatment of Opioid Addiction: Medication-Assisted Treatment (MAT)

Prior to widespread appreciation of the prescription opioid epidemic and focusing on illicit (e.g., heroin) abuse, a National Institutes of Health consensus panel in 1997 [40] advised:

> a commitment to offer effective treatment for [opioid addiction] for Federal and State efforts to reduce the stigma attached to MAT and to expand MAT through increased funding, less restrictive regulation, and efforts to make treatment available in all States.

With the rise of the prescription opioid epidemic, further support for implementation of MAT has been provided at a congressional level with the passage of the 2008 Mental Health Parity and Addiction Equity Act (MHPAEA) and the 2010 Patient Protection and Affordable Care Act (ACA.) The Substance Abuse and Mental Health Services Administration (SAMHSA), National Institute on Drug Abuse (NIDA), ASAM and international organizations such as the World Health Organization all champion the use of MAT as part of a comprehensive recovery/rehabilitation strategy in appropriately selected patients [38, 41–43].

Systematic reviews performed within the last decade have shown that MAT is effective in attenuating opioid use disorder, whether illicit or prescription [44–47]. Studies addressing efficacy generally consider the outcome of reduction in opioid use (other than medications used in treatment) as evidenced by self-report and/or urinalysis or the outcome of retention in treatment. However, in this author's opinion, these outcomes should be "taken with a grain of salt" or at least evaluated in the context of greater multivariate analysis, as compliance with substitution therapy or retention in programs offering essentially low- or no-cost maintenance of dependence/addiction may not accurately reflect improvement in opioid use disorder. Timko et al. [47] reported increased treatment retention for methadone compared to buprenorphine and heroin compared to methadone. This begs the question, of course, of what we are really trying to accomplish with MAT. A recent thought-provoking article exploring different perspectives on treatment duration/retention highlighted the importance of considering outcomes of sobriety/"freedom [from] dependence" and self-determination when evaluating MAT strategies [48].

The ASAM National Practice Guideline for MAT [38] recommends that when considering MAT, triage and referral for intoxication or serious withdrawal, as well as other psychiatric urgency/emergency, take place initially. Assuming no such critical situation, comprehensive assessment as described above, with history, physical examination, and routine laboratory screening (complete blood count and differential, liver function tests, hepatitis C and human immunodeficiency virus serology, and pregnancy testing in females of childbearing age), should occur at initial consultation. Decision as to treatment pathway, which includes both overall venue (e.g., office-based with outpatient counseling vs. "methadone clinic" as discussed below vs. residential facility or hospitalization) as well as specific medication(s) for facilitation of treatment, should then be discussed with the patient. These medications are discussed below in greater detail.

Methadone Maintenance Therapy

Methadone has long been favored for opioid addiction maintenance/substitution treatment as it is inexpensive, has a very long half-life, and seems to show relative resistance to the development of tolerance [49, 50]. Treatment retention appears to be optimized with daily doses between 60 and 100 mg [51–54].

As discussed in Chap. 4, numerous studies support the efficacy of "methadone maintenance therapy (MMT)" in reducing illicit opioid use and reducing both biomedical and societal harms associated with such [55–58]. Two longitudinal studies from the 1980s and 1990s, the Drug Abuse Reporting Program (DARP) and the Treatment Outcome Perspective Study (TOPS) both showed roughly a 40% reduction in illicit opioid use at the end of 1 year after methadone maintenance treatment [59, 60]. A Cochrane review from the previous decade evaluating the effectiveness of MMT compared to no MAT [61] showed superiority of MMT in facilitating decreased heroin use but no evidence of reductions in either criminal activity or mortality.

Methadone (or any opioid besides buprenorphine, discussed below) prescribing for the purposes of maintenance/substitution therapy is only permissible in the United States by federally licensed opioid treatment programs (OTPs.) Specific instructions/guidelines are available through the Department of Health and Human Services [62] and are outside the scope of this book.

In the 1990s, its increasing therapeutic use in pain management in the United States paralleled an increase in the overall push toward greater opioid prescriptions discussed previously. However, increasing evidence of its disproportionate dangers began to amass with increased prevalence of use, and up to one-third of opioid-related deaths have been attributed to methadone in some samples [63, 64]. The need for extreme caution and selectivity is now recognized, and in fact many of the more recent national-level opioid CPGs advise that only those practitioners well-educated and experienced with methadone treatment should initiate and continue it [65–67].

Methadone-specific clinical practice guidelines (CPGs) have recently been published from both the pain management and addictionology communities [67–69], and methadone prescription for chronic pain is discussed in Chap. 8. Both pain management and addictionology/MMT expert consensus statements express homogenous recommendations to "start low and go slow." Most methadone-related deaths occur within the first 2 weeks of initiating therapy [64, 70], and a major factor thought to be associated with this phenomenon is the long half-life as discussed in Chap. 3, which results in insidious buildup of plasma levels over days to weeks even at a consistent dose regimen. As such, starting doses of no more than 5–10 mg/day in the naïve, with increases of 5–10 mg every 5–7 days are recommended.

In addition, the contribution to mortality from co-prescribed (or abused) sedatives and other CNS depressants, especially benzodiazepines, is very significant, and extreme caution, including consideration of discontinuation, is warranted in these situations.

One of the main considerations in its use is the recently highlighted risk of ventricular dysrhythmias (especially torsades de pointe) related to QT interval prolongation, as discussed in greater detail in Chap. 3. Methadone treatment should not be instituted or should be weaned/discontinued at corrected QT intervals greater than 500 ms, and treatment is discouraged at intervals greater than 450 ms. Baseline electrocardiography (ECG) is recommended for all patients being considered for initiation of methadone therapy, with subsequent surveillance ECG performed at intervals determined by baseline QT interval, medical history (including syncopal history), co-prescribed medications, and dose/rate of methadone treatment; in addition, follow-up ECG is recommended at thresholds of 30–40 mg/day and again at 100 mg/day if daily dose reaches those numbers [68].

Buprenorphine

Since 2000, buprenorphine (as the monoproduct with brand name Subutex® or combination buprenorphine-naloxone best known as Suboxone®) has been increasingly used for medication-assisted treatment of opioid addiction and possesses advantages over methadone of increased safety (as discussed in Chap. 3) and also increased access, as the DATA 2000 and recent CARA2016 legislation have allowed for physicians and now mid-level practitioners to prescribe buprenorphine for office-based treatment (OBT) of opioid dependence pending federally approved training completion and Drug Enforcement Agency waiver ("X-number").

Evidence for efficacy of buprenorphine in the treatment of opioid abuse, whether prescription or illicit, has been shown in numerous trials [45, 46, 71–73]. A Cochrane review [71] reported high-quality evidence showing superiority of any dose to placebo in achieving treatment retention but also moderate-quality data suggesting that only high doses (greater than or equal to 16 mg/day) effectively suppressed illicit use compared to placebo. By many metrics, buprenorphine has been shown to be equivalent to methadone [46, 71, 72, 74, 75] in the treatment of opioid addiction. To date, no studies have shown superiority of buprenorphine in terms of traditional outcomes (retention, decreased illicit opioid use), but there remains tremendous rationale for its preferential use in OUD given its improved safety profile, unparalleled MOR dissociation coefficient (opioid-blocking effect) among agonists, and, again, increased access.

As with any form of MAT, it should be clarified between provider and patient at the outset of treatment whether the goal is abstinence/sobriety/freedom from opioid dependence or indefinite maintenance. Both approaches have strong supportive arguments, and individual risk factors should be taken into account when crafting a plan, consonant with the concept of multidimensional assessment.

Numerous studies have compared outcomes from indefinite buprenorphine maintenance vs. tapering/wean-down and discontinuation [76–78]. While no study has yet to (nor likely will) demonstrate the optimal treatment duration with buprenorphine in terms of facilitating recovery, a general theme in the literature is that longer durations seem to correlate with improved outcomes [76–78]. However, none of these investigations (nor any addressing methadone treatment duration for that matter) have included transition to injectable naltrexone, as discussed below, which may be a "game changer." It is conceivable that (successful) accelerated transition to injectable naltrexone may yield superior efficacy in facilitating recovery/sobriety.

The ASAM National Practice Guideline for MAT [38] recommends careful multidimensional assessment and selectivity when considering buprenorphine OBT, as comorbid psychiatric (including other substance abuse disorders) conditions or diversion risk may require a higher echelon of care. Withdrawal from opioids prior to initiation of buprenorphine OBT is necessary to prevent severe "precipitated" withdrawal from premature introduction of this powerful displacing agent with its unparalleled dissociation coefficient. Specific suggested withdrawal durations as well as standardized instruments (e.g., Clinical Opioid Withdrawal Score) are discussed in greater detail within the guidelines.

In-office monitored induction is recommended by ASAM as well as SAMHSA [79], and several hours should be dedicated to a slow titration to optimal dose while observing for precipitated withdrawal and also over-sedation. In general, maintenance doses fall within the range of 8–16 mg/day while initiating treatment, and despite the long half-life of the agent, anecdotal evidence shows that dividing the dose throughout the day seems to provide improved attenuation of cravings as well as analgesia.

The process of discontinuation (with recommended transition to antagonist therapy, i.e., naltrexone) is an individualized one, and ASAM recommends maintaining OBT for at least several months while jointly assessing with the patient readiness for weaning based on several indicators including motivation and psychosocial stability and support.

Naltrexone

Naltrexone, a long-acting mu-opioid receptor (MOR) antagonist has been used increasingly orally or more recently intramuscularly (depot injection) in abstinence-based approaches to opioid addiction recovery, as well as in pharmacotherapeutic support for alcohol dependence which is outside the scope of this book. Like naloxone (discussed below), naltrexone's competitive antagonistic properties at the MOR can confer significant "precipitated" opioid withdrawal if patients are physiologically opioid dependent. Prior to initiation of treatment with naltrexone, it has been recommended that patients be abstinent from opioids for 7–10 days prior to treatment, and most treatment protocols recommend point of care urine immunoassay for opioids followed by an observed oral naltrexone challenge with sufficient time elapsing (generally 1 h) to rule out precipitated withdrawal prior to regular oral administration or injection of depot naltrexone (discussed below.) In addition, comprehensive metabolic panel to evaluate renal and hepatic function and point-of-care hCG testing for pregnancy are also advised prior to treatment. Hepatic dysfunction is frequently cited as a relative contraindication for naltrexone therapy; however, actual case reports of significant hepatocellular injury are rare and generally occur at doses greater than 300 mg/day or greater [80]. Several recent studies have shown corroborating evidence of safety in cases of mild to moderate liver disease from both alcohol-related and viral hepatic diseases [81–83].

Once-daily oral dosing (typically 50 mg) is possible due to the long elimination half-life of 13 h, but this still requires considerable commitment to daily maintenance dosing on the part of the patient, or the MOR may be quickly available again for agonism within a matter of a day or two. As such, the development of a sustained, long-term delivery system has been pursued for decades, and recently extended-release naltrexone (XR-NTX) has been brought to market as both intramuscular depot injection (Vivitrol®) and also as surgically implanted polymer capsules (not approved in the United States). Obvious advantages of these systems include greater potential adherence with fewer potential opportunities to defeat the system by simply stopping daily pill ingestion, as well as fewer reported adverse effects than from oral naltrexone [84]. The proposed reason for this latter phenomenon is the avoidance of higher (albeit intermittent) plasma levels due to sustained release pharmacokinetics from XR-NTX systems, as well as obviation of the need for large (oral) doses to overcome first-pass hepatic metabolism [84].

Several earlier studies and systematic reviews including a 2011 Cochrane Review [85] showed that oral naltrexone with or without psychosocial intervention did not perform better than placebo or other MAT in terms of preventing relapse to opioid use; this correlated with poor adherence/treatment retention rates.

The Phase III clinical trial for Vivitrol® was performed in Russia between 2008 and 1010 [86]. Two hundred and fifty opioid-dependent patients, the vast majority of which were intravenous heroin users, were randomized to treatment with Vivitrol® or placebo for 24 weeks; both groups also underwent behavioral health intervention. Retention was significantly higher in the treatment group (median 168 days with Vivitrol® compared to 96 days in the placebo group) with correspondingly significantly increased abstinence as well as craving for opioids.

A follow-up 1-year open-label extension trial was performed subsequently in the same population [83], and over 60% of patients completed the trial with 50% of them abstinent from opioids during the study period.

An initial Cochrane Review was performed in 2008 but was limited by a paucity of data; no conclusions could be drawn. Lobmaier et al. [87] in 2011 reported on four studies involving Vivitrol® and 42 involving surgical implants, "a few of which" comprised randomized controlled trials (RCTs); the pooled data suggested that XR-NTX led to significant reductions in relapse compared to no MAT, placebo injections or oral naltrexone. Further large trials and systematic reviews are currently in process at the time of this writing [88, 89].

Provision of prophylactic naloxone (as discussed in greater detail below) is recommended by many as the patient undergoing naltrexone therapy for any length of time, whether oral or injectable will be essentially opioid naïve after as little as 1–2 weeks of treatment and as such is at significantly higher risk of apnea and death from opioid overdose than they were prior to naltrexone therapy, which in fact may not be apparent to them.

Behavioral Treatment

It must be remembered and communicated to patients, society, and policymakers that the most important point of consideration of MAT is that the "MA" (medication-assisted) component is supportive of "T" (treatment) and is neither the primary recovery modality nor an end in itself. The ASAM National Practice Guideline for MAT [38] spells out in no unclear language:

> Addiction should be considered a bio-psycho-social-spiritual illness, for which the use of medication(s) is but only one component of overall treatment.

Similarly, a recent SAMHSA publication [90] states:

> All medications for the treatment of the opioid use disorder should be prescribed as part of a comprehensive treatment approach that includes counseling and other psychological therapies delivered by a psychiatrist, psyschologist, or professional counselor, as well as social support through participation in… mutual help programs.

Furthermore, as stated unequivocally by SAMHSA [91] pharmacotherapy without behavioral treatment is not an adequate treatment plan for individuals with comorbid psychiatric conditions ("dual diagnoses").

Despite limited evidence, as mentioned below, essentially all relevant authorities including the currently highly biologic addiction model-centric NIDA acknowledge the efficacy of pure behavioral approaches to addiction recovery in many situations, and also advocate the addition of psychosocial treatment to pharmacotherapy.

While most of the attention to psychosocial therapy occurs during "maintenance" phases of addiction treatment, the benefit of these interventions (with acceptance and commitment therapy in particular showing promise) toward patients undergoing the highly vulnerable detoxification period where the majority of relapses have historically occurred due to the discomfort of withdrawal should not be overlooked [92].

Attaching psychosocial-spiritual approaches to the biologic at every stage of addiction treatment, from detoxification through post-recovery management, is only logical and consonant with the greater wisdom beyond the medical community.

In what is likely the largest systematic review to date [93] examining the use of psychosocial interventions in conjunction with MAT, the authors report overall evidence of benefit for combination behavioral/medication-assisted treatment, but note highly variable efficacy depending upon specific intervention (both behavioral and medical) and also upon outcomes measured. They also contend that the often contradictory literature likely reflects artificially inflated (compared to typical community treatment programs) counseling effects upon control groups, diluting out experimental effect. While numerous reports suggest failure of behavioral therapy to increase the efficacy of pharmacotherapeutic approaches, many of the control groups in these investigations receive a substantial degree of counseling [78], and furthermore the heterogeneity of psychosocial-spiritual offerings renders any conclusions a gross generalization.

Along those lines, the majority of interventions in the behavioral treatment arms likely receive limited therapy focusing on certain aspects of treatment traditionally perceived as "high-yield" (e.g., trigger identification, relapse prevention, stress management, etc.) while neglecting more in-depth and rigorous aspects requiring cultivation of longer-term therapeutic relationship and guidance toward true psychological and spiritual growth and development. Bona fide, sustained change takes considerable effort and time, and many grassroots/mutual support organizations such as Alcoholics Anonymous recognize the indefinite timetable of commitment required for successful sobriety. In the DATOS study [13], those individuals who maintained sobriety/recovery were almost four times more likely than those who relapsed to perceive improved overall personal growth including:

- Ability to handle responsibility
- Ability to recognize and express feelings
- Improved relational and social skills
- Improved self-efficacy perception in health maintenance
- Ability to lead a constructive and contributing life

Instillation or at least facilitation of these maturation indicators requires considerable time and effort on the part of the various practitioners involved as well, but by available evidence as well as common sense is well worth the effort if recovery is to be sustained. In our experience, substitution of one chemical coping method for another or merely expressing intellectual assent to a set of principles or practices is not nearly as effective in producing long-term change as is a gradual (yet radical) apprenticeship in life skills and the pursuit of personal development.

As discussed above, to overlook the tremendous success of spirituality-focused and faith-based programs upon substance misuse reduction [13, 30–35] is precariously unwise and a disservice to people who are by definition multidimensional and diverse and whose psychosocial-spiritual faculties and needs far exceed the scope and expertise of the medical (including psychiatric) community.

Overdose Education and Naloxone Distribution

While possessing no role in the prevention of opioid use disorder (and conversely accused of potentially hindering prevention and treatment in that it may confer a false sense of security), prophylactic prescription of *naloxone* (a shorter-acting mu-opioid receptor antagonist than naltrexone) has become an increasingly recommended and adopted component of an overall effort to reduce mortality from opioid overdose. Although community-based programs offering *overdose education and naloxone distribution* (*OEND*) have been functioning to this end since 1996, it has only been within the past few years that *Narcan kits* consisting of either injectable or more recently intranasal naloxone has become a widespread and accessible option for harm reduction. The American Medical Association in 2012 [94], and numerous federal organizations over the next few years, most notably SAMHSA in 2013 and the Office of National Drug Control Policy in 2014, began to promote OEND, recognizing that formal emergency response may not be rapid enough to intervene in the case of opioid overdose, responders may be prohibited by law in some states to administer naloxone, and in situations involving illicit use many parties might be hesitant or even unwilling to involve the authorities.

As a result of these increased publicity campaigns, Narcan kit prescriptions to patients at risk of overdose, or to third-party associates, have become much more widely accepted and practiced, and more recently thanks to federal and other grant monies, in many states, Narcan kits are distributed without the direct order of a physician. OEND programs have concomitantly multiplied throughout the country for the purpose of training interested laypersons in recognizing signs of opioid overdose and administering naloxone and other supportive care while awaiting emergency response service.

A survey of 140 known Narcan kit distributing organizations in the United States was carried out in 2014, and for the time period from 1996 to 2014 (with the vast majority of incidents occurring between 2013 and 2014), over 150,000 kits were dispensed and over 26,000 overdose reversals were recorded [95].

Clark et al. reviewed the literature on community OEND programs and reported on 19 articles with almost 1950 reported naloxone administrations. The majority of the articles reviewed reported 100% successful resuscitation, with the lowest survival rate among the reports being 83% [96]. The literature reviewed also suggests that OEND programs confer significant and effective education to laypersons regarding overdose recognition and response.

Giglio et al., in another review [97], reported on the results of bystander naloxone administration and also the effectiveness of training of laypersons in its use. They found that naloxone administration by bystanders was associated with a significantly increased odds of survival compared with no naloxone administration. Sixty-six witnessed overdoses were reported in the pooled literature, 39 of which received naloxone at the hands of bystanders, and 100% of which survived. Conversely, 3 of the 27 overdose victims who did not receive naloxone died, yielding an odds ratio of 8.58 (95% CI = 3.90–13.2) for bystander naloxone effect on survival. They also found that laypersons trained in overdose recognition and naloxone administration performed markedly better in test scenarios of overdose recognition, EMS activation, and naloxone administration.

McDonald and Strang performed another review of the literature, examining most of the same publications reviewed by Clark previously [98] but with a specific aim to evaluate likelihood of opioid overdose survival resulting from bystander naloxone administration. Over 2300 naloxone administrations were documented, with over 2200 successful resuscitations (>96%). In the absence of prospective randomized trial data, observational epidemiologic (augmented Bradford Hill) criteria were used to evaluate the data, and the authors concluded there was sufficient evidence in favor of causality.

Until recently, legal barriers at the state level have stood in the way of implementation of these programs across the nation. While direct prescription of naloxone to a patient by a licensed provider has never been in direct contention, prescriber fears (and unfamiliarity, lack of "standard of care" precedent, etc.) have retarded adoption of the practice. With significant federal and other stakeholder backing, state laws addressing increased access (*Naloxone Access Laws*) have recently multiplied, with 44 States having passed such laws at the time of this writing [99, 100]. The two main innovations within this legal arena include provision for direct prescription of Narcan kits to third-party family members, other associates, etc. by the practitioner and also "standing order" prescriptions by the state's chief medical officer or other appointed officials that allow for dispensation through traditional pharmacy channels or community programs independently of any direct physician evaluation/ therapeutic relationship. Laws protecting bystanders/third parties from civil or criminal charges for both administration of naloxone and/or summoning of emergency response services (*Good Samaritan Laws*) have also been passed in the majority of states at the time of this writing [101].

Given the staggering and relentless increases in opioid-related deaths and the increasing pressure on prescribers to provide at-home naloxone (as discussed below), it will undoubtedly soon be considered tantamount to malpractice to prescribe opioids (perhaps with the exception of low-dose/limited postoperative prescriptions) without provision for OEND. Individual state laws however still display such heterogeneity of requirements, restrictions, and nuance that, as with all professional matters, up-to-date familiarity with one's state laws is imperative.

Multiple clinical practice guidelines including the recent CDC Guidelines on opioid prescription for non-cancer pain [102] and The American Society of Addiction Medicine [38] both advocate the prescription of naloxone (directly or third-party) to high-risk individuals, whether in the context of opioid therapy for pain or for dependence treatment. Such high-risk individuals include those with comorbid pyschiatric diagnoses including substance abuse disorders, those being treated with methadone, those receiving synergistic respiratory depressants such as benzodiazepines, and even those simply receiving higher doses of opioids (the recent CDC guidelines suggest 50 morphine milligram equivalents per day [102]). In addition, and in the context of this section on tertiary prevention it bears specific mention that patients in the process of detoxification and those achieving sobriety may be at particularly increased risk of opioid overdose, as reduction in tolerance to the respiratory depressive effects of opioids has likely ensued with reduction or elimination of chronic exposure.

As with any rescucitative intervention, simple provision of tools is insufficient for optimal results and it is incumbent upon the prescriber and the healthcare community to provide education on naloxone kit use. Many of the state laws referenced above include or imply requirements for education as conditions for medicolegal immunity [99, 100].

Summary

The public health concepts of primary, secondary, and tertiary prevention are increasingly discussed in the context of the opioid abuse epidemic. Primary prevention seeks to avert the onset of disease or injury, secondary prevention comprises screening for/identifying and if possible reversing early effects of the disease or injury state, and tertiary prevention attempts to attenuate the consequences of established disease as well as strive for cure. To continue the infectious disease metaphor used throughout the book, behavioral "immunity" toward opioid-seeking and misuse must be cultivated at every stage of prevention, and the enhancement of motivation for avoidance comprises the strategic goal for both individuals and populations. Both negative and positive motivation—healthy respect for and fear of opioid adverse effects—and a desire to address underlying physical and psychological discomfort and distress with alternate and multimodal means including prevention are essential.

As individuals are not islands unto themselves, addressing the environment (beyond the concept of vectors as explored in detail in Part III of the book) is critical. Social pressures and norms exert powerful sway upon individual behaviors, and harnessing these forces from the level of domiciles and families to nationwide public awareness and education efforts is imperative if this epidemic is to be staunched and reversed.

Weaning and discontinuation require careful attention to underlying sources of discomfort and distress and to facilitating resilience and self-efficacy. Substitution (e.g., methadone, buprenorphine) and antagonist (e.g., naltrexone) pharmacotherapies in conjunction with psychosocial-spiritual treatment have been shown to be effective in harm reduction but also in assisting recovery from addiction. It must be remembered that medication-assisted treatment requires much more than medication to be successful in accomplishing recovery from opioid dependence. Attending to the complex psychosocial-spiritual needs of human beings and facilitating self-development is critical to that goal. This is reflected in the understanding and statements of multidimensional assessment and treatment/placement guidelines provided by organizations such as the American Society for Addiction Medicine.

Finally, overdose education and naloxone distribution are increasingly championed as effective efforts in reducing mortality, and it must be recognized that given frequent relapse behaviors, opioid-dependent individuals are at greatly increased risk of overdose and death compared to never users, as they are accustomed to risky practices but may have achieved unappreciated reductions in tolerance by periodic abstinence.

References

1. Kolodny A, Courtwright DT, Hwang CS, Kreiner P, Eadie JL, Clark TW, et al. The prescription opioid and heroin crisis: a public health approach to an epidemic of addiction. Annu Rev. Public Health. 2015;36:559–74.
2. Alexander GC, Frattaroli S, Gielen AC, editors. The prescription opioid epidemic: an evidence-based approach. Baltimore, MD: Johns Hopkins Bloomberg School of Public Health; 2015.
3. Pravetoni M, Pentel PR, Potter DN, Chartoff EH, Tally L, LeSage MG. Effects of an oxycodone conjugate vaccine on oxycodone self-administration and oxycodone-induced brain gene expression in rats. PLoS One. 2014;9(7):e101807. doi:10.1371/journal.pone.0101807.
4. Laudenbach M, Baruffaldi F, Vervacke JS, Distefano MD, Titcombe PJ, Mueller DL, et al. The frequency of naïve and early-activated hapten-specific B cell subsets dictates the efficacy of a therapeutic vaccine against prescription opioid abuse. J Immunol. 2015;194:5926–36.
5. Ohler N. Blitzed. London: Penguin Books Ltd; 2016.
6. Schaller M, Park JH. The behavioral immune system (and why it matters). Curr Dir Psychol Sci. 2011;20:99–103.
7. Dostoevsky F. Notes from underground (vintage classics). New York: Random House; 1994.
8. Janz NK, Becker MH. The health belief model: a decade later. Health Educ Q. 1984;11:1–47.
9. Bandura A. Self-efficacy: toward a unifying theory of behavioral change. Psychol Rev. 1977;84:191–215.
10. Simpson DD, Joe GW. Motivation as a predictor of early dropout from drug abuse treatment. Psychotherapy. 1993;30:357–68.
11. DeLeon G, Melnick G, Kressel D, Jainchill N. Circumstances, motivation, readiness, and suitability (the CMRS scale): predicting retention in therapeutic community treatment. Am J Drug Alc Abuse. 1994;20:495–515.
12. Miller WR, Rollnick S. Motivational interviewing: helping people change. 3rd ed. New York: Guilford Press; 2013.
13. Flynn PM, Joe GW, Broome KM, Simpson DD, Brown BS. Recovery from opioid addiction in DATOS. J Subst Abus Treat. 2003;25:177–86.
14. Blankenship J, Dansereau DF, Simpson DD. Cognitive enhancements of readiness for corrections-based treatment for drug abuse. Prison J. 1999;79:431–45.
15. Joe GW, Simpson DD, Broome KM. Retention and patient engagement models for different treatment modalities in DATOS. Drug Alcohol Depend. 1999;57:113–25.
16. Farrelly MC, Niederdeppe J, Yarsevich J. Youth tobacco prevention mass media campaigns: past, present, and future directions. Tob Control. 2003;12:i35–47.
17. McAfee T, Davis KC, Alexander RL Jr, Pechacek TF, Bunnell R. Effect of the first federally funded US antismoking national media campaign. Lancet. 2013;382:2003–11.
18. Veehof MM, Trompetter HR, Bohlmeijer ET, Schreurs KM. Acceptance- and mindfulness-based interventions for the treatment of chronic pain: a meta-analytic review. Cogn Behav Ther. 2016;45:5–31.
19. Louw A, Diener I, Butler DS, Puentedura EJ. The effect of neuroscience education on pain, disability, anxiety, and stress in chronic musculoskeletal pain. Arch Phys Med Rehabil. 2011;92:2041–56.

20. Louw A, Zimney K, Puentedura EJ, Diener I. The efficacy of pain neuroscience education on musculoskeletal pain: a systematic review of the literature. Physiother Theory Pract. 2016;32:332–55.
21. Halpern J. Empathy and patient-physician conflicts. J Gen Intern Med. 2007;22:696–700.
22. Elder N, Ricer R, Tobias B. How respected family physicians manage difficult patient encounters. J Am Board Fam Med. 2006;19:533–41.
23. Beckman HB, Markakis KM, Suchman AL, Frankel RM. The doctor-patient relationship and malpractice: lessons from plaintiff depositions. Arch Intern Med. 1994;154:1365–70.
24. Levinson W, Roter D, Mullooly J, Dull V, Frankel R. Physician-patient communication: the relationship with malpractice claims among primary care physicians and surgeons. JAMA. 1997;277:553–9.
25. Hegan T. The importance of effective communication in preventing litigation. Med J Malaysia. 2003;58(Suppl A):78–82.
26. Depression and other common mental disorders: global health estimates. Geneva: World Health Organization; 2017. Accessed from: http://apps.who.int/iris/bitstream/10665/254610/1/WHO-MSD-MER-2017.2-eng.pdf?ua=1
27. Gorsuch RL, Butler MC. Initial drug abuse: a review of predisposing social psychological factors. Psychol Bull. 1976;83:120–37.
28. Bromet E, Moos RH. Environmental resources and the posttreatment functioning of alcohol patients. J Health Soc Behav. 1977;18:326–38.
29. Blechman EA. Conventional wisdom about familial contributions to substance abuse. Am J Drug Alc Abuse. 1982;9:35–53.
30. Hater JJ, Singh BK, Simpson DD. Influence of family and religion on long-term outcomes among opioid addicts. Adv Alcohol Subst Abuse. 1984;4:29–40.
31. Cook CCH. Addiction and spirituality. Addiction. 2004;99:539–51.
32. Shields JJ, Broome KM, Delany PJ, Fletcher BW, Flynn PM. Religion and substance abuse treatment: individual and program effects. J Sci Study Relig. 2007;46:355–71.
33. Geppert C, Bogenschutz MP, Miller WR. Development of a bibliography on religion, spirituality and addictions. Drug Alc Rev. 2007;26:389–95.
34. Monitoring the future. Accessed from: www.monitoringthefuture.org
35. Schoenthaler SJ, Blum K, Braverman ER, Giordano J, Thompson B, Oscar-Berman M, et al. NIDA-drug addiction treatment outcome study (DATOS) relapse as a function of spirituality/religiosity. J Reward Defic Syndr. 2015;1:36–45.
36. Manchikanti L, Manchukonda R, Damron KS, Brandon D, McManus CD. Does adherence monitoring reduce controlled substance abuse in chronic pain patients? Pain Physician. 2006;9:57–60.
37. The American Society of Addiction Medicine. The ASAM standards of care for the addiction specialist physician. Chevy Chase, MD: The American Society of Addiction Medicine; 2014.
38. The American Society of Addiction Medicine. The national practice guideline for the use of medications in the treatment of addiction involving opioid use. Chevy Chase, MD: The American Society of Addiction Medicine; 2015.
39. Mee-Lee D, editor. The ASAM criteria: treatment criteria for addictive, substance-related, and co-occurring conditions. Carson City, NV: The Change Companies; 2013.
40. National Institutes of Health (NIH). Effective medical treatment of opiate addiction. NIH Consens Statement. 1997;15(6):1–38.
41. https://www.samhsa.gov/medication-assisted-treatment. Accessed 20 May 2017.
42. National Institute on Drug Abuse. Principles of drug addiction treatment: a research-based guide. 3rd ed. Bethesda, MD: National Institutes of Health; 2012. NIH Publication No. 12–4180
43. World Health Organization. WHO guidelines for the psychosocially assisted pharmacological treatment of opioid dependence. Geneva, Switzerland: WHO; 2009.

44. Amato L, Davoli M, Perucci CA, Ferri M, Faggiano F, Mattick RP. An overview of systematic reviews of the effectiveness of opiate maintenance therapies: available evidence to inform clinical practice and research. J Subst Abus Treat. 2005;28:321–9.
45. Connery HS. Medication-assisted treatment of opioid use disorder: review of the evidence and future directions. Harv Rev. Psychiatry. 2015;23:63–75.
46. Nielsen S, Larance B, Degenhardt L, Gowing L, Kehler C, Lintzeris N. Opioid agonist treatment for pharmaceutical opioid dependent people. Cochrane Database Syst Rev. 2016;5:CD011117. doi:10.1002/14651858.CD011117.pub2.
47. Timko C, Schultz NR, Cucciare MA, Vittorio L, Garrison-Diehn C. Retention in medication-assisted treatment for opiate dependence: a systematic review. J Addict Dis. 2016;35:22–35.
48. Vogel M, Dürsteler KM, Walter M, Herdener M, Nordt C. Rethinking retention in treatment of opioid dependence-the eye of the beholder. Int J Drug Policy. 2017;39:109–13.
49. Parrino MW, editor. State methadone treatment guidelines. Treatment improvement protocol (TIP) series 1. Rockville, MD: Substance Abuse and Mental Health Services Administration; 1993.
50. Substance Abuse and Mental Health Services Administration. Treatment of persons with co-occurring disorders. Treatment improvement protocol (TIP) series 42. HHS publication no. (SMA) 08–3992. Rockville, MD: Department of Health and Human Services; 2004.
51. Strain EC, Stitzer ML, Liebson IA, Bigelow GE. Dose-response effects of methadone in the treatment of opioid dependence. Ann Intern Med. 1993;119:23–37.
52. Strain EC, Bigelow GE, Liebson IA, Stitzer ML. Moderate- vs high-dose methadone in the treatment of opioid dependence. A randomized trial. JAMA. 1999;281:1000–5.
53. Faggiano F, Vigna-Taglianti F, Versino E, Lemma P. Methadone maintenance at different dosages for opioid dependence. Cochrane Database Syst Rev. 2003;3:CD002208.
54. Fareed A, Casarella J, Amar R, Vayalapalli S, Drexler K. Methadone maintenance dosing guideline for opioid dependence, a literature review. J Addict Dis. 2010;29:1–14.
55. Marsch LA. The efficacy of methadone maintenance interventions in reducing illicit opiate use, HIV risk behavior and criminality: a meta-analysis. Addiction. 1998;93:515–32.
56. Mattick RP, Breen C, Kimber J, Davoli M. Methadone maintenance therapy versus no opioid replacement therapy for opioid dependence. Cochrane Database Syst Rev. 2003;2:CD002209.
57. Metzger DS, Woody GE, McLellan AT, O'Brien CP, Druley P, Navaline H, et al. Human immunodeficiency virus seroconversion among intravenous drug users in- and out-of-treatment: an 18- month prospective follow-up. J Acquir Immune Defic Syndr. 1993;6:1049–56.
58. Gowing L, Farrell M, Bornemann R, Ali R. Substitution treatment of injecting opioid users for prevention of HIV infection. Cochrane Database Syst Rev. 2004;4:CD004145.
59. Simpson DD, Sells SB. Effectiveness of treatment for drug abuse: an overview of the DARP research program. Adv Alcohol Subst Abuse. 1982;2:7–29.
60. Condelli WS, Dunteman GH. Exposure to methadone programs and heroin use. Am J Drug Alcohol Abuse. 1993;19:65–78.
61. Mattick RP, Breen C, Kimber J, Davoli M. Methadone maintenance therapy versus no opioid replacement therapy for opioid dependence. Cochrane Database Syst Rev. 2009;3:CD002209. doi:10.1002/14651858.CD002209.pub2.
62. Substance Abuse and Mental Health Services Administration. Federal guidelines for opioid treatment programs. HHS publication no. (SMA) PEP15-FEDGUIDEOTP. Rockville, MD: Substance Abuse and Mental Health Services Administration; 2015.
63. National Drug Intelligence Center. Methadone diversion, abuse and misuse: deaths increasing at alarming rate. No. 2007-Q0317–001. Johnston, PA: Drug Enforcement Administration; 2007.
64. Webster LR, Cochella S, Dasgupta N, Fakata KL, Fine PG, Fishman SM, et al. An analysis of the root causes for opioid-related overdose deaths in the United States. Pain Med. 2011;12(Suppl 2):S26–35.
65. Dowell D, Haegerich TM, Chou R. CDC guideline for prescribing opioids for chronic pain–United States, 2016. MMWR. 2016;65:1–49.

66. Manchikanti L, Abdi S, Atluri S, Balog CC, Benyamin RM, Boswell MV, et al. American society of interventional pain physicians (ASIPP) guidelines for responsible opioid prescribing in chronic non-cancer pain: part 2- guidance. Pain Physician. 2012;15(Suppl 3):S67–116.
67. American Academy of Pain Medicine. Methadone for Pain Management: Improving Clinical Decision Making; 2016. Available from: http://www.painmed.org/files/methadone-for-pain-management-improving-clinical-decision-making.pdf. Accessed 23 Nov 2016.
68. Chou R, Cruciani RA, Fiellin DA, Compton P, Farrar JT, Haigney MC, et al. Methadone safety: a clinical practice guideline from the American pain society and college on problems of drug dependence, in collaboration with the heart rhythm society. J Pain. 2014;15:321–37.
69. Baxter LE Sr, Campbell A, Deshields M, Levounis P, Martin JA, McNicholas L, et al. Safe methadone induction and stabilization: report of an expert panel. J Addict Med. 2013;7:377–86.
70. Modesto-Lowe V, Brooks D, Petry N. Methadone deaths: risk factors in pain and addicted populations. J Gen Intern Med. 2010;25:305–9.
71. Mattick RP, Breen C, Kimber J, Davioli M. Buprenorphine maintenance versus placebo or methadone maintenance for opioid dependence. Cochrane Database Syst Rev. 2014;(2):CD002207.
72. Feelemyer J, Des Jarlais D, Arasteh K, Abdul-Quader AS, Hagan H. Retention of participants in medication-assisted programs in low- and middle-income countries: an international systematic review. Addiction. 2014;109:20–32.
73. Thomas CP, Fullerton CA, Kim M, Montejano L, Lyman DR, Dougherty RH, et al. Medication-assisted treatment with buprenorphine: assessing the evidence. Psychiatr Serv. 2014;65:158–70.
74. Potter JS, Marino EN, Hillhouse MP, Nielsen S, Wiest K, Canamar CP, et al. Buprenorphine/naloxone and methadone maintenance treatment outcomes for opioid analgesic, heroin, and combined users: findings from starting treatment with agonist replacement therapies (START). J Stud Alc Drug. 2013;74:605–13.
75. Canadian Agency for Drugs and Technologies in Health. Suboxone versus methadone for the treatment of opioid dependence: a review of the clinical and cost-effectiveness. Ottawa: The Agency; 2013. Available from: http://www.cadth.ca/media/pdf/htis/dec-2013/RC0495_Suboxone%20for%20opioid%20dependence_Final.pdf
76. Kornor H, Wall H, Sandvik L. Time-limited buprenorphine replacement therapy for opioid dependence: 2 year followup outcomes in relation to programme completion and current agonist therapy status. Drug Alc Rev. 2007;26:135–41.
77. Sigmon SC, Dunn KE, Saulsgiver K, Patrick ME, Badger GJ, Heil SH. A randomized, double-blind evaluation of buprenorphine taper duration in primary prescription opioid abusers. JAMA Psychiat. 2013;70:1347–54.
78. Weiss RD, Rao V. The prescription opioid addiction treatment study: what have we learned. Drug Alc Depend. 2017;173:S48–54.
79. Center for Substance Abuse Treatment. Clinical guidelines for the use of buprenorphine in the treatment of opioid addiction. Treatment improvement protocol (TIP) series 40. DHHS publication no. (SMA) 04–3939. Rockville, MD: Substance Abuse and Mental Health Services Administration; 2004.
80. Center for Substance Abuse Treatment. Incorporating alcohol pharmacotherapies into medical practice. Treatment improvement protocol (TIP) series 49. HHS publication no. (SMA) 13–4380. Rockville, MD: Substance Abuse and Mental Health Services Administration; 2009.
81. Tetrault JM, Tate JP, McGinnis K, Goulet JL, Sullivan LE, Bryant K, et al. Hepatic safety and antiretroviral effectiveness in HIV-infected patients receiving naltrexone. Alcohol Clin Exp Res. 2012;36:318–24.
82. Mitchell MC, Memisoglu A, Silverman BL. Hepatic safety of injectable extended-release naltrexone in patients with chronic hepatitis C and HIV infection. J Stud Alcohol Drugs. 2012;73:991–7.

83. Krupitsky E, Nunes EV, Ling W, Gastfriend DR, Memisoglu A, Silverman BL. Injectable extended-release naltrexone (XR-NTX) for opioid dependence: long-term safety and effectiveness. Addiction. 2013;108:1628–37.
84. Kunoe N, Lobmaier P, Ngo H, Hulse G. Injectable and implantable sustained release naltrexone in the treatment of opioid addiction. Br J Clin Pharmacol. 2014;77:264–71.
85. Minozzi S, Amato L, Vecchi S, Davoli M, Kirchmayer U, Verster A. Oral naltrexone maintenance treatment for opioid dependence. Cochrane Database Syst Rev. 2011;(4):CD001333. doi:10.1002/14651858.CD001333.pub4.
86. Krupitsky E, Nunes EV, Ling W, Illeperuma A, Gastfriend DR, Silverman BL. Injectable extended release naltrexone for opioid dependence: a double-blind, placebo-controlled, multicentre randomised trial. Lancet. 2011;377:1506–13.
87. Lobmaier PP, Kunoe N, Gossop M, Waal H. Naltrexone depot formulations for opioid and alcohol dependence: a systematic review. CNS Neurosci Therap. 2011;17:629–36.
88. National Institute on Drug Abuse. Extended-release naltrexone vs. buprenorphine for opioid treatment (X:BOT); 2013. http://ctndisseminationlibrary.org/protocols/ctn0051.htm. Accessed 14 May 2017.
89. Dennis BB, Naji L, Bawor M, Bonner A, Varenbut M, Daiter J, et al. The effectiveness of opioid substitution treatments for patients with opioid dependence: a systematic review and multiple treatment comparison protocol. Syst Rev. 2014;3:105.
90. Substance Abuse and Mental Health Services Administration. Clinical use of extended-release injectable naltrexone in the treatment of opioid use disorder: a brief guide. HHS publication no. (SMA) 14-4892R. Rockville, MD: Substance Abuse and Mental Health Services Administration; 2015.
91. Substance Abuse and Mental Health Services Administration. General principles for the use of pharmacological agents to treat individuals with co-occurring mental and substance use disorders. HHS publication no. SMA-12-4689. Rockville, MD: Substance Abuse and Mental Health Services Administration; 2012.
92. Ramsey SE, Rounsaville D, Hoskinson R, Park TW, Ames EG, Neirinckx VD, et al. The need for psychosocial interventions to facilitate the transition to extended-release naltrexone (XR-NTX) treatment for opioid dependence: a concise review of the literature. Subst Abuse Res Treat. 2016;10:65–8.
93. Dugosh K, Abraham A, Seymour B, McLoyd K, Chalk M, Festinger D. A systematic review on the use of psychosocial interventions in conjunction with medications for the treatment of opioid addiction. J Addict Med. 2016;10:91–101.
94. Mueller SR, Walley AY, Calcaterra SL, Glanz JM, Binswanger IA. A review of opioid overdose prevention and naloxone prescribing: implications for translating community programming into clinical practice. Subst Abus. 2015;36:240–53.
95. Wheeler E, Jones TS, Gilbert MK, Davidson PJ. Opioid overdose prevention programs providing naloxone to laypersons – United States, 2014. MMWR. 2015;64:631–5.
96. Clark AK, Wilder CM, Winstanley EL. A systematic review of community opioid overdose prevention and naloxone distribution programs. J Addict Med. 2014;8:153–63.
97. Giglio RE, Li G, DiMaggio CJ. Effectiveness of bystander naloxone administration and overdose education programs: a meta-analysis. Inj Epidemiology. 2015;2:10.
98. McDonald R, Strang J. Are take-home naloxone programmes effective? Systematic review utilizing application of the Bradford Hill criteria. Addiction. 2016;111:1177–87.
99. Brodrick JE, Brodrick CK, Adinoff B. Legal regimes surrounding naloxone access: considerations for prescribers. Am J Drug Alc Abuse. 2016;42:117–28.
100. Davis C, Carr D. State legal innovations to encourage naloxone dispensing. J Am Pharm Assoc. 2017;57(Suppl 2):S180–4.
101. Davis C, Carr D. Legal changes to increase access to naloxone for opioid overdose reversal in the United States. Drug Alcohol Depend. 2015;157:112–20.
102. Centers for Disease Control and Prevention. CDC guideline for prescribing opioids for chronic pain — United States, 2016. MMWR. 2016;65(1):1–49.

Conclusion

> "How oft, in nations gone corrupt,
> And by their own devices brought down to servitude,
> That man chooses bondage before liberty.
> Bondage with ease before strenuous liberty."
> "They who have put out the people's eyes reproach them of their blindness."
>
> – John Milton

Twenty years ago a complex constellation coalesced to catalyze the current opioid epidemic in America. Frequently cited factors include an increased emphasis on pharmacotherapeutic intervention on undertreated chronic pain and aggressive marketing by certain pharmaceutical companies. The temporally parallel rise in chronic pain complaints and care seeking is widely appreciated. Generally peripheral to the discussion, however, is the widespread and more difficult to measure increase in psychopathology and social structure breakdown. A significant national decrease in self-efficacy and health mindset (with concordant increases in fear-avoidance behaviors, disability mindset, etc.) is obvious to "those with eyes to see" but remains much more difficult to quantitate and analyze.

The classic epidemiologic model involving agent, environment/vector, and host has been applied to the opioid epidemic herein, with the drugs conceptualized as agent, prescribers as vector, and the population as host. From the standpoint of descriptive statistics, we are told that over a hundred people a day die from an opioid overdose and that despite a downturn in prescribing, enough are prescribed annually to supply every American with at least one bottle of prescription opioids. The agent is ubiquitous, the environment is ripe, and the hosts seem to grow increasingly vulnerable.

Opioids, both endogenous and manufactured, serve an important role beyond the simple analgesic—our understanding of their complex interweavings with the neuroimmunoendocrine system is nascent and rudimentary. Elimination of the *agent*, however, is neither possible nor feasible, nor would it be beneficial to us. Rendering the host impervious to their effects carries similar disadvantage (and yet may be necessary in tertiary prevention when their harms outweigh their benefits).

H.B. McAnally, *Opioid Dependence*, DOI 10.1007/978-3-319-47497-7

Opioids are no more malicious in the sense of sentient harmful intent than are microbes; the havoc they wreak on individuals and populations is motivated by no self-interest nor species preservation instinct. We need not fear them in that regard, but we must respect them. Ignorance of their destructive power and our vulnerability to their seductive and injurious grip are to be feared.

There is demonstrable benefit to attenuating the virulence of the agent, so to speak. Altering "likability" by reduced hedonic reward properties (which may correlate with phasic dopaminergism in the mesolimbic pathway) must be pursued. Abuse-deterrent/tamper-resistant reformulations are only logical. Further pharmacoengineering to more closely approximate the balanced properties of the endogenous opioid system is worth the effort and will certainly expand our understanding of our own physiology, likely generating new and complimentary, if not more effective, therapeutic approaches. None of these modifications, however, can eliminate all risks associated with their use, nor can they prevent a simple shift in "drug of choice."

Altering *vector* (prescriber) transmission is certainly a national and professional priority and has received much welcome attention within the past several years. Both increased regulatory oversight and numerous (and proliferating) clinical practice guidelines seem to be making a difference by many metrics, although whether these interventions simply result in drug of choice shifting again remains to be seen. Care must be taken as with all aspects of medicine and healthcare to adhere to the best of our ability to an evidence-based foundation; while it is increasingly clear that chronic opioid therapy for chronic non-cancer pain is generally a bad idea, overreaction in pendulum fashion is inevitable and runs the risk of harming some individuals, if not directly then again by diversifying their pathology (psychological as well as physical). This may be most salient in the arena of acute pain management, where evidence exists that aggressive and effective analgesia may prevent the development of chronic pain.

Nonetheless, pain management, whether acute or chronic, must begin and continue with comprehensive biopsychosocial-spiritual assessment and treatment. Failure of the physician to attend to the underlying somatic and emotional discomforts and distress that encourage people to seek opioids is failure indeed. Multimodal, prevention-oriented, and self-efficacy-instilling therapy, with specific attention paid to the nonphysical, is incumbent upon those who purport to treat pain.

Ultimately, however, as with all epidemics, this one will end only when we—the *host*—as a species are able to cultivate sufficient (behavioral) immunity to overuse and misuse of these powerful and pernicious agents. Unlike historic infectious disease epidemics, where hosts generally shun the agent and environment/vector, this epidemic is characterized by an unprecedented (excepting the obesity epidemic) flocking to the agent. Education, a cornerstone of primary prevention, is essential to turning the tide, but must include far more than negative motivation toward chronic opioid use. Preferable (and viable) alternatives to opioids for chronic pain management must be taught. Prevention of chronic pain—which has been errantly regarded by both populace and practitioners as a primarily somatic issue—must be practiced within every arena of healthcare and must address the full spectrum of biopsychosocial-spiritual needs of the patient.

The prescription of opioids must always follow thorough assessment of these needs, with specific attention paid to the psychological, as the literature consistently identifies psychopathology (especially comorbid substance abuse disorders, anxiety, and PTSD) as the main risk factors for opioid use disorder/dependence. Opioids should always be prescribed on a trial basis, as "rescue medications" for severe pain refractory to more conservative measures, and in this author's opinion, with clear and plausible organic pathology that correlates with the complaint. Diligent education of the patient as to the long-term harms of continued use, including hyperalgesia with perpetuation or worsening of pain, is incumbent at every visit, with discussion of the inadvisability of disruption of normal healing and adaptation—psychological, if not physical. Compassion and empathy for the patient's suffering are paramount and part of our oath. It must, however, never be forgotten that we swore to first do no harm, and mounting evidence reveals the harms of chronic opioid use in non-cancer pain. Reassurance, with fostering of resilience and self-efficacy while promoting and coaching personal health and wholeness maintenance, is the job of every physician and mid-level practitioner.

Tertiary prevention or damage control/harm reduction is a developing science and art. Addiction has long been a polarizing concept, with staunch advocates insisting that it is either a primarily moral issue (weakness of character and discipline) or, more recently, a biological disease, perhaps even genetically inherited. Elements of both are likely true in almost all cases, and the understanding of both neurophysiology and human motivation is essential to the understanding and successful treatment of opioid dependence. What is clear is that addiction generally follows a two-phase course with initial hedonic/reward motivation followed by negative motivation comprising avoidance of withdrawal once physical dependence has gripped the individual.

National authorities have provided a framework and guidelines for biopsychosocial-spiritual ("multidimensional") assessment and treatment of opioid dependence, with a combined medication-assisted psychosocial approach recommended whenever appropriate. Data seem to support a more successful recovery when agonist replacement or antagonist pharmacotherapy is combined with a behavioral approach; data also show that those who succeed most often endorse increased personal growth and maturation in resilience, coping skills, responsibility, communication skills, etc. Not all approaches work for all individuals, but acknowledgement and presentation of spiritual and faith-based components are consonant with a biopsychosocial-spiritual model, and decades of data (e.g., Alcoholics Anonymous and more recent investigations of polysubstance abuse) support their invaluable contribution. When considering the likelihood (with at least strong temporal correlation evidence) of the association between widespread social structure breakdown, increasing distress, and increasing "chemical coping," it seems evident that supreme strategic disadvantage and illogic, from a public health standpoint if none other, is ours from failure to recruit allies whose expertise and purpose comprise healthy minds, souls, relationships, families, and communities.

Regardless of the individual patient's alignment or resonance with any of these treatment "axes," we have found essentially universal acquiescence to and, in many cases, efficacy from championing the following ideal. Pharmacotherapy is beneficial, a change in environment (e.g., from a "using" community to one of sobriety and mutual encouragement) is essential and professional help is required, but all of these interventions are insufficient in bringing about sustained change and recovery without replacement of the desire for opioids with a greater and higher desire. Thus, only will the opioid epidemic end.

Index

H.B. McAnally, *Opioid Dependence*, DOI 10.1007/978-3-319-47497-7

CPSIA information can be obtained
at www.ICGtesting.com
Printed in the USA
LVOW06*0724231017
553425LV00002B/11/P